Management of Ambulance Services

Prepared by the

National EMS Management Association

Text Editor

Skip Kirkwood, M.S., J.D., NREMT-P, EFO, CEMSO

National EMS Management Association

Wake Forest, North Carolina

EMS Management Series

SERIES EDITOR, *Jeffrey T. Lindsey, PhD, PM, EFO, CFO*
Distance Education Coordinator
for the Fire and Emergency Services Programs
University of Florida
Gainesville, Florida

PEARSON

Boston   Columbus   Indianapolis   New York   San Francisco   Upper Saddle River
Amsterdam   Cape Town   Dubai   London   Madrid   Milan   Munich   Paris   Montreal   Toronto
Delhi   Mexico City   São Paulo   Sydney   Hong Kong   Seoul   Singapore   Taipei   Tokyo

Publisher: Julie Levin Alexander
Publisher's Assistant: Regina Bruno
Editor-in-Chief: Marlene McHugh Pratt
Product Manager: Sladjana Repic
Program Manager: Monica Moosang
Development Editor: Kay S. Peavey, iD8-TripleSSS
Editorial Assistant: Kelly Clark
Director of Marketing: David Gesell
Executive Marketing Manager: Brian Hoehl
Marketing Specialist: Michael Sirinides

Project Management Lead: Cynthia Zonneveld
Project Manager: Julie Boddorf
Full-Service Project Manager: Munesh Kumar, Aptara®, Inc.
Editorial Media Manager: Amy Peltier
Media Project Manager: Ellen Martino
Creative Director: Jayne Conte
Cover Designer: Suzanne Behnke
Cover Image: Shutterstock/B Calkins
Composition: Aptara®, Inc.
Text Font: Times Ten LT Std

Credits and acknowledgments borrowed from other sources and reproduced, with permission, in this textbook appear on the appropriate pages within text.

Copyright © 2015 by Pearson Education, Inc. , All rights reserved. Manufactured in the United States of America. This publication is protected by Copyright, and permission should be obtained from the publisher prior to any prohibited reproduction, storage in a retrieval system, or transmission in any form or by any means, electronic, mechanical, photocopying, recording, or likewise. To obtain permission(s) to use material from this work, please submit a written request to Pearson Education, Inc., Permissions Department, One Lake Street, Upper Saddle River, New Jersey 07458, or you may fax your request to 201-236-3290.

Notice: The authors and the publisher of this volume have taken care that the information and technical recommendations contained herein are based on research and expert consultation, and are accurate and compatible with the standards generally accepted at the time of publication. Nevertheless, as new information becomes available, changes in clinical and technical practices become necessary. The reader is advised to carefully consult manufacturers' instructions and information material for all supplies and equipment before use, and to consult with a health care professional as necessary. This advice is especially important when using new supplies or equipment for clinical purposes. The authors and publisher disclaim all responsibility for any liability, loss, injury, or damage incurred as a consequence, directly or indirectly, of the use and application of any of the contents of this volume.

Many of the designations by manufacturers and sellers to distinguish their products are claimed as trademarks. Where those designations appear in this book, and the publisher was aware of a trademark claim, the designations have been printed in initial caps or all caps.

Library of Congress Cataloging-in-Publication Data
Kirkwood, Skip.
 Management of ambulance services / Skip Kirkwood from NEMSMA.
  pages cm
 ISBN-13: 978-0-13-502829-2
 ISBN-10: 0-13-502829-9
 1. Ambulance service. 2. Emergency medical services. I. Title.
 RA995.5.K57 2015
 362.18—dc23   2013011275

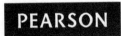

ISBN-13: 978-0-13-502829-2
ISBN-10:   0-13-502829-9

Dedication

This book is dedicated to the men and women who provide emergency medical services throughout the United States each and every day. Many times, we identify our best paramedics, and we promote them to supervisory and managerial positions without the necessary skills, tools, and information to be successful in their new roles. Along with the group of subject-matter experts that authored this book's chapters, I dedicate the hours and labors that went into its production to the future leaders of ambulance services throughout the country. May you lead well, by example, from out in front.

I would like to express my thanks to those who suffered through my work on this project: my colleagues at the Wake County Department of Emergency Medical Services; the members of the Board of Directors of the National Emergency Medical Services Management Association; and most of all my wife, Natalie, and my daughters, Elizabeth and Devin, who fended for themselves as I drafted, edited, and chased down copyright permissions. Last, I'd like to acknowledge two world-class emergency services leaders who have served as sources of inspiration and motivation to me: first, the late James O. Page, J.D., whose leadership and dedication to the improvement of emergency medical services over more than three decades inspired me to pursue the path that led to a place where I, too can make a small contribution to the cause; and second, Dr. Jay Fitch, who provided guidance, opportunity, and sometimes painfully frank professional feedback that has helped me to stay on track through times good and not so good.

Contents

Chapter 3

Chapter 4

Chapter 5

Medical Transportation–Scheduled
Matt Zavadsky, MS-HSA, EMT   96

Chapter 6

Air Ambulance and Air Medical Transportation   *Edward R. Marasco, M.P.M., CMTE, EMT-P (Ret.)*   106

Chapter 7

Deployment and Staffing Models

Chapter 8

Human Resources Administration   *Chris*

Chapter 9

Ambulance Specification and Procurement *Jonathan A. Olson, M.B.A., M.H.A., NREMT-P, EFO* 183

Chapter 10

Patient Care Reporting Documentation and Documentation Systems *Kevin M. T. Sullivan, M.S., NREMT-P* 213

Chapter 11

Marketing, Media, and Community Relations *Keith Griffiths and Tom Tornstrom, M.B.A., EMT-P* 245

Chapter 12

Ambulance Service Dispatch and Radio Communications *Barry Furey* 266

Chapter 15

The Regulatory Environment of Ambulance Services   *Sean M. Caffrey, M.B.A., CEMSO, NRP, and D. Randy Kuykendall, M.L.S., NREMT-P*   321

Chapter 16

Legal and Compliance Issues for Ambulance Services   *David M. Shotwell Jr., J.D., NREMT-P*   340

Chapter 17

Safety Considerations for Ambulance Services   *Peter Dworsky, M.P.H., EMT-P*   354

Chapter 18

Ambulance Service Activities in Support of the Community   *Skip Kirkwood, M.S., J.D., NREMT-P, EFO, CEMSO*   395

Chapter 19

Ambulance Operations in Support of Disaster Operations   *Lawrence Nelson, M.Sc., EMT-P (Ret.), NMCEM*   405

Foreword

JAY FITCH, PH.D.

Throughout the history of EMS there has been a push-pull relationship between rapid change and the desire for stability. As leaders, we often struggle to achieve balance in our systems, with our caregivers and personally.

Being among the early groups of paramedics trained in America and having had the unique opportunity to both lead and design multiple types of EMS systems, I've witnessed periods of revolution, evolution, and stagnation along our professional journey. Some observers would say that EMS doesn't accept or manage change well.

EMS organizations now operate in an environment that is substantially more volatile, uncertain, and complex than in their early years. Leaders must cope with clinical, operational, and financial issues while at the same time transforming those with whom we work to adapt to nonstop change. You could say that leading an EMS system is like building a bicycle while riding it—*downhill.*

The dramatic effects of rising complexity compel EMS executives to lead their teams with bold creativity, connect with customers in imaginative ways, and design the agency's operations for speed and flexibility. So how does that happen?

Leaders must continually acquire new knowledge and skills. In *The Seven Habits of Highly Effective People*, Steven Covey suggests, "Begin with the end in mind." If EMS leaders are to successfully prepare others for the future, we must be prepared for the future ourselves.

If you are reading this book, then your career (bicycle) is already moving forward. And if you are working on your degree, then you've realized that in a complex environment having a broad perspective is a distinct advantage. And if you've already graduated, then use this text as a resource for being a lifelong learner.

A number of your colleagues have volunteered their time to put together in this book detailed explanations of complex concepts and practical ideas for your benefit. I couldn't resist sharing seven action-oriented thoughts for your leadership journey:

Understand the stories. Each of those with whom you interact has an important story to share. By listening well, you gain insight and context. Both are required to make good decisions.

Reach beyond silos. Pull creative ideas and elements of your organization out of compartments and integrate them. Transcend the obvious to form unconventional partnerships. Proactively exchange knowledge and collaborate with internal and external stakeholders, eliminating every communication barrier to improve your ability to handle the unknown.

Utilize breakthrough thinking. Practice and encourage experimentation at all levels of the organization. Forge ahead with rule-breaking innovation to set your EMS agency apart. Study and question what others do—scour technology and customer trends. Build scenarios to plan responses to a range of possible futures.

Act despite uncertainty. Fight the natural urge to wait for clarity and stability, taking calculated risks—while others hesitate—will pay off. Find a creative way to turn complexity into an advantage. Rely on deeply felt values and a well-defined vision to provide the confidence and conviction required to open the windows of opportunity.

Strengthen your ability to persuade and influence. Even if it feels uncomfortable, lead others by working together toward a shared vision. Dare to relinquish some control in favor of building more mutual trust throughout the organization. Don't present your answers and logic—discover the logic and best answer with your leadership team.

Consistently coach. Spark others' imagination. Instill the pursuit of quality into your EMS organization's mission through informal and formal training. Challenge every team member to be creative, supporting, and rewarding caregivers who step outside their comfort zones to innovate.

Use a wide range of communications approaches. More than before, supplement top-down organizational communications with less formal, more innovative channels. New and innovative forms of communication are often faster. Be more open in giving stakeholders access to you.

When considering a career as an EMS leader, Steven Covey's admonition to "begin with the end in mind" is wonderful guidance. It is not a contradiction to encourage you to enjoy the journey. The journey—including the people you meet, the incredible things you will learn, and the gifts you share along the way—are as important as your ultimate career destination. I hope we have the opportunity to meet personally and share the stories of your journey and success.

Dr. Fitch is the founding partner of the emergency services consulting group Fitch & Associates. Throughout his career he has written extensively about EMS leadership and was the primary author of one of the first management textbooks utilized in EMS.

Introduction

Skip Kirkwood, M.S., J.D., NREMT-P, EFO, CEMSO

Management of Ambulance Services was created as a textbook to support a survey course on that subject: the management of ambulance services. It has been a group effort—by a group of hard-working, dedicated subject matter experts who agreed to serve as chapter authors, and by the officers, the board of directors, and the members of the National EMS Management Association, who have patiently supported and encouraged this project.

Managing this project was filled with challenges. The EMS environment is continuously changing, and the 2 years during which this book was created were no exception. The release of the National EMS Education Standards and the continually evolving titles and "levels of certification" made terminology a moving target. Throughout the book, we have retained the current (some may think of it as "old") levels of certification because the majority of states have not yet changed the titles, licenses, and patches. If the new levels take hold, we will address them in future chapters.

Another limitation of the project was maintaining the scope. The title of the book is *Management of Ambulance Services*, which is not the same thing as managing an EMS system. Thus, omissions of topics such as *first response agencies* is by design, not a result of oversight. We also quickly discovered that some topics don't lend themselves to being addressed in a single chapter and are better served by texts and courses of their own. For this reason, there is no chapter on quality management in ambulance services, or on the role and education of medical directors.

Ambulance services in the United States are at a crossroads. Over the last 40 years, many have become one-trick ponies, offering only a single service: the response to a request for service, followed by transportation to a hospital. Why? Because it's easy to get paid for it. The model is totally predictable. However, its future is limited because our emerging workforces are composed of employees who want a variety of professional challenges. If our ambulance services don't evolve to provide that variety, they will have an even more difficult time attracting and retaining sufficient employees to do the job—and some other organization will step up to hire those employees.

We at NEMSMA believe that a quality ambulance service is an essential element of every community—just like good streets, good schools, and low crime rates. We hope that this text provides a foundation for the next generation of ambulance service executives to build the community ambulance service of the twenty-first century, where paramedics of all levels provide essential mobile health intervention services to their communities and, where necessary and appropriate, transportation to a medically appropriate venue.

National EMS Management Association
a professional association of EMS leaders dedicated to the discovery, development, and promotion of excellence in leadership and management in EMS systems, regardless of EMS system model, organizational structure or agency affiliation.

Preface

Ambulance services are ubiquitous throughout the United States. They range in size from one ambulance operated by volunteers and managed by a community board of directors, through large governmental agencies and even larger private, for-profit corporations—and everything in between. There have been few opportunities for individuals to undertake formal coursework that covers all of the subject matter that the manager of an ambulance service, large or small, needs to have at his command in order to understand the operation and to successfully make the myriad decisions that must be made to keep the business solvent, in good standing in the community, staffed, and providing competent, compassionate, and clinically excellent service to the community protected by that ambulance service.

This text offers nineteen chapters of "best practices" information about the management of an ambulance service. Each chapter was written by someone who is a recognized expert in that area of ambulance service operation. Most have written on their topic elsewhere, some of those extensively. Many have taught their subject matter at national conferences, training programs, and academies. They have each provided living examples and "best practices" for EMS agencies that wish to improve in a particular area.

ORGANIZATION OF THIS TEXT

Management of Ambulance Services is intended to support an upper-division baccalaureate course in the Fire and Emergency Services Higher Education (FESHE) Consortium baccalaureate degree program. Information about this program can be found at www.usfa.fema.gov/nfa/higher_ed/feshe/feshe_direction. shtm. The FESHE program's mission is to establish an organization of postsecondary institutions that promote higher education and to enhance the recognition of the fire and emergency services as a profession that reduces loss of life and property from fire and other hazards. Currently more than a hundred institutions participate in the FESHE program at the associates level, thirty-eight at the baccalaureate level, and thirteen that offer graduate degrees.

Chapter 1 begins the text with a history of ambulance services in the United States, and it stretches back to precolonial times to examine the military medicine roots of today's ambulance services. Chapter 2 explores the various levels of ambulance service commonly found in the United States, then Chapter 3 examines the possibilities for corporate structures of those services.

Chapter 4 provides an academic examination of the ambulance market, which is not a common consideration except at the large corporate level—but it is something about which every ambulance executive and manager should be aware.

Chapter 5 looks at the nonemergency, scheduled medical transportation business, which is markedly different from the 9-1-1 or "emergency" business. In Chapter 6, the air medical business is explored.

The next group of chapters examines some specialty areas in which ambulance service managers must have familiarity, if not expertise. Chapter 7 looks at the science of demand analysis, deployment, and scheduling of ambulance resources, and Chapter 8 looks at the complex world of human resources from the eyes of an ambulance service human resources executive. Chapter 9 provides detailed information about the specification and procurement of ambulance vehicles, and Chapter 10 addresses the complex world of patient care reporting documentation and documentation systems.

Chapter 11 explores the not-well-understood world of marketing, media, and community relations. Chapter 12 focuses on ambulance service dispatch and radio communications. Chapter 13 provides useful guidance on technology in support of ambulance operations.

Chapters 14, 15, and 16 address the finance and accounting functions, the regulatory environment, and related legal and compliance issues for ambulance services. Chapter 17 examines the many safety considerations that must be addressed by a successful ambulance service.

Chapter 18 illustrates some non-transportation activities that represent best practices in terms of the support an ambulance service can provide to its community, and Chapter 19 reviews the roles of an ambulance service in support of disaster operations.

Subjects that are *notably* not addressed in this textbook are two:

First, the role of the medical director in an ambulance service is not discussed. We believe that this subject is well described in other publications, particularly those of our colleagues at the National Association of EMS Physicians.

Second, we have not addressed the topic of quality improvement, for two reasons: (1) Doing that topic justice would probably require a full textbook to do it justice. (2) We feel that the topic is well addressed in other resources.

FEATURES

Chapter Objectives: Objectives are identified at the beginning of each chapter and outline the material the reader should understand upon completion of the chapter.

Key Terms: Key terms are listed at the beginning of each chapter and are boldfaced where introduced in the chapter. Each chapter's terms are defined at the end of the chapter, and all terms are included in the comprehensive glossary at the end of the book.

What Would You Do? Case Study: Every chapter starts with an EMS manager tackling some issue related to public information and education that is related to the content of the chapter. How he resolved the issue based on information in the chapter is presented in the **What Would You Do? Reflection** feature at the end of the chapter.

Best Practice: Every chapter includes a real-world example that illustrates information from the chapter having been used successfully by an EMS agency.

Sidebars: This feature relates interesting information that corresponds very closely to text discussion.

Review Questions: Students are required to draw on the knowledge presented in the chapter to answer the questions.

References: A list of bibliographical references appears at the end of each chapter.

ROAD MAP/HOW TO USE THIS TEXT

This text is designed to support a survey course in ambulance service management. It is constructed such that each chapter addresses an important area of consideration for an ambulance service manager. Individual chapters may serve as resources for middle managers with responsibility for that area, or the entire text may be a helpful reference for senior ambulance service executives who desire a refresher reference for a particular functional part of their service.

TEACHING AND LEARNING RESOURCES

For information on instructor resources, including PowerPoint presentations and assessment tools, please contact your Brady sales representative.

Acknowledgments

Several individuals were extremely helpful to me throughout this long process. In addition to Monica Moosang and Kay S. Peavey, I would like to thank Chief Josh Holloman, M.H.S., EMT-P, of Johnston County (NC) EMS, and Rob Luckritz, J.D., EMT-P, of Liberty Health Systems and the Jersey City (NJ) Medical Center, for their editorial assistance. When the going got tough, these two guys did not hesitate to pick up and provide content and editorial assistance that helped to get the job done.

I also appreciate the unwavering moral support and advice provided by Keith Griffiths, NEMSMA's Executive Director; Gary Wingrove, who preceded me as NEMSMA president; and Troy Hagen, who succeeded me as NEMSMA president. These gentlemen are truly EMS leaders who live and breathe the NEMSMA mission—they are professional EMS leaders "dedicated to the discovery, development, and promotion of excellence in leadership and management in EMS systems, regardless of EMS system model, organizational structure or agency affiliation."

About the Text Editor

Skip Kirkwood, M.S., J.D., NREMT-P, EFO, CEMSO

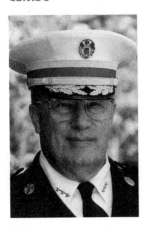

Skip Kirkwood, this text's editor and author of Chapters 3, 13, and 18, served as the Chief of the Wake County, North Carolina, Emergency Medical Services Division from April 2005 through June 2013 and currently holds the position of EMS Director at Durham County, North Carolina. He has been involved in EMS since 1973, as an EMT, paramedic, supervisor, educator, manager, consultant, state EMS director (Oregon), and chief EMS officer. Over the course of his career, he has served in EMS systems in Virginia, Connecticut, Hawaii, New Jersey, Oregon, Florida, Iowa, and North Carolina—the last four as chief of the department.

Chief Kirkwood holds a Master of Science in Health Services Administration from Central Michigan University and a Juris Doctorate from the Rutgers University School of Law. He is a graduate of the U.S. Fire Administration's Executive Fire Officer program, and was recently recognized by the Commission on Public Safety Excellence as one of the first five credentialed Chief EMS Officers (CEMSO) in the United States.

Chief Kirkwood has served (2011–2012) as President of the National EMS Management Association, having served on its board of directors since 2004, and he currently serves as Immediate Past President. He also has served as chair of the Leadership Development Project Group (2008–2011) and as principal author of NEMSMA's leadership agenda white paper, "EMS Management and Leadership Development in the United States: An Agenda for the Future." Chief Kirkwood's current and future NEMSMA projects include chairing the Emergency Medical Services Field Training and Evaluation Program and championing the NEMSMA Violence Against Paramedics initiative.

In addition to his NEMSMA activities, Chief Kirkwood is a member of the National Association of EMTs and the International Association of Fire Chiefs.

About the Chapter Authors

The following individuals served as chapter authors for this textbook. It is their work that brings value to it, for they are truly subject matter experts.

Vincent D. Robbins, FACHE (Chapters 1, 3)—Mr. Robbins is the President and Chief Executive Officer of MONOC, New Jersey's single-largest EMS and medical transportation service. MONOC is a consortium of more than a dozen hospitals in the state that provides shared services for its members. He holds a master's degree in Healthcare Administration, is a Fellow with the American College of Healthcare Executives, and has lectured, authored, and consulted on EMS and medical transportation systems for more than 30 years. He formerly served in the administration of Temple University Hospital, in Philadelphia, Pennsylvania, and with the New Jersey State Department of Health's Office of Emergency Medical Services. He began his career in EMS as a cadet member of his local volunteer EMS agency and was among the first group of EMTs and paramedics certified in the state.

Matt Zavadsky, MS-HSA, EMT (Chapters 2 and 5)—Mr. Zavadsky is the Public Affairs Director at MedStar Mobile Healthcare, the self-operated public utility model system providing emergency and nonemergency EMS and mobile health care services for Fort Worth and fourteen surrounding cities in North Texas. He holds a master's degree in Health Service Administration and has 32 years of experience in EMS, including volunteer, fire department, public sector, and private sector EMS agencies. He is a frequent speaker at national conferences and has done

consulting in numerous EMS issues, specializing in high-performance EMS system operations, public/media relations, public policy, employee recruitment and retention, data analysis, costing strategies, and EMS research. Mr. Zavadsky is an adjunct faculty for the University of Central Florida's College of Health and Public Affairs teaching courses in Healthcare Economics and Policy, Healthcare Finance, Ethics, Managed Care, and U.S. Healthcare Systems.

Skip Kirkwood, M.S., J.D., NREMT-P, EFO, CEMSO (Chapters 3, 13, 18)—See "About the Text Editor."

Robert Luckritz, J.D., NREMT-P (Chapter 3)—Mr. Luckritz has served in various capacities in EMS since 1996. He has worked across the northeastern United States in EMS Management, overseeing various clinical, operational, and educational programs. He recently completed his tenure overseeing EMS operations for Jersey City Medical Center's EMS, an award-winning EMS agency running over 90,000 calls per year. During his time at the department, the service became the first EMS agency in the nation to be triply accredited by the Commission on Accreditation of Ambulance Services, the National Association of Emergency Dispatch, and the Commission on Accreditation of Allied Health Education Programs. He currently serves as the Director of Government Relations for Liberty Health Systems, Jersey City Medical Center.

Art Groux, B.S., EMT-P (Chapter 3)—Mr. Groux is currently the Chief of Service for Suffield Volunteer Ambulance in Suffield, Connecticut, the region's largest volunteer

EMS service provider. Chief Groux has been involved in EMS for over 20 years from field provider, with experience in both U.S. and Israeli systems, to service chief. Chief Groux developed and implemented the only true third service in northern Connecticut. Chief Groux is a founding member and currently serves as the Vice President of the Connecticut EMS Chiefs Association, the Deputy Planning Section Chief for Connecticut IMT-3, and EMS section leader for the Capital Region Emergency Planning Commission.

Robert K. (Bob) Waddell II, EMT-P (Ret.) (Chapter 3)—Mr. Waddell has been actively involved in various aspects of EMS since the age of 15. His service to the profession includes being an EMT-Basic in rural Wyoming, a paramedic in Front Range Colorado, the president of an international health care education company, National EMS Systems Director for the EMS for Children's program, and co-author of an evidence-based triage model. Mr. Waddell has chaired and/or served on numerous state, national, and international committees. He has authored, contributed, or reviewed more than twenty chapters, articles, and books. He is a member of NAEMSE and NAEMT, and is past international chair and founding development team member of NAEMT's Emergency Pediatric Care (EPC) program.

Dave Shrader (Chapter 4)—Mr. Shrader is president of The Polaris Group, an ambulance, EMS, and public safety consulting firm. The Polaris Group was formed in 1997 and serves public clients and hospitals in EMS system design and contracting. Mr. Shrader has nearly 40 years of experience in the ambulance industry, having served as an EMT, paramedic, flight medic, and SWAT medic and in various senior management roles in public, private, public utility model, hospital, and fire-based EMS systems. He is also an experienced firefighter and fire officer, and currently serves as Deputy Chief of the Southern Shores (NC) Fire Department.

Mike Touchstone, M.A., EMT-P (Chapter 3)—Mr. Touchstone is currently the Philadelphia Fire Department (PFD) Fire Service Paramedic Chief in charge of EMS Training. He has been involved in EMS since 1980, and he was certified as an EMT-P in 1983 and as an instructor in 1996. He has served in a third-service ALS ambulance corps, in a hospital-based ALS 9-1-1 service, and with the PFD since 1989. Chief Touchstone has experience as a field supervisor and as a CQI officer, and he has more than 10 years in EMS training. Chief Touchstone has presented on leadership and education topics at local, regional, national, and international conferences and symposia. He has authored numerous articles, including a twelve-part professional development series for *EMS Magazine* (now *EMS World*) and a series for EMS1.com. He holds a bachelor's degree from George Washington University in Health Sciences/EMS Management. He is the current (2013–2014) President-Elect of the National EMS Management Association.

Edward R. Marasco, M.P.M., CMTE, EMT-P (Ret.) (Chapter 6)—Mr. Marasco is currently the Vice President of Business Development for Quick Med Claims, a nationally recognized medical transportation billing and reimbursement agency. He has been involved in prehospital care since 1979 and has extensive experience managing air medical services operations. He has served on and chaired numerous committees and councils throughout the prehospital care community over the years. Mr. Marasco serves as a member of the Board of Regents for the Medical Transport Leadership Institute (MTLI), a comprehensive leadership training program offered through the Association of Air Medical Services (AAMS). He is also an adjunct instructor in the Emergency Medicine Program at the University of Pittsburgh School of Health and Rehabilitation Sciences (SHRS).

Steven Cotter, M.B.A., NREMT-P (Chapter 7)— Mr. Cotter is the Director of Emergency

Medical Services for Piedmont EMS, a division of the Piedmont Medical Center Healthcare System in Rock Hill, South Carolina. He has been involved in Emergency Medical Services since 1992, beginning his career in a rural setting. He then joined Greenville County EMS and spent the next 13 years there. During that time, he held the positions of Paramedic, Field Training Officer, Rescue Specialist, and Shift Supervisor. Mr. Cotter became the EMS Director for Laurens County EMS in 2005 and, in 2007, became the Director of EMS for Sedgwick County in Wichita, Kansas. In 2010, he returned to EMS in South Carolina.

Mr. Cotter holds a dual B.S. in finance and accounting, an M.A. in business administration, and is currently pursuing a Ph.D. in health care administration. He is an author for *EMS World Magazine* and has contributed to both EMS paramedic and EMS management and leadership textbooks. Mr. Cotter currently serves as faculty teaching EMS leadership and management at Spartanburg Community College in South Carolina and has previously taught operations management and statistics at the undergraduate level. He also frequently speaks on EMS leadership, EMS operations efficiencies, and EMS system design at both the state and national levels. Mr. Cotter is the Chairman of the Board of Directors for the Midland EMS Council in Columbia, South Carolina, serves on the Advisory Board for the PULSE Emergency Medical Update, and serves on the Data Committee for South Carolina DHEC EMS.

Chris Colangelo, M.S.H.R., NREMT-P (Chapter 8)—Chief Colangelo currently serves as the Executive Officer of the Wake County EMS System. In this position, he is primarily responsible for system budget administration, human resource administration, and contract/franchise oversight. Chief Colangelo has worked in public safety since 1988 in varied roles from a volunteer EMT/firefighter to EMS Operations Chief for Wake County EMS Division to his current position. He earned his master's degree in Human Resources from Western Carolina University. Chief Colangelo serves as an at-large member of the Board of Directors of the International Association of EMS Chiefs, and he is a member of the National EMS Management Association and The Society for Human Resource Management.

Forrest ("Woody") Wood, EMT-P (Chapter 8)—Mr. Wood currently serves as a Training Manager for the Texas A&M paramedic program. He has served the university and its extension service for the past 10 years. Prior to joining the Texas A&M system, he held a variety of positions with the Rural/Metro Corporation, where he also served for 10 years. Mr. Wood is a past member of the Board of Directors of the National EMS Management Association, where he chaired the Education Committee.

Ernesto Rodriguez, EMT-P (Chapter 8)—Chief Ernesto Rodriguez currently serves as the Chief of the Austin-Travis County (TX) EMS system. He has over 25 years of experience in EMS. He began his career as a volunteer firefighter and migrated into the paid fire service. His experience encompasses 10 years in the fire service as a paramedic and firefighter. He also served for 4 years as Assistant State EMS Director (TX), during which time he managed the EMS development programs such as local projects grants, the Emergency Medical Services for Children grant program, and disaster preparedness. Mr. Rodriguez has several years of experience in the private sector in clinical oversight, operations management, and deployment. He served for a combined 10 years with MedStar in Fort Worth, Texas, where he served as Assistant to the Medical Director and Director of Operations. Chief Rodriguez is currently chief of the Austin–Travis County EMS. In 2010 he was recognized as the EMS Executive of the Year by the National EMS Management Association.

Jonathan A. Olson, M.B.A, M.H.A, NREMT-P, EFO (Chapter 9)—Chief Olson holds multiple fire service certifications and currently serves in the role of Chief of Operations with Wake County EMS. He has been a volunteer firefighter in Wake County since 1986 and has been paid staff there since 1990. In addition to overseeing field and special operations, Chief Olson is the lead on ambulance and support vehicle specification and procurement. He has been directly involved with fleet procurement at Wake County since 1992. Prior to moving to operations, Chief Olson served as Management Services Chief, controlling budget, logistics, and capital facility planning. He served as an EMS District Chief from 1994 to 2001, and he has held a National Registry Paramedic credential since 1990. He was recently conveyed the Executive Fire Officer credential by the US Fire Administration. He is a Type III All Hazards Incident Commander, Operations Section Chief, and Planning Section Chief. Chief Olson holds a Bachelor of Science from Western Carolina University and Master of Business Administration and Master of Health Administration degrees from Pfeiffer University, as well as an Executive Fire Officer certificate from the U.S. Fire Administration.

Kevin M. T. Sullivan, M.S., NREMT-P (Chapter 10)—Mr. Sullivan is currently the Vice President of Operations at STAT Medical Solutions, a company that specializes in providing corporate medical services and EMS medical director solutions. Mr. Sullivan began his EMS career at Georgetown Emergency Response Medical Service (GERMS) and has held leadership positions in several EMS departments, including serving as the Deputy Chief of Grady EMS in Atlanta, before transitioning to the private sector. He holds a master's degree in Emergency Health Services from the University of Maryland–Baltimore County.

Keith Griffiths (Chapter 11)—Mr. Griffiths has more than three decades of experience in editing, writing, publishing, marketing, and conference production in the EMS and public safety professions, including the startup of Jems Communications in 1980, where as executive editor he helped lead the creation of multiple trade magazines, research journals, trade shows, newsletters, books, videos, and online resources for the emergency care market. With his partner, the late Jim Page, Mr. Griffiths arranged the sale of Jems in 1993 to the Times Mirror Corporation and continued to head the Jems Division for Times Mirror for the next 4 years. He left to form his own consulting organization in 1997 and continues to serve as a contributing editor for *JEMS*, the *Journal of Emergency Medical Services*. He serves as chair of the Alliance Committee on the College of Fellows for the National Academies of Emergency Dispatch and on the advisory boards of several national organizations, including EPIC Medics and the National 911 Educational Coalition. He is the chair of the James O. Page Charitable Foundation and serves on the board of the Western Publishing Association. Mr. Griffiths also has served as the editor-in-chief of the newsletter *Best Practices in Emergency Services* since 2009. As President of the RedFlash Group, he helps nonprofit, commercial, and government organizations "tell their story" to constituents through research, marketing, advertising, and public relations. He received a Presidential nomination to the U.S. Naval Academy, which he attended for 2 years and has a bachelor of arts degree in journalism from San Diego State University where he later studied marketing, advertising, accounting, and management as a graduate student in its MBA program.

Tom Tornstrom, M.B.A., EMT-P (Chapter 11)—Mr. Tornstrom is currently the Executive Director of Tri-State Ambulance, a wholly owned, not-for-profit subsidiary of Gundersen Lutheran Health System based in La Crosse, Wisconsin. Tri-State Ambulance provides 9-1-1 and interfacility ambulance service to thirty communities and nearly 3,000 square miles in Wisconsin, Minnesota, and Iowa. Mr. Tornstrom has been involved in EMS for more than 20 years and has extensive experience in business development, information technology, and ambulance service regionalization. He serves as a board member of the Professional Ambulance Association of Wisconsin and is passionate about providing high-quality patient care while maintaining efficiency and fiscal responsibility.

Barry Furey (Chapter 12) — Mr. Furey is currently the Director of the Raleigh-Wake County (NC) Emergency Communications Center, which has been designated an Accredited Center of Excellence by the National Academy of Emergency Dispatch and is the first agency in the state to receive CALEA Accreditation. Director Furey has been involved in public safety since 1970 as a director of four multijurisdictional 9-1-1 centers, a consultant, and a fire-rescue officer. A life member of APCO, he has chaired or served on numerous national committees, authored portions of *The Fire Chief's Handbook*, and is a Contributing Editor for *Firehouse* magazine, columnist for *9-1-1 Magazine* online, and communications editor for Firefighterclosecalls. com.

Sean Caffrey, M.B.A., CEMSO, NRP (Chapters 14 and 15) — Mr. Caffrey has been involved in EMS for 25 years and currently serves as the EMS System Development Coordinator for the State of Colorado. His duties with the state EMS office include policy analysis, project management, and technical assistance to local EMS services. He has previously served in EMS leadership positions in public, hospital-based, nonprofit, private, and volunteer EMS organizations in Colorado, Virginia, and the District of Columbia. Mr. Caffrey has an undergraduate degree in EMS Administration from George Washington University and a graduate degree in business administration from University of

Denver. He is currently the Treasurer of the National EMS Management Association and has a strong interest in the financial management of EMS and rural EMS delivery systems.

Asbel Montes, B.S. (Chapter 14) — Asbel Montes is the Vice President of Governmental Relations & Reimbursements at Acadian Ambulance Service, headquartered in Lafayette, Louisiana, with operations throughout the southeastern United States.

D. Randy Kuykendall, M.L.S., NREMT-P (Chapter 15) — Chief Kuykendall leads the Health Facilities & EMS Division (and former state EMS director) of the Colorado Department of Public Health and Environment. He is the Immediate Past President of the National Association of State EMS Officials.

David M. Shotwell Jr., J.D., NREMT-P (Chapter 16) — Mr. Shotwell is currently an attorney and Corporate Compliance Officer for Monmouth Ocean Hospital Service Corporation (MONOC), Wall Township, New Jersey, where he also serves as a paramedic. A graduate of the University of Delaware and Rutgers University Law School, his public safety career began in 1976 on the New Jersey shore, where he continues to serve as a seasonal lifeguard and member of the United States Lifesaving Association. Mr. Shotwell has served as Chief of the Ocean Grove Fire Department (New Jersey) and legal advisor to EMS agencies and fire protection districts.

Peter Dworsky, M.P.H., EMT-P (Chapter 17) — Mr. Dworsky is the Corporate Director of Support Services for MONOC Mobile Health Services, New Jersey's largest EMS provider. He is responsible for risk management and reduction and injury prevention and safety programs. Previously, he was the Director of EMS and Disaster Preparedness for St. Barnabas Medical Center (New Jersey). He is a member of the EMS Safety Foundation and NAEMT's Health and Safety Committee. He also serves as the Safety Officer for the New Jersey State EMS Task Force and as subchair for the New Jersey State EMS Safety Committee. In addition, he is the Secretariat for International Paramedic. He has been working in EMS and emergency management for more than 25 years and has published numerous articles and book chapters related to EMS and emergency management. He has spoken at national and international conferences, including those sponsored by JEMS, NFPA, and the AAA. Mr. Dworsky holds a Master of Public Health in EMS Management and is an OSHA-certified Safety Professional.

Lawrence (Larry) Nelson, M.Sc., EMT-P (Ret.), NMCEM (Chapter 19)—Mr. Nelson is currently the Director of the online BAAS EMS Management and Emergency Management concentrations at Eastern New Mexico University in Portales. In addition, he is an adjunct instructor for the New Mexico Department of Homeland Security and Emergency Management, teaching Intermediate and Advanced ICS and Community Emergency Response Team courses throughout the state. He has 35 years of public safety response and public health emergency management, administration, and teaching experience, including response to four Presidentially Declared Disasters. He remains a practitioner as an Exercise Planner for the campus emergency management program and a volunteer with the Melrose, New Mexico, Fire-EMS Department.

About the Series Editor

JEFFREY T. LINDSEY, PH.D., PM, EFO, CFO

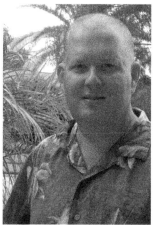

Dr. Jeffrey Lindsey has served in a variety of roles in the fire and EMS arena for the past 30 years. He has held positions of firefighter, para-medic, dispatcher, educator, coordi-nator, deputy chief, and chief. He started his career in Carlisle, Penn-sylvania, as a volunteer firefighter/EMT. In 1985 Dr. Lindsey pioneered the first advanced life support service in Cumberland County, Pennsylvania. He is retired as the Fire/EMS Chief for Estero Fire Rescue, where he served as the South Division Incident Commander during major events. He was also part of the Area Command for Lee County EOC. Currently he is the Distance Education Coordinator for the Fire and Emergency Services Programs at the University of Florida.

He has served as an inaugural member on the National EMS Advisory Council, represent-ing fire-based EMS, and is a past member of the State of Florida EMS Advisory Council, where he served as the firefighter/paramedic represent-ative. He currently serves as representative to the Fire and Emergency Services Higher Education EMS degree committee. He has been active in the IAFC, serving as liaison to ACEP and attend-ing various meetings representing fire-based EMS, and as the inaugural chair of the Commu-nity Paramedic committee, and he is an associate member of the Prehospital Research Forum.

He was a monthly columnist on product reviews for 3 years for *The Journal of Emergency Medical Services (JEMS)*, a national EMS journal. He is a columnist for Firerehab.com and has authored numerous fire and EMS texts for Brady/Pearson. He is currently the Chief Learning Officer for the Health and Safety Institute, which produces *24-7 EMS* and *24-7 Fire* videos. He also was an EMS pro-fessor for St. Petersburg College (Florida).

Dr. Lindsey has been involved in a number of large events and has served within the inci-dent command system at the upper level, includ-ing during a number of wildland fires and Hurricane Charley. He has also been involved in the preparations for a number of other hurri-canes and tropical storms.

He holds an associate's degree in para-medicine from Harrisburg Area Community College, a bachelor's degree in Fire and Safety from the University of Cincinnati, a master's degree in Instructional Technology from the University of South Florida, and a Ph.D. in Instructional Technology/Adult Education from the University of South Florida.

In addition, Dr. Lindsey has completed the Executive Fire Officer Program at the National Fire Academy. He has designed and developed various courses in fire and EMS. Dr. Lindsey is accredited with the Chief Fire Officer Designa-tion. He also is a certified Fire Officer II, Fire Instructor III, and paramedic in the state of Florida; holds a paramedic certificate for the state of Pennsylvania; and is a certified instruc-tor in these and a variety of other courses.

Dr. Lindsey has an innate interest in alter-native health. He is a certified nutritional counselor, a master herbalist, and a holistic health practitioner.

Reviewers

Thank you to the following individuals who gave generously of their time and expertise in reviewing the content of this first edition of *Management of Ambulance Services*.

David S. Becker, MA, EFO, EMT-P
EMS Program Director
Sanford-Brown College
Fenton, MO

Sam Bradley, BS, EMT-P, EMT-D
Paramedic/Firefighter Educator and QI
Specialist
Sam Bradely and Associates
Pittsburg, CA

Christopher Ebright, B.Ed., NREMT-P
EMS Education Coordinator
National EMS Academy
Covington, LA

Wally Grooms, M.S., CEP, NREMT-P
EMDI, EMS Instructor
Central Arizona College
Chandler, AZ

George A. Hettenbach, BBA, MS
Havertown, PA

Peggy Lahren, B.S., NREMT-P
Central Arizona College
Coolidge, AZ

Gregg Lander, B.S., NREMT-P
Program Chair/Instructor
Chemeketa Community College
Salem, OR

M. Ryan Maloney, B.S., EMS
Clinical and Educational Services
American Medical Response
San Diego, CA

Mark Stevens, B.A., NREMTP
Division Chief
Tualatin Valley Fire & Rescue
Tigard, OR

About FESHE

Fire and Emergency Services Higher Education (FESHE) is a dedicated group of individuals from around the country. It is hosted by the U.S. Fire Administration through the National Fire Academy. The mission of this group is to develop a uniform model curriculum for associate, bachelor, and master degrees. In December 2006 a group of EMS educators convened as the inaugural EMS committee for FESHE. The mission was to develop a model curriculum in EMS management at the bachelor's degree level. It was the consensus of leaders across the United States that the committee focus on the management issues of EMS. The clinical portion of the industry is addressed through the National EMS Education Standards and is mainly focused at the associate's level.

This text is written to meet the needs of the national model curriculum for EMS management at the bachelor's level. The EMS management curriculum includes six core courses and seven elective courses. Following are titles in Brady's *EMS Management Series*, designed to meet the FESHE curriculum.

CORE

- Foundations of EMS Systems
- Management of EMS
- EMS Community Risk Reduction
- EMS Quality Management and Research
- Legal, Political and Regulatory Environment in EMS
- EMS Safety and Risk Management

ELECTIVE

- Management of Ambulance Services
- Foundations for the Practice of EMS Education
- EMS Special Operations
- EMS Public Information and Community Relations
- EMS Communications and Information Technology
- EMS Finance
- Analytical Approaches to EMS

The History of Ambulance Services and Medical Transportation Systems in the United States

VINCENT D. ROBBINS, FACHE

Objectives

After reading this chapter, the student should be able to:

1.1 Explain the origins of ambulance services in the United States.
1.2 Discuss the development of key components of emergency medical services and the role played by ambulance services.
1.3 Describe the importance of milestones in the maturation of American emergency medical services.
1.4 Explain the impact of military conflict on the creation of ambulance and emergency medical systems.
1.5 Identify the most important national developments that advanced emergency medical services in the United States.
1.6 Summarize critical legislations that led to America's current state of emergency medical services delivery.

Overview

Ambulance services in the United States range in size from one ambulance operated by volunteers and managed by a community board of directors to large governmental agencies and even larger, private, for-profit corporations. This text presents information that the manager of an ambulance service, large or small, needs in order to keep the business solvent and provide clinically excellent service to the community.

Key Terms

"Accidental Death & Disability: The Neglected Disease of Modern Society"

ambulance

American Red Cross

Baron F. P. Percy

delivery models

Dominique-Jean Larrey

emergency medical services (EMS)

EMS Systems Act of 1973

Eugene Nagel, M.D.

hospital

J. Frank Pantridge, M.D.

Jonathan Letterman, M.D.

medical transportation systems

Medicare

Mickey Eisenberg, M.D.

National Highway Safety Act

National Highway Traffic Safety Act (NHTSA)

National Street and Highway Safety Conferences

National Traffic and Motor Vehicle Safety Act

President's Commission on Highway Safety system

U.S. Public Health Service

WHAT WOULD YOU DO?

To better orient its new employees, XYZ Ambulance Service included a presentation during orientation that reviewed the inception and evolution of **emergency medical services (EMS)** in America.

EMS in America evolved slowly at first and didn't actually become visible until the Civil War. Prior to that, health care in the United States was very much a local issue and stemmed primarily from the individual care that physicians rendered to their patients, primarily in the patient's home or the physician's individual office or what in those days was considered surgery. No systems existed that provided a cohesive and comprehensive way to expeditiously care for persons struck by sudden illness or injury, nor to ensure their recuperation and rehabilitation.

During the Civil War, the Union Army adopted many aspects of modern-day EMS, which were first applied by Emperor Napoleon Bonaparte's surgeon, Dominique-Jean Larrey. These included triage, in-field medical treatment, transportation in specialized vehicles, and definitive care at health care institutions. As the country changed, EMS became embodied in civilian life and was provided in different ways through various delivery models and agencies.

Beginning in the 1960s and continuing for the next 25 to 30 years, EMS in North America matured in sophistication, resulting in disparate, yet highly functional systems that include multiple levels of prehospital care, specialty health care treatment centers for different acute illnesses and injuries, precise resource management capabilities, and complex triage mechanisms, which include surge capacity components.

1. What is an EMS system?
2. What landmark events helped shape our modern perception of an EMS system?

3. How did the American Revolution, the Civil War, and American Military conflicts of the later twentieth century influence EMS in the United States?

■ INTRODUCTION

This chapter provides a history of EMS, from its origins in ancient medicine to its development and maturation in the United States. It is intended to provide the reader with a basic knowledge of how EMS began and evolved into what exists today. This history shows the impact of specific events, as well as the gradual growth of technical and scientific knowledge, on the advancement of EMS in the United States.

■ DEFINITIONS

As with any technical subject matter, the history of EMS and **medical transportation systems** in the United States must begin with an understanding of its unique vocabulary. The lexicon for this topic includes the following terms.

SYSTEM

The term **system** can have many meanings based on its context, but for the purpose of ensuring that the discussion of the subject at hand is lucid, it is initially interpreted in this chapter to mean a group of objects or subsystems interacting in an organized manner to produce an intended outcome.

The meaning of *system* will change during the course of this chapter and become more honed as the discussion approaches the late 1960s and early 1970s. At that point, it will reach its definitive meaning, which was established by description in federal P.L. 93-154

(usually referred to as the **EMS Systems Act of 1973**). This law determined that an EMS system "provides for the arrangement of personnel, facilities, and equipment for the effective and coordinated delivery of health care services in an appropriate geographical area under emergency conditions. These emergency conditions may occur as a result of the patient's condition, a natural disaster, or similar situation." It also identified the following fifteen components as essential to an EMS system: communications, training, manpower, mutual aid, transportation, accessibility, facilities, critical care units, transfer of care, consumer participation, public education, public safety agencies, standard medical records, independent review and evaluation, and disaster linkage (Sayad, 2005).

Disagreement exists among experts in the field regarding whether an EMS system includes the medical activities and facilities associated with patient care within the **hospital** setting. Some contend that "proper" EMS is concerned only with the prehospital environment, as envisioned early on by the federal government and described in the **National Highway Traffic Safety Act (NHTSA)** of 1966.[1] Others believe the intent of the federal government changed over time and eventually included every aspect of medical care, from incident detection

---

[1]The Highway Safety Act of 1966 established the office of Emergency Medical Services within the National Highway Traffic Safety Administration (NHTSA) of the Department of Transportation and outlined six core aspects, or system functions, of emergency medical services: detection, reporting, response, on-scene care, care in transit, and transfer to definitive care.

through post-discharge rehabilitation, but most especially the emergency departments and critical care units of hospitals. This position is supported by the federal EMS Systems Act of 1973, some components of which are clearly part of hospitals or posthospital entities.

AMBULANCE

For the purposes of this chapter, an **ambulance** is a vehicle (automotive, airborne, or waterborne) used for transporting medical personnel and equipment to the location of a sick or injured person, and for transporting sick or injured individuals to a location where further care can be provided.

In early (prior to the eighteenth century) military terms, *ambulance* referred to a mobile hospital, not a vehicle, that stayed with an army in the field to provide for the collection, triage, treatment, and care of the wounded and sick until they could be moved to stationary hospitals farther away. The term *ambulancias*,[2] from which *ambulance* derives through the Spanish language, related militarily to special tents where medical supplies and equipment were brought and stored, and where soldiers received care for their wounds or illness. King Ferdinand and Queen Isabella of Spain used it in this way as early as the fifteenth century. Today, we refer to such facilities as *field hospitals* or *MASHs* (*Mobile Army Surgical Hospitals*).

HOSPITAL

In the framework of the modern-day EMS system (which began after 1966[3]), a hospital is a physical facility, whether permanent or temporary (such as a field hospital), where sick or injured persons are examined, diagnosed, treated, and rehabilitated from illness or injury. The system usually includes the building, the equipment therein, and the health care and other personnel who work to provide a spectrum of health care services.

Hospitals may be categorized into several levels based on their ability, or inability, to adequately deal with patients who have specialized medical or trauma needs.[4] They are often referred to by the suffix "Center" to designate their advanced ability to provide medical care in a designated area of expertise. These types of hospitals include trauma centers, burn centers, spinal cord centers, children's hospitals, and, more recently, chest pain centers[5] and stroke centers.[6]

EMERGENCY MEDICAL SERVICES

The term *emergency medical services* did not exist as a familiar expression defining a specific

---

[2]It is believed that the word *ambulance* was first used by King Ferdinand and Queen Isabella of Spain in the fifteenth century.

[3]Virtually all medical authors and EMS experts agree that modern-day U.S. emergency medical services began in September 1966 with the publication of "Accidental Death and Disability: The Neglected Disease of Modern Society," a report by the Committees on Trauma and Shock of the Division of Medical Sciences, National Academy of Sciences/National Research Council.

[4]While hospitals began specializing at their very inception in the United States (circa 1750), the concept of categorizing hospitals based on their ability to meet the needs of emergency patients was first "officially" elucidated, albeit in a rudimentary way, in the landmark white paper by the NAS/NRC entitled "Accidental Death and Disability," referenced earlier.

[5]The Society of Chest Pain Centers (SCPC) was established on September 18, 1998. It is a professional society that claims to be dedicated to "patient advocacy and focusing on ischemic heart disease." Central to its mission, the SCPC promotes standardized medical treatment based on established protocols, delivered through chest pain centers, to care for patients affected by acute coronary syndromes and heart failure. They also promote the adoption of "process improvement science" by health care providers.

[6]The Joint Commission (www.jointcommission.org) now recognizes and has established a criteria-based assessment process, the Primary Stroke Center Certification Program, which is based on recommendations from the Brain Attack Coalition and the American Stroke Association. According to the Joint Commission, achievement of this certification signifies that the services provided by a named hospital have the critical elements necessary to achieve long-term success in improving outcomes.

application of medical care prior to the 1960s. Generally, it now means the provision of medical care by specially trained and authorized personnel to the suddenly ill or injured prior to, and in the absence of, a hospital setting. Contemporarily, it refers to any one of a variety of clinically different levels of medical care, provided to those who become unexpectedly incapacitated, whether from a chronic or acute illness or injury.[7]

MEDICAL TRANSPORTATION

Medical transportation (MT) in current parlance refers to the movement of patients to, from, or between medical facilities of any kind, including physicians' offices, ambulatory care centers, and specialized medical facilities, such as dialysis centers and hospitals. It usually concerns patients who are not experiencing emergent medical conditions, although not always. Some individuals requiring transport to a higher level of definitive medical care may be moved from one hospital to another, including a tertiary care hospital, and may be in a critical and/or unstable state. The mode of transport may vary according to the level of medical attention and care needed during movement. The patient's medical status dictates not only the type of vehicle used (e.g., mobility assistance van,[8] ambulance, helicopter, airplane, etc.) but also the number and training of personnel accompanying them (e.g., EMT, paramedic, nurse, respiratory therapist, etc.). The term *medical transportation* typically does not refer to EMS activities and is almost exclusively relegated to describing the activities of

patient movement that occur after the patient is initially treated at a hospital.

LEVELS OF MEDICAL PROFESSIONALS

The maturation of EMS in the United States has created a categorization of medical caregivers known as prehospital or EMS personnel. They are separated by the degree of their medical education and clinical training and, thus, their level of certification or licensure. This classification determines the extent of treatment they may provide, the medical devices and supplies they may use, and the specific titles that denote their roles. While each state has developed its own distinctive catalog of providers, the following groups of providers tend to correspond with the National Scope of Practice EMS Provider levels:

> *Emergency Medical Responder (EMR)* normally refers to police or fire department personnel who have received minimal first aid or limited basic emergency medical care training. They are nominally educated to provide rescue breathing,[9] CPR, and defibrillation using AEDs,[10] as

---

[7]The sophistication of the medical care included in EMS today is separated into multiple levels of expertise. From bystander first aid, through emergency medical responder, EMT, advanced EMT, to paramedic, prehospital medicine is regulated in virtually all states and includes specific categories of training and certification that delineate the role, responsibility, and type of care an individual may provide.

[8]Also known as invalid or wheelchair coach.

---

[9]Formerly called *artificial respiration*, invention of the term *rescue breathing* is attributed to the American Heart Association.

[10]Automatic external defibrillators (AEDs) were developed to ease the use of administering a regulated electric shock to the victim of sudden cardiac arrest for the purpose of resuscitation. They have been simplified to a point that even untrained civilians are able to use them adequately. Originally, AEDs were reserved for use by hospital and trained EMS personnel, but have now been modified substantially to allow use from bystanders. Today they are lightweight, durable, and equipped to give audible instructions to the operator. Once applied, they sense and interpret the patient's EKG rhythm and discharge an appropriate electric shock to the patient. Intervention by the operator is minimal. Because of this, and studies dating back to W. Douglas Weaver et al. in the *New England Journal of Medicine* (1988) that revealed speed to defibrillation within the first 10 minutes of SCA (sudden cardiac arrest) dramatically improved a patient's survival, AEDs have become part of the care given by first responders.

well as to control bleeding, administer oxygen, and stabilize fractures.

Emergency Medical Technician: Basic or Defibrillator (EMT-B/D) refers to individuals who are trained to meet a national standard of EMS[11] care that subsumes that of the first responder, and, in addition, includes a more thorough education in anatomy and physiology; rudimentary assessment of a patient's condition; splinting of fractures; application of cervical spine immobilization devices; various forms of victim extrication, lifting and movement; airway management and maintenance; various specific treatments of a variety of medical and trauma conditions; care of the obstetrical patient; and delivery of babies. These professionals also receive training in triage and fundamental management of mass casualty incidents.

Emergency Medical Technician: Intermediate (EMT-I) or Advanced Emergency Medical Technician (AEMT) is more highly trained than EMTs but less than paramedics. Beyond the ability of the EMTs, AEMTs can administer a few medications that are time critical in truly life-threatening situations. These usually include intravenous lines (IV) for either fluid replacement in patients suffering from traumatic shock or as a direct route to the circulatory system for the administration of vital drugs, such as epinephrine (adrenaline) in anaphylactic shock (severe allergic reaction) cases, and dextrose for critically symptomatic diabetics. Also, some

---

[11]This national standard was first developed in 1968 by The Task Force of the Committee on EMS of the NAS/NRC. Published by Dunlop and Associates, it was called "Training of Ambulance Personnel and Others Responsible for Emergency Care of the Sick and Injured at the Scene and During Transport." This was superseded in 1971 by the American Academy of Orthopedic Surgeons' text *Emergency Care and Transportation of the Sick and Injured*. The standard training program for Basic and Advanced EMS is now promulgated by the National Highway Traffic Safety Administration of the U.S. Department of Transportation.

AEMTs are permitted to insert devices, such as endotracheal tubes, to secure a patient's airway and provide artificial ventilation in those individuals who have stopped breathing on their own (respiratory arrest) and to use blood-glucose analysis devices (glucometers).

Paramedics receive far more extensive education in the biological processes of the human body, as well as advanced medical treatment techniques, than do EMRs or EMTs. In addition to the skills and drugs available to other certification levels, paramedics can administer an extensive variety of medications (in some locales more than sixty) via several routes, including subcutaneous, intramuscular, intravenous, endotracheal, and intraosseous (access in children and adults through bone). Often, paramedics are allowed to provide other forms of therapy previously reserved for the clinical setting of a hospital, such as nebulizer treatments (medication delivered by aerosol mist for respiratory disorders), external cardiac pacing (minor external electric shocks given to control dangerous heart activity), chest decompression (insertion of a needle into the chest cavity to re-expand a collapsed lung), and cricothyrotomy (insertion of a needle into the throat to bypass a blocked airway).

Specialty Care Transport Paramedics and Nurses is a relatively new provider level. These individuals are trained in and allowed to perform certain duties beyond their respective normal scope of practices. They usually staff advanced medical care transport ambulances that specialize in the transfer of patients needing sophisticated monitoring and treatment between medical facilities and potentially for extended time frames. These providers maintain a continuum of care, by virtue of their additional skill sets and use of complex medical equipment, as identical as possible to the patient's hospital of origin. Their operation is similar in function to EMS in that they operate in the out-of-hospital (EMS) setting, but usually these providers are utilized to perform interfacility medical transports.

HISTORY OF EMS AND MEDICAL TRANSPORTATION

To comprehend and fully appreciate the history of EMS and medical transportation in the United States, it is important to understand the nature of medicine (in particular the state of hospitals, prehospital emergent medical care, and patient transportation) around the world from the beginning.

MEDICINE BEFORE AMERICA

Throughout ancient times, civilizations around the world developed their own specific medical cultures, often derived from, or in tandem with, their evolving religious beliefs. A lack of reference or documentation indicates that little attention was paid to the movement of patients from the location of incipient need to the physician or, later, to the hospital. Historical records mention, rarely and with generalized descriptions, some apparatus used during these times to transport ill or injured individuals. However, even early on, certain people designed specific, customized devices to provide efficient, or at least convenient, movement of the incapacitated.

Stories from the early Roman and Greek epochs mention the use of chariots and two-wheeled carts as vehicles for the transport of injured soldiers (University of Pittsburgh, 2004). In some cases, soldiers were carried off the battlefield on their own shields. None of these instruments were especially designed with the transport of the ill or injured in mind. They were simply used, on an ad hoc basis, because they were readily available and conveniently suited to the task. There seems to be no special focus at this time in history on specializing a transport device specific to the needs of the incapacitated.

In Homer's *Iliad* and *Odyssey*, circa 1250 B.C., descriptions of battlefield wounds and treatment clearly indicate that the severely wounded were not moved from the site of their injury. Rather, medical personnel, usually surgeons, came to the scene and treated patients where they laid, prior to transport. Medical care would be administered even during the fighting (Homer, 2004).[12] This is substantiated by ancient artwork and pottery images. As an example, a kylex[13] dated at about 490 B.C., by the Greek artist Euphronios (c. 520–470 B.C.),[14] depicts Achilles bandaging the arm wound of Patroclos, another soldier, apparently on the field of battle (Major, 1954).

The first known institutions that focused on providing cures for illnesses were recorded as Egyptian temples, circa 4000 B.C. Treatment was mostly self-directed, incorporating religious beliefs of the culture, such as prayers to specific gods. Later, Greek temples dedicated to the physician god Asclepius (Latin, *Aesculapius*) served in a similar way but also allowed the ill to stay overnight while they awaited guidance in the context of dreams (Encyclopædia Britannica, n.d.–a) Many of these temples eventually expanded into Asklepieia (pl., Asclepieion), which consisted of a group of buildings constructed on adjoining, staggered terraces, the higher retaining their religious function and the lower acting as what would now be considered a hospital. The lower sections of the Asklepieia maintained rooms for hydrotherapy, physical therapy, and treating fractures (Major, 1954).

The earliest known facilities that were dedicated solely to admitting and treating

---

[12]A detailed analysis of the *Iliad* and the *Odyssey* by Frohlich revealed that of the 147 wounds mentioned in the great works, 106 were inflicted by spears with a fatality rate of 80%, 17 by sword with 100% mortality, 12 by arrow with 42% fatal, and 12 by slingshot, 66% resulting in death.

[13]An ancient Greek drinking vessel.

[14]Euphronios was a Greek artist who spent his early career as a painter, working mainly in the red-figure style. Later, he was known primarily as a potter.

the sick or injured were hospitals that arose by 431 B.C. in Sri Lanka (or Ceylon as it was known before 1972) and are referred to now as Brahmanic hospitals (Encyclopædia Britannica, n.d.–b). At about the same time, Hippocrates (c. 460–377 B.C.) taught and published the concepts of medical ethics and basic medical philosophy in Greece (Garrison, 1966). He used the foundations of medicine previously espoused by Empedocles of Acragas (c. 490–430 B.C.) in 450 B.C. that four bodily humors—blood, phlegm, choler (yellow bile), and melancholy (black bile)—must be maintained in balance to result in health (Encyclopædia Britannica, n.d.–b). During this period Greek surgeons built and maintained their own offices, *iatreia* (Cavallo, 1997), which were often separate from their personal residences.

The first mention of a system of medical facilities, however, does not occur until the second century B.C. and is generally credited to the Buddhist King Ashoka (also, *Asoka*) (273–232 B.C.), ruler of the Mauryan dynasty in India.[15] He issued a series of edicts, inscribed on rocks and pillars throughout his kingdom, some of which described two kinds of hospitals and medical care, one for humans and the other for animals. The edicts also memorialized that healing herbs were imported, grown, and made available for medical treatment purposes throughout the empire. Before he was done, Ashoka had established a series of eighteen hospitals throughout Hindustan,

many staffed with doctors and nurses and all supported by state funds (Major, 1954).[16]

Around 100 b.c., Romans established *valetudinaria* (Encyclopædia Britannica, n.d.–b) or military medical treatment facilities, for slaves, gladiators, and soldiers. These facilities were located and moved with the armies they served. Citizens not in military service sought out care from physicians individually, either at special offices the doctor had established or by summoning him to their home.

Beginning in about 1080 A.D., a sect of monks who would eventually become a military fraternity provided evacuation from the field of battle, medical aid, and convalescent comfort for both pilgrims and crusading knights as a primary function of their order.[17] The exact method they used to extricate the injured is not readily documented, but it probably involved traditional conveyances of the time. It is one of the first validated examples of what could be called, in today's terms, a regional EMS system, incorporating the basic

---

[15]Inscriptions dating from the third century B.C. by Ashoka include statements that hospitals had been established. According to his scribe, Samhita, there were elaborate dispensaries in their own compounds, set apart from state buildings. One of the hospital structures was usually a maternity facility where patients could stay throughout delivery and postpartum care. A second contained distinct areas where apprentices examined patients before reporting to the court physician, a pharmacy for the preparation and dispensing of medications, and an operating room away from areas that patients frequented.

---

[16]Some dispute this claim, citing works by King Duttha Gamani, a later ruler of the same region, in which he takes credit for establishing a group of eighteen hospitals.

[17]A hospital was founded in Jerusalem, in about 1080 A.D., by the Brothers of the Benedictine Monastery of Saint Mary Latina to provide medical aid and comfort for the throngs making pilgrimage to the Holy Land. This group of monks, being granted gradual sovereignty by a succession of popes, eventually became the Knights of St. John. They transformed from a religious order into a military group, fighting on behalf of Christianity during the Crusades. It is reported that they also took on the role of evacuating injured colleagues and enemies from the battlefield and rendering medical aid to them, including long-term hospital care. Their emblem eventually became the Maltese Cross, the universal insignia of fire departments around the world, supposedly because they extinguished fires caused by the enemies' use of naphtha and provided rescue and emergency medical care to victims. The hospital was purported to have operated along contemporary Greek theories of medicine and was divided into wards. It may have had as many as two thousand beds during the height of Christian control. The introduction of advanced Arab medicine to the hospital enhanced western European knowledge of medical care considerably.

elements of detection, response, assessment, treatment, transport, and definitive care.

MEDICAL TRANSPORTATION BEFORE AMERICA

Prior to the 1600s, several methods of moving the debilitated were in use around the world. In what would become the United States, Native Americans used the travois (Answers.com, n.d.), which was essentially a stretcher affixed at one end to a horse or large dog to pull and use as a conveyance for matériel or disabled people. In India, dhoolies (Free Dictionary, n.d.),[18] or covered stretchers, were used to transport the sick or injured. In Egypt, camel stretchers called panniers (Wikipedia, n.d.–a) were the method of choice, even through the Napoleonic period,[19] to move the nonambulatory. Panniers also were used in many other regions around the world with alternate beasts of burden, such as mules.

As mentioned earlier, in the fifteenth century, King Ferdinand and Queen Isabella of Spain were instrumental in the deployment of *ambulancia* (mobile field hospitals) to provide rapid medical aid to their soldiers. They were staffed by physicians and surgeons and were primarily used for the storage of medical supplies and the treatment of the wounded. *Ambulancia* were relocated often to follow the army and maintain a close geographical relationship to the battlefield in order to reduce transport time from the site of injury to the point where medical intervention could take place. As the conveyance for the wounded, used to transport them to the strategically placed field hospital, the Spanish Army employed horse-drawn carts or wagons, with attendants, as early as April 1487 during the 40 days Siege of Malaga.[20]

THE AMERICAN COLONIAL PERIOD

Beginning with the landing of the *Mayflower* on November 11, 1620, in Provincetown, Cape Cod, the Colonial Era of American history began. Even though two of the settlers were physicians (Captain Myles Standish and Dr. Samuel Fuller[21]), American medicine did not enjoy a propitious beginning. At first, and for a significant period of time thereafter, early Americans did not emulate their ancestors from Europe regarding medicine or medical technology. In fact, colonial medicine was significantly less advanced than what could be found in Europe during this period. While hospitals and medical schools had been well established for decades in England, France, Italy, the Middle East, and even Russia, none existed in America until L'Hôpital des Pauvres de la Charité (also known as St. John's Hospital of the Poor)[22] opened its doors on May 6, 1736, in New Orleans[23] (Pennsylvania Hospital, depicted in

---

[18]A dhooly, or doolie, is a covered litter, from the Hindi *doli*. It consists of a cot or frame, suspended by its four corners from a bamboo pole, and it is carried by two or four men.

[19]Side-saddle panniers were used to carry patients in Baron Jean Dominique Larrey's (1766–1842) camel ambulance during Napoleon's years of war.

---

[20]A fifteenth-century Muslim seaport city and province located on the Mediterranean coast of Spain.

[21]Samuel Fuller, a physician and surgeon, did not have an opportunity to significantly influence the development of medicine in America since he succumbed to the smallpox epidemic of 1633.

[22]Established by the bequeath of Jean Louis, a French boat building seaman, in 1735, it eventually became known as Charity Hospital and remains operational at printing.

[23]Disagreement exists about this fact. Most authors cite Pennsylvania Hospital, which began operations in 1752 in Philadelphia, as America's earliest hospital because it was the first in the colonies proper. Some believe Bellevue Hospital of New York was first since it began service on March 31, 1736, with a six-bed facility located on the second floor of a prison ("public workhouse and house of correction"). Others refute this claim because it was not originally a building dedicated to solely serve the sick. Lastly, some insist that Master Jacob Hendrickszen Varrevanger, a surgeon with the Dutch West India Company, established a small hospital that served the one thousand inhabitants of New Amsterdam (later New York City) in 1658.

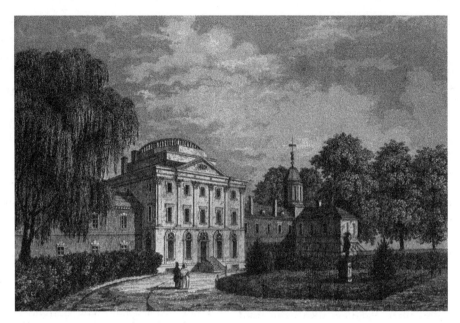

FIGURE 1.1 ■ L'Hôpital de Pensylvanie (Pennsylvania Hospital) circa 1751. *Source: National Library of Medicine copyright.*

Figure 1.1 and established by Benjamin Franklin and Dr. Thomas Bond in 1751, was the earliest hospital in the colonial states of America.)

Likewise, early Americans did not receive medical care to the standard available elsewhere in "modern societies" around the world. In this regard, America could be considered a developing country. Physicians were among a group of medical practitioners who were neither traditionally schooled nor in possession of any formal degrees from established colleges. Other medical caregivers of the time included apothecaries, herbalists, midwives, quacks, surgeons, and barbers.[24]

Patients were more often than not treated and cared for by their own families or neighbors. If someone saw a physician (or other

practitioner), it was usually in the patient's home or at the site of an accident. Medical practitioners would frequently travel to the scene of an injured person, rather than have the injured person transported, since virtually no dedicated treatment facilities existed.

With few hospitals or other specialized facilities for medical care available in North America, little need existed for a structured transport system or even medically specialized movement apparatus. Even though in some cases patients would be housed in their physician's personal residence when their condition warranted, no specialized means of transport developed for some time. If injured or taken suddenly ill away from their home or other shelter, patients needed to arrange for their own transport. Usually, if a significant distance were involved, the victim, or family or neighbors, would use any available cart, buggy, or wagon.

American medicine at this time was quite primitive by today's standards. Physicians and

---

[24]Surgeons and barbers were both in the same guild until they separated in 1745. Prior to that, both used a red and white striped pole to advertise their *professional* place of business

surgeons could do little in emergent circumstances and focused mostly on longer-term illnesses. Although they would set simple fractures and periodically amputate limbs affected by multiple breaks, they mostly prepared herbal remedies, bled patients, and provided comfort and advice.

THE AMERICAN REVOLUTION

The American Revolution marked the beginning of the development of EMS systems in what would become the United States. While the Civil War is often cited as this inauguration, it is the American Revolution that rightly holds the distinction because it brought two critical elements of EMS to the forefront for the first time. First, it was recognized by the successive Director Generals of the Continental Army's Hospital Department (Drs. Benjamin Church, John Morgan, William Shippen, and John Cochran) that a significant need existed for extensive and rapid transportation of the medically needy, especially the battle wounded, to designated medical facilities.[25] Second, a categorization of hospitals, between "camp" and "regimental/general," was devised as a means to sort patients according to the intensity of their medical needs, urgency of medical care required, and their burden upon local armies' medical capabilities and battle readiness.

At the outset, and during the course of the American Revolution, documents reveal that much thought, and sometimes debate, centered on the proper design of the medical services system for the army. This system included mobile and stationary hospitals and their design, location in proximity to battle areas, staffing, sanitation, supply and medical

capability designation; response of appropriate medical care to the wounded on the battlefield, including a rudimentary triage process; extrication of the injured to remote treatment sites/facilities; and eventual transportation of patients, based on their needs, between immediate (*camp* or *flying* hospitals) and regional, individual colonial military hospitals (*regimental*) or Continental Army (*general*) hospitals[26] (Gillett, 1981).

George Washington recognized early on that the diversified, individual colonial armies' hospitals and their personnel needed to be incorporated into an overall command structure and operational system.[27] The Continental Congress enacted a series of laws designed to formulate a national military medical system, repetitively and increasingly detailing the components, composition, and organizational structure of that system.[28] It became the Director General's responsibility to ensure that the regimental physician/surgeon was supplied with sufficient quantities "of large strong tents, beds, bedding, medicines, and hospital

---

[25]Their arguments later convinced General George Washington, who forcefully pursued their concepts. In fact, Washington became involved in issuing orders to clarify or modify the Continental Congress's edicts in an attempt to organize the army's medical department, which was in significant disarray.

[26]An argument persisted throughout the development of the Continental Army medical system whether locally controlled colonial "state" hospitals or regional Continental "federal" hospitals were superior. George Washington sided with the "national" concept of general over regimental hospitals.
[27]Washington wrote "Disputes and Contentions have arisen and must continue until it is reduced to some system." When Washington arrived at Cambridge, Massachusetts, on July 3, 1775, to take command of the Continental Army, the hospitalized sick and wounded, most of whom were from Massachusetts, were being cared for by Massachusetts regimental surgeons in Massachusetts facilities. It was obvious to all concerned, however, that this approach would be inadequate when units from other colonies became involved and when the fighting spread beyond the confines of that colony. Washington pointed out that, already, "Disputes and Contentions have arisen and must continue until it is reduced to some system" (http://history.amedd.army.mil/booksdocs/rev/gillett1/ch2.html, which cites to "The Medical Administrators of the American Revolutionary Army," *Military Affairs 25* (1961), which in turn cites to the original document).
[28]The Continental Congress's Laws of July 27, 1775; July 17, 1776; April 7, 1777; February 6, 1778; and September 30, 1780.

stores" and with "wagons and drivers" whenever patients needed "conveyance" to the general hospital.[29] The latter constitutes the first recorded recognition of need and attempt to establish an EMS and/or medical transportation system.

In January 1777, George Washington instructed the army's Hospital Department Director General, Dr. John Cochran, to consult with another well-known physician of the day and his future successor, Dr. William Shippen,[30] to reorganize the medical system, including the "flying hospitals," to accompany his armies in the field. Flying hospitals were equivalent to today's Mobile Army Surgical Hospitals (MASHs). They were semitransient field hospitals[31] that moved with the regiment or divisional army, providing immediate care to postbattle wounded and for the medically ill. Directly after combat they would either dispatch physicians and surgeons from their base camp to the battlefield to triage and treat the wounded or they would send assigned wagons to retrieve the injured for transport back to the flying camp for medical aid. Once initially treated at the camp hospital, certain soldiers, depending on their need for continued care or convalescence, would be moved again, this time to a regimental or general medical institution.

Throughout the war, however, this military medical care system remained in disarray, never being completely or appropriately organized despite increasingly detailed infrastructure design and operational instructions from the Continental Congress, the Hospital Department's Director General, and George Washington himself. With little financial support and a poor initial outline of organizational authority from the Continental Congress, along with few commanders in the field who paid sufficient attention to directives being handed down on how to configure medical care delivery, build and maintain hospitals, staff facilities, and store needed supplies, the condition of the military hospitals and the care received by the soldiers suffered greatly.

In spite of innovative concepts such as tiered, specialized medical care and priority assignment of wagons as ambulances,[32] the Continental Army was unable to effectuate efficient medical operations. In fact, it was not even possible to adequately maintain a decent standard of medical care. Military hospitals were notoriously unsanitary, understaffed, and poorly supplied. Medical transport wagons were never specially designed or equipped (other than the supplies and instruments their occasional physician/surgeons carried) to handle the ill or injured. However, during what would be classified today as "interfacility transports," physicians or surgeons did sometimes accompany the medically incapacitated during large movements of patients from camp hospitals to regimental or general hospitals. It is arguable that the soldiers of the American Revolution

---

[29]Law of 7-8 April 1777 of the United States Continental Congress.

[30]Shippen was the personal choice and favorite of Washington from the very beginning of the revolution for the position of Director General of the Hospital Department. However, it wasn't until April 11, 1777, that Shippen became the third to hold the post.

[31]According to Weedon's *Valley Forge Orderly Book* (General George Weedon of the Continental Army, under command of General George Washington, in the campaign of 1777–1778,), p. 191: "The Flying Hospitals are to be 15 feet wide and 25 feet long in the clear and the story at least 9 feet high to be covered with boards or shingles only without any dirt, windows made on each side and a chimney at one end. Two such hospitals are to be made for each brigade at or near the center and if the ground permits of it not more than 100 yards distance from the brigade."

---

[32]From the Continental Congress documents; LAW OF 30 SEPTEMBER 1780: "That the quartermaster general furnish the Hospital Department, from time to time, as occasion may require, with such a number of horses and wagons as may be necessary for removing the sick and wounded, and for transporting the hospital stores; but that no other horses than those belonging to the officers of the department, for which forage may be herein allowed, be kept separately and at the expense of the department."

received worse medical care than their civilian counterparts, even though the soldiers lived with a more primitive health care system.

BETWEEN WARS: THE AMERICAN REVOLUTION–THE CIVIL WAR

Following the Treaty of Paris in 1783, the Continental Army, along with its Hospital Department, was disbanded. Essentially no medical structure remained active in the military of the United States between the end of the American Revolution and the period just prior to the War of 1812. Although laws and military regulations existed on paper, virtually none were in force. No advancements in prehospital care or transportation took place during this time, despite continued combat activity during the military campaigns of the American Indian Wars of the 1790s.

While America was stagnating in the arena of EMS system development and continued to fail to recognize the need for the creation of effective, customized medical transport mechanisms, others in the world were moving forward. In 1788, a Royal Ordinance was passed in France that required the creation of improved transportation for those wounded in battle. In addition, on November 12, 1792, the French National Convention declared the need to construct "suspended carts for the transportation of the sick and wounded of the armies" (Ortiz, 1996).[33]

Despite a landmark in world history regarding EMS and medical transportation

in 1793, the United States took little notice and failed to incorporate any of its components for decades. **Dominique-Jean Larrey (1766–1842)**, Napoleon Bonaparte's chief physician and surgeon, conceptualized and implemented a cogent, comprehensive prehospital care system that, for the first time, triaged the injured; provided immediate, temporary medical care;[34] and transported the injured from the battlefield to strategically placed medical aid stations in a formal, regulated way using special apparatus. Larrey's *ambulance volante* (flying ambulances [field hospitals]) were comprised of a corps of surgeons and nurses who accompanied armies into battle and rendered care to soldiers' wounds both on the battlefield and in mobile field hospitals. Responding to the site of injury (usually the field of battle) and often under continuing enemy fire, they determined who was the most seriously hurt and treated them first. They utilized new, advanced medical techniques for the time (also invented by Larrey), and then moved those in need of continued, or more definitive care, to temporary medical facilities, which were especially equipped and supplied

---

[33]A prize was offered for the design that complied the best with the commission's specifications. The criteria included a requirement for the vehicle to be "light, solid, suspended, and comfortable for carrying four or six casualties lying down, eight at most." However, after 8 months of considering over 29 designs, the commission decided its specifications were unrealistic. Political leaders, nonetheless, forced the committee to pursue a design. The result: an ambulance that was too heavy and impractical for the battlefield. These efforts coincidentally delayed the implementation of Larrey's ambulance design, which had already been successfully field-tested.

[34]From Dominique-Jean Larrey's writings (*Memoir of Baron Larrey*, http://books.google.co.uk/books?id=bH wIAAAAIAAJ&printsec=frontcover&source=gbs_ge_ summary_r&cad=0#v=onepage&q&f=false): "The best plan that can be adopted in such emergencies, to prevent the evil consequences of leaving soldiers who are severely wounded without assistance, is to place the ambulances as near as possible to the line of the battle, and to establish headquarters, to which all the wounded, who require delicate operations, shall be collected to be operated upon by the surgeon-general. Those who are dangerously wounded should receive the first attention, without regard to rank or distinction. They who are injured in a less degree may wait until their brethren-in-arms, who are badly mutilated, have been operated and dressed, otherwise the latter would not survive many hours; rarely until the succeeding day. Besides with a slight wound, it is easy to repair to the hospital of the first or second line, especially for the officers who generally have means of transportation. Finally, life is not endangered by such wounds."

to handle battle trauma. This corps used customized wagons that Larrey designed, which constituted the first specialized and practical conveyance devices to move the injured from point of incapacitation to medical facilities (what we now refer to as ambulances, that he subsequently modified to meet local demands of terrain and specific transport obstacles[35]).

Larrey's memoirs reveal how he came to realize the need for and first conceptualized the idea of a specialized medical transport vehicle: "I now first discovered the inconveniences to which we were subjected in moving our ambulances or military hospitals. The military regulations required that they should always be one league[1] distant from the Army. The wounded were left on the field, until after the engagement, and were then collected at a convenient spot, to which the ambulances speeded as soon as possible; but the number of wagons interposed between them and the Army, and many other difficulties so retarded their progress that they never arrived in less than 24 or 36 hours, so that most of the wounded died for want of assistance. . . . this suggested to me the idea of constructing an ambulance in such a manner that it might afford a ready conveyance for the wounded during battle. I was unable to carry my plans into execution until sometime later" (Ortiz, 1996).

Larrey considered several designs for the transport vehicle he had determined was needed to rapidly evacuate the injured to a field hospital. One included stretchers affixed to the sides of horses, as in the fashion of saddlebags, which he was to later utilize in the deserts of Egypt, replacing the horse with a camel. However, at the outset he settled on covered wagons drawn by horses, with either one (for level ground) or two (for rough terrain) sets of wheels (Ortiz, 1996). His flying-ambulances were also designed to carry medical equipment, supplies, and medicines to aid in the evacuation and in-transit care of the patient.

At the same time that Dominique-Jean Larrey invented and deployed his revolutionary prehospital care system, another French surgeon, **Baron F. P. Percy**, formulated his own concept of EMS. Percy's system resembled more of a mobile emergency room than an ambulance–field hospital system. Baron Percy introduced the idea of a regular corps, specially trained in and equipped for the transport of injured, using stretchers and educated in a formal, regimented course of instruction. The corps' task was to accompany a large medical wagon,[36] capable of treating a large number of patients, to the scene of the battle wounded, and to strike out radially to rapidly retrieve the injured. Once the wounded were returned to the mobile hospital wagon, the surgeons would immediately provide medical care, treating patients sufficiently until they were either ambulatory or could be transported in the wagon.

Back in America, on July 16, 1798, President John Adams signed into law the Act for the Relief of Sick and Disabled Seamen, which created the Marine Hospital Service[37] that we now know as the **U.S. Public Health Service**. A year later the law was extended to cover all officers and sailors serving in the U.S. Navy. Initially, this law established a network of medical care, with a system of hospitals, for the aid of American merchant seamen. Beginning along the northeast coast,

---

[35]Larrey altered his ambulance design from a covered wagon to a pannier or saddle-bag type that was affixed to camels in Egypt.

[36]It could carry as many as ten persons (surgeons and assistants), with equipment, to critical points in a fluid battlefield. A corps of stretcher-bearers then brought the wounded by foot to the surgeons. Such duty was not only quite strenuous and dangerous, but also was militarily significant: It relieved the common infantrymen of the arduous task of caring for their own wounded. While these were great innovations of this time, Percy's ambulance system never saw widespread battlefield implementation and, thus, never achieved the operational significance of Larrey's system.

[37]This was the first prepaid medical care program in the United States, financed through compulsory employer tax and federally administered. Twenty cents were deducted every month from each seaman's wages to fund the system.

it would proliferate to the Great Lakes as well as the Gulf and Pacific coasts. However, it relied on local mechanisms of transportation to move its patients until the system acquired ambulances of its own, circa 1900. Emergent medical care was still provided onboard ship when a seaman became ill or injured. The Maritime Hospital System primarily provided definitive care and convalescence, not EMS.

In the U.S. Army, the period between the American Revolution and the War of 1812 brought no significant improvement, enhancement, or expansion of medical care or medical transportation. In fact, during this time, what already had been designed and established generally atrophied. The leaders of the country were still reticent concerning an organized military and thus reluctant to enlarge America's forces. Despite three successive War Department secretaries who were physicians and some laws still in effect concerning a military Medical Department, the state of medical care in the land militia of the United States regressed.

Legislation in 1799 that created the post-revolution Medical Department did, however, codify some lessons learned during that war. Namely, a lesson learned was the need for the purveyors (purchasers of medical supplies and equipment) and the regimental surgeons to be under the control of the physician-general of the Medical Department and the senior hospital surgeon of an army district. This legislation further detailed patient care assignment responsibilities, hospital staffing schedules and discipline rules, camp sanitation requirements, and examination boards for candidates seeking positions within the department. Thus, the importance of having a structure for governing the provision of medical care, at least in urgent circumstances such as battle, was realized. A medical care system had become an integral part of the American military establishment, albeit mostly on paper for the time being (Gillett, 1981).

Undedicated, unspecialized wagons and carriages were still being used during this time to move the wounded and nonambulatory ill.

These vehicles were not particularly outfitted to provide comfortable transport or allow for the convenient rendering of medical care in transit. Excerpts from historical documents of the time—for example, the August 20, 1794, Battle of Fallen Timbers near Fort Defiance in the Northwest Territories—reveals, "The wounded . . . were considered fortunate to be moved from the battlefield in a carriage"; however, "Doctor Carmichael, through neglect, had the wounded men of the artillery and cavalry thrown into wagons, among spades, axes, picks, etc." (Gillett, 1981).

The introduction of predefined, unit-specific medical supply packages occurred now. They were created to organize and improve supply distribution within the land militia's hospital system. Dr. James Mease, followed by Dr. Francis LaBaron, delineated standardized medical supply and drug inventories, designed and built "medicine chests," and packaged the caches for distribution to the various military hospitals of the army.[38]

Little changed in American EMS during the early part of the nineteenth century, even though medicine in general was maturing, both in the United States and around the world. Advances in health care, preventative and definitive, were taking place at a rapid pace. The use of anesthesia for surgeries was introduced;[39] the stethoscope was born (Whonamedit, 2011); and Addison, Bright, Hodgkin, Graves, and Parkinson disease were all discovered. Rudolph Virchow, a German pathologist, broke radical new ground by displacing the traditional

---

[38]Each "medicine chest" was designed to serve 500 men and be carried on a baggage wagon 3.5 feet long.

[39]In 1842, the American physician Crawford Long discovered the anesthetic effects of ether. In 1844 dentist Horace Wells used nitrous oxide as an anesthetic for the first time. Also in the United States, a dentist named William Morton used ether during a tooth extraction in 1846. Anesthetics were shown to reduce surgical mortality and allow surgeons to perform longer, more complex operations.

humoral,[40] Boerhaave,[41] and Cullen[42] theories of medicine predominant in the United States, showing instead that all disease was based on disorders of the cells. Despite these extraordinary steps forward, no significant changes occurred regarding prehospital emergent care or transportation.

During the War of 1812, dedicated, specially equipped wagons were still not in use for the transport of wounded or sick. The procedures used to retrieve and treat patients were the same they had been during the American Revolution. The structure of the army's Medical Department was unchanged, and the designation of field versus general hospitals was identical to that of the Continental Army. It is interesting to note that, in spite of their knowledge of Dominique-Jean Larrey's pioneering work for Napoleon in emergency medicine circa 1790, the military doctors of the American Army failed to implement any of his innovations (Gillett, 1981).

In other places, however, EMS development was occurring. Around 1840, a specialized medical transport vehicle was introduced for use in Scotland (Science & Society Picture Library, n.d.). It was a converted Growler or Clarence (Science & Society Picture Library)

carriage and could carry two to three patients at a time with an attendant nurse. This coupe coach was equipped with large elliptic springs from which the carriage itself was suspended, providing a relatively comfortable ride. It was modified with pneumatic tires to provide an even smoother ride for the patients it was transporting. It became known as the Clarence Ambulance.[43] In addition, its interior was lined with highly polished butternut wood paneling to facilitate sanitary washing. It remained in use until the beginning of the twentieth century.

THE CIVIL WAR

The next significant development of American EMS and medical transport was to take place during the Civil War (1861–1865). In finally adopting some of the ideas put forth by Larrey, the Union Medical Department implemented the use of committed, customized horse-drawn wagons as ambulances as well as stretcher-litters and pack animal cacolets (Figure 1.2).[44] In addition, a dedicated group of stretcher-bearers and ambulance wagon attendants/drivers was formed and received specialized training by the Medical Department in their tasks (Dammann and Bollet, 2008) and a tiered transport system was developed.

The level of medical care afforded soldiers was separated based on intensity needed and the fundamentals of triage. At the location of injury, rudimentary assessment of wound severity was performed and rapid transportation, usually by stretcher, was provided

---

[40]Aristotle developed the Humoral theory in the fourth century. It described four principal fluids (or humors) existing within the body: blood, choler (yellow bile), melancholy (black bile), and phlegm. An equal balance between the four was necessary for good health. The theory conjectured that one or more humors predominate in most people, giving rise to particular temperaments, characters, and illnesses.

[41]Herman Boerhaave believed that disease was based on chemical and physical qualities, such as acidity and alkalinity, or tension and relaxation, not the four humors. A main tenet of his theory was that nature should be permitted to aid in any cure.

[42]William Cullen believed either an excess (characterized by fever) or an insufficiency (characterized by chill) of nervous tension underlaid all disease. Excess was to be treated by depleting regimens including bleeding, a restricted diet, purging, rest, and sedation. Insufficiency, excess's opposite, called for restorative measures.

---

[43]Named after the Duke of Clarence (1765–1837), who later became King William IV of England. The duke had designed a light carriage in the fashion of the Brougham coach, a popular transport device of the time resembling American stagecoaches of the West.

[44]Cacolets were a pair of rigid chairs that hung over the back of mules or other pack animals, in saddlebag fashion, for the purpose of carrying the sick or wounded in a sitting position. They were in use in other parts of the world prior to the American Civil War, such as in Crimea during a conflict in that area.

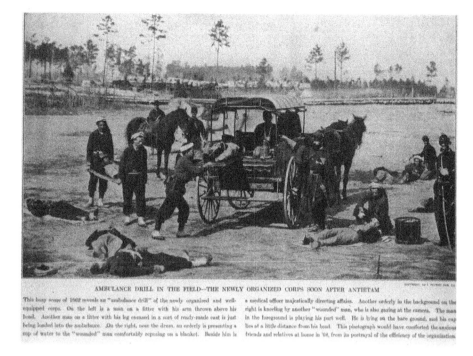

AMBULANCE DRILL IN THE FIELD—THE NEWLY ORGANIZED CORPS SOON AFTER ANTIETAM

This busy scene of 1862 reveals an "ambulance drill" of the newly organized and well-equipped corps. On the left is a man on a litter with his arm thrown above his head. Another man on a litter with his leg encased in a sort of ready-made cast is just being loaded into the ambulance. On the right, near the drum, an orderly is presenting a cup of water to the "wounded" man comfortably reposing on a blanket. Beside him is a medical officer majestically directing affairs. Another orderly in the background on the right is kneeling by another "wounded" man, who is also gazing at the camera. The man in the foreground is playing his part well. He is lying on the bare ground, and his cap lies at a little distance from his head. This photograph would have comforted the anxious friends and relatives at home in '62, from its portrayal of the efficiency of the organization.

FIGURE 1.2 ▪ A Civil War ambulance squad conducting training. *Source: National Library of Medicine copyright.*

to the field dressing stations. These stations were located very close to battle, sometimes on the battlefield itself, and were where the first medical intervention was made. Medical personnel attended to the wounded, applying bandages and administering pain-killing medication (predominantly whiskey and morphine).[45] Then the patient was moved by ambulance to the field hospital (Figure 1.3). Once in the field hospital, soldiers were formally triaged and separated into one of three categories: wounded, surgical cases, and mortally wounded. The nonfatally wounded were treated with more secure dressings, splints for simple fractures, and so on. Surgical cases were usually those requiring amputations that were performed on site using either chloroform or ether, if available, as anesthetics. Postsurgical cases and the wounded requiring further care were then transported to the general hospital, located well behind the lines, often in major cities or towns. Here soldiers were provided some definitive medical attention, as well as follow-up and convalescent care.

While the organization of the Medical Department became more structured and effective over time, it initially did not provide for the removal of wounded from the battlefield or their transport to aid stations or hospitals. Surgeon General William A. Hammond expressed his concern with the lack of this needed component of the military medical care system in a letter to Secretary of War Edwin Stanton on September 7, 1862: "attention to the frightful state of disorder existing in the arrangement for removing the wounded

---

[45]It is interesting to note that throughout the Civil War, both the Union and Confederate medical services provided care for the opponent not only on the battlefield but often for a significant time thereafter. Triage was did not consider on which side of the conflict a soldier was engaged.

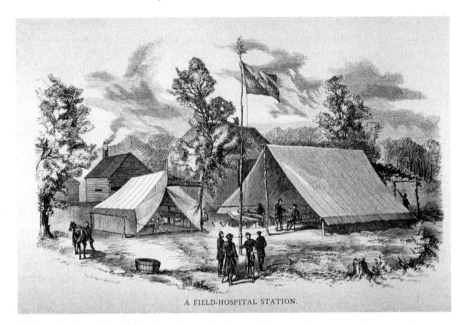

A FIELD-HOSPITAL STATION.

FIGURE 1.3 ■ A Civil War field hospital. *Source: National Library of Medicine copyright.*

from the field of battle. The scarcity of ambulances, the want of organization . . . the total lack of ambulance attendants," concluding, "An ambulance corps should be organized and set in instant operation. . . . " (Munson, Thompson, and Deering, 1911).[46]

The disorganization that burdened the Medical Department is evidenced by events that occurred during and immediately after the Seven Days Battle (Peninsular Campaign of April–July 1862). In the aftermath of fighting, the injured were sent to hastily established gathering points and field hospitals, the ambulance system that did exist quickly failed, and many of the wounded piled up untreated for days (Air University, n.d.).

_____

[46]Hammond's contemporary, but subordinate, Dr. Charles Tripler (Medical Director of the Army of the Potomac prior to Jonathan Letterman) is also given credit for implementing dedicated ambulance wagons and training attendants.

On June 19, 1862, Hammond appointed **Jonathan Letterman, M.D.** as the new Medical Director of the Army of the Potomac. Letterman was instrumental in putting Hammond's concepts into practice and honed them even further. Letterman established an effective ambulance corps and included techniques in the loading and unloading of patients on stretchers into and out of ambulance wagons. He ordered that all ambulances be staffed with dedicated attendants at all times and prepared to move immediately and quickly when called upon. Letterman fine-tuned the use of ambulances by separating their duties based on their capabilities. He determined that light, two-wheeled ambulance carts should be used to retrieve and move the wounded from the battlefield to the dressing station or field hospital, while the larger, four-wheeled wagon ambulances should be held in reserve to move patients to more definitive facilities, such as general hospitals rear of the lines. Further,

Letterman made it clear that ambulance vehicles were expressly for the sick and wounded and could not be used for other reasons.

At the battle of Fredericksburg, Hammond's and Letterman's reorganization of the Medical Department's EMS operations demonstrated its effectiveness. In stark contrast to previous engagements, at Fredericksburg over 9,000 soldiers were transported, treated, and hospitalized within 24 hours.

In addition, Letterman contributed to many other improvements of the medical system. He streamlined the supply process and established, for the first time in America, automatic delivery to medical facilities of medical provisions on a large scale, at predetermined levels, and according to a specified timetable. He also categorized his medical staff, organizing them by ability and assigning them thusly to dressing stations, collection points (triage stations), field hospitals, and rear definitive-care facilities. He also implemented protocols of triage and echeloned medical care, and maintained the use of detailed medical statistical data throughout his tenure.[47]

As word within the Union Army spread about the efficacy of the ambulance system, other divisions adopted the concept. Finally, on March 11, 1864, President Abraham Lincoln signed into law "An Act to Establish a Uniform System of Ambulances in the Armies of the United States," legislation passed by Congress that established a standardized system of ambulance service throughout the military. The law also mandated the use of special uniforms for the ambulance corps and special signs for the ambulances. Regulations issued during the war by both sides, and incorporated into this law, also conventionalized

specific insignia and signage for recognition of ambulances and hospitals (Figure 1.4).[48]

Aside from litters, cacolets, and wagons, trains and boats were also employed on a regular basis as medical transportation vehicles. Ambulance wagons may have taken the wounded and sick from field hospitals to trains or hospital ships[49] instead of directly to the general hospital. This would have occurred if the general hospital was too far to allow for reasonable transport by wagon and conveyance by train or ship was more convenient. Thus, a stratified system of medical transport and transport vehicles came into existence.

The military significantly influenced the enhancement of medical care during the war as seen in creation of the Sanitary Commission (modeled after the English Sanitary Commission of the same era), later to become the **American Red Cross**. The Sanitary Commission was a private organization, founded by the first woman physician in America, Elizabeth Blackwell, along with Dr. Henry Bellows, serving as its first president, and influenced by Clara Barton. It provided necessary items, such as blankets, food, medicines, and so on and aided in the establishment of field hospitals. In addition, the commission trained and provided nurses for the army. Its most important contribution may have been its codifying of criteria to be used by medical personnel for the maintenance of sanitary

---

[47]Letterman's record-keeping activity resulted in the renowned, and massive, six-volume *Medical and Surgical History of the War of the Rebellion*, which provided a wealth of information on morbidity and mortality associated with the war.

[48]Adopted from its use as early as 1699 by ordinance in Philadelphia, Pennsylvania, to mark ships with contagious occupants, and its use to identify U.S. marine hospitals established in 1798, a yellow flag was used by both the Union and Confederate armies to designate hospitals during the Civil War. The flag was changed to include a centered green "H" and varied in size to designate field from general hospitals. Ambulances and their depots were initially marked by red flags, later by smaller yellow flags, and eventually by yellow flags with green borders.

[49]The USS *Red Rover* was the first ship dedicated and commissioned as a hospital during the Civil War, in December 1862. It was a captured confederate ship (the CSS *Red Rover*), refitted, equipped, and staffed to act as a floating, mobile hospital and transport vessel.

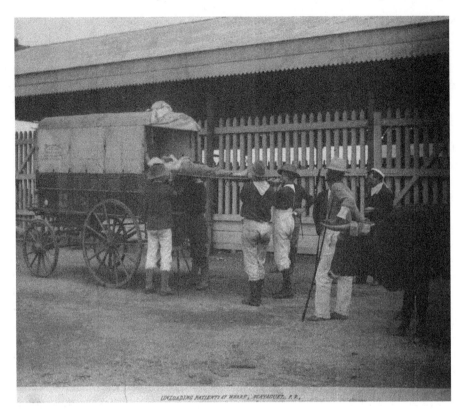

UNLOADING PATIENTS AT WHARF, MAYAGUEZ, P. R.

FIGURE 1.4 ■ An ambulance in use during the Spanish-American War. *Source: National Library of Medicine copyright.*

conditions in the treatment of soldiers and the environment of the hospitals.

Around that time (1863–1864), the Geneva Convention was held in Switzerland. This international meeting of sixteen nations and four philanthropic groups was convened to negotiate agreement among world powers for the treatment during conflicts of wounded combatants, medical personnel on battlefields and at hospitals, and affected civilians. Those in attendance at the convention promulgated a treaty that conferred neutrality upon the injured and their caregivers of all countries involved or affected by wars. Provisions of the treaty, which the world's nations agreed to follow, included requirements governing sanitary and medical supplies, equipment, and ambulances. The

convention also led to the establishment of the International Committee of the Red Cross and the use of the red cross symbol to signify persons or places of neutrality. Over time, the scope of the Geneva Convention broadened to include the sick at sea, prisoners of war, and protection of civilians (NobelPrize.org, n.d.).

THE PREMODERN, INDUSTRIAL ERA

Following the Civil War, several hospitals throughout the United States maintained the ambulance services they had created to transport soldiers during the conflict. In Ohio, Commercial Hospital (founded in 1820 as Commercial Hospital & Lunatic Asylum, now known as Cincinnati General Hospital) established what is generally considered as the first regular ambulance service for the general public in 1865.[50] This service is now operated by the city's fire department. Other ambulance services immediately followed at Grady Hospital in Atlanta and Charity Hospital in New Orleans (the same hospital established in 1736 and considered by many as the first hospital in America).

In New York City, Bellevue Hospital initiated its ambulance service in 1869[51] (Wikipedia, n.d.–b). It was organized by Dr. Edward L. Dalton, a former U.S. Army surgeon. His ambulance service is notable because it was staffed with physicians and included a significant amount of specialized equipment for the treatment of patients not only at the scene of the emergency but also during transit to the hospital.[52] The carriage was relatively lightweight, between six hundred and eight hundred pounds, and had a moveable floor that could be pulled out to receive the patient. The horses used to pull the ambulances were stabled nearby the hospital with quick application harnesses to expedite their response, similar to the procedures and apparatuses used by fire departments of the day. This service also used an alarm system of sorts to notify the drivers and physicians assigned to the ambulance of an emergency request: A released weight would fall to trigger the lighting of a lamp to awaken the sleeping crew. By 1870, the telegraph was used to send requests to Bellevue's Center Street branch, where ambulances would then be dispatched (NewYorkCity.gov, n.d.).[53]

Arguably, the design and establishment of the first civilian prehospital emergent care system provided by trained nonphysician, nonmilitary personnel in the world, occurred in Great Britain in 1872 and is credited to Surgeon-Major Peter Shepard. He invented a special vehicle to transport the sick and injured, called a St. Johns Ambulance after the altruistic order of knights who provided medical aid to crusaders and pilgrims in the eleventh century. Shepherd[54] instructed a group of civilians in the use of the ambulance and also trained them to care for patients both at the scene and in transit to hospitals through a formalized educational program with a standardized curriculum. This group formally organized in 1877, calling itself the St. Johns Ambulance Association.

The first civilian-manufactured ambulance (i.e., a specialized medical transport vehicle) in the United States was produced in 1890 and was built by the Hess-Eisenhardt Company of Cincinnati, Ohio (O'Gara-Hess, 2005).[55] It was a horse-drawn wagon specifically designed to move the incapacitated in need of medical care. Shortly thereafter, the first motorized

---

[50]It is generally believed that this was the first hospital-based ambulance service in the world. Records from the hospital for the year ending February 28, 1866, name an employee, number 27, James A. Jackson, as "driver of ambulance" at an annual salary of $360.

[51]Bellevue's service completed 74 calls in 1869. A total of 1,466 calls were answered in 1870, and by 1891 that number increased to 4,392. While this increase is noteworthy, five other hospitals in New York City also provided ambulance service by 1891.

[52]The equipment included stretchers, handcuffs, and straitjackets and under the driver's seat were a box with brandy, two tourniquets, six bandages, sponges, splint material, and a small bottle of persulfate of iron.

---

[53]By 1893, Bellevue maintained a fleet of nine ambulances. Four drivers and two surgeons were assigned full time to the ambulance service. Requests for their service were received from the New York City Fire or Police Departments by telephone or telegraph.

[54]In 1878 Shepard, of the Royal Herbert Military Hospital (Woolwich, London), and another Aberdeenshire military officer, Colonel Francis Duncan, joined forces to teach first aid skills to civilians. Shepard conducted the first class in the hall of the Presbyterian school in Woolwich using a comprehensive first aid curriculum that he had developed.

[55]Founded in 1876 as the Sayer-Scovill Company, the company initially built custom coaches and carriages. It is also recognized as producing the first motorized ambulances in 1906, and the first with air conditioning in 1937. The company no longer manufactures ambulances, specializing now in armored vehicles, including limousines for the President of the United States.

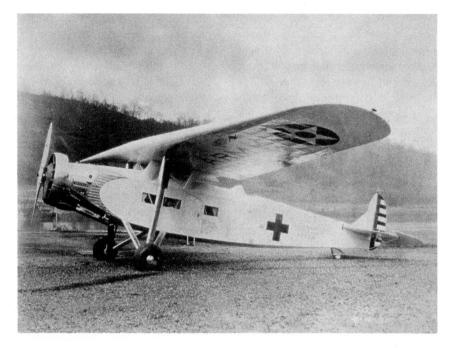

FIGURE 1.5 ■ An early air ambulance. *Source: National Library of Medicine copyright.*

ambulance was made in Chicago and donated to the Michael Reese Hospital by five local businessmen in 1899. This was quickly followed by St. Vincent's Hospital of New York, which began operating an automobile ambulance in 1900.[56, 57]

In 1910, the first known aircraft ambulance (a plane modified to carry a supine patient) was built in North Carolina and tested in Florida. It failed shortly following take-off and crashed after flying only 400 yards in Fort Barrancas, Florida. Captained by George H. R. Gosman

and Lieutenant A. L. Rhodes, it flew just 100 feet off the ground before blowing an oil line.

By 1929, the U.S. Army Air Corps had been organized and had designed three planes to perform as ambulances. They were built and equipped to carry two patients on stretchers: a pilot and an attendant (Figure 1.5).

At the dawn of the twentieth century, local governments and hospitals in America were continuing to assume the responsibility for the provision of EMS to the public.[58] No particular pattern developed and no standards became customary as each locale invented its own, homegrown version of EMS. The military, likewise, continued to develop and modernize its EMS operations. By the outbreak of

---

[56]The first motorized ambulances were equipped with two-horsepower electric engines able to travel about 20 to 30 miles. The physician attending the patient in the back of the vehicle communicated with the driver through a speaking tube. These ambulances had electric lights, inside and out, and their intensity was typically measured in candlepower.

[57]On September 6, 1901, the first U.S. president ever transported in an ambulance was the dying William McKinley after he was shot by an assassin at the Pan-American Exposition in Buffalo, New York.

---

[58]Examples during this period include Phoenix, Arizona, Fire Department . initiates answering "inhalator" calls; Los Angeles County, California, and Columbus, Ohio, Fire Department begin providing medical response service; and Yale–New Haven Hospital begins ambulance operations.

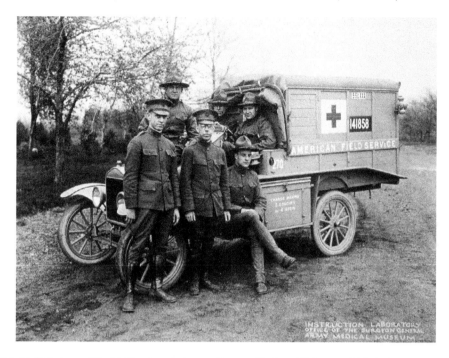

FIGURE 1.6 ■ U.S. Army World War I ambulance. *Source: National Library of Medicine copyright.*

World War I (1914–1918), the U.S. Army was well prepared, including a fleet of specially designed, motorized ambulances (Figures 1.6 and 1.7). The core concepts of emergency prehospital medicine remained fundamentally unchanged within the military from those espoused by Larrey and Letterman, while those in civilian America had yet to be fashioned.

Beginning in 1928 with the inauguration of the Roanoke (Virginia) Life Saving and First Aid Crew, founded by Julien Stanley Wise,[59]

civilian, nonhospital-based EMS became a thriving option in the United States. Even though municipally sponsored services, such as fire department rescue squads, were multiplying around the country, no independent, volunteer organizations had been established until Wise's Roanoke experiment. Throughout the 1920s and 1930s, numerous volunteer EMS groups incorporated and began serving local areas.

A significant milestone in EMS system development in the United States was reached by 1936. By that year the American Red Cross (ARC) had established nearly 900 dedicated posts, spread along the country's highways, with the purpose of aiding those involved in motor vehicle accidents. These emergency first aid stations were usually housed in existing facilities such as stores, inns, gas stations, and firehouses. Local ARC chapters provided the first aid training to the volunteers who staffed the posts, were responsible for first

[59]Julian Stanley Wise was a leading pioneer in the development of the volunteer EMS in the United States. His idea stemmed from a 1909 accident that occurred when he was nine years old and watched helplessly, with some friends, from the banks of the Roanoke River while two canoeists drowned. It is reported that he resolved on the spot to become a "lifesaver." From 1928 on, he devoted his life to spreading the volunteer EMS concept across the nation and thereby created a movement of international significance.

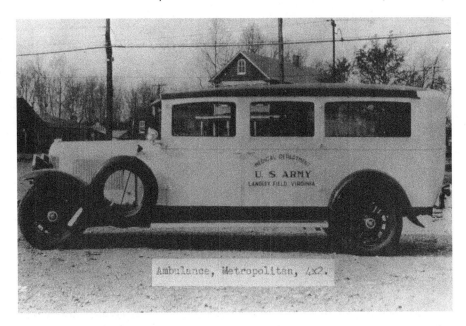

FIGURE 1.7 ■ Another early U.S. Army ambulance. *Source: National Library of Medicine copyright.*

aid kits and medical supplies, and guaranteed that the stations met sanitation requirements. Mobile aid units, composed of fleets of trucks, highway patrol cars, and other vehicles, were also organized as adjuncts to the stations. The posts, which were required to respond to appeals within their designated region, maintained lists of doctors and ambulances available in the area to be summoned as necessary. By 1939, there were almost 5,000 posts and mobile aid units with trained volunteers (American Red Cross, 2013).

During this period, and prior to World War II, hospitals were substantially involved in providing ambulance service in many large cities throughout the country. But during the war, consequent to the severe manpower shortages that resulted, many hospitals found it difficult to maintain these operations. City governments were forced to seek solutions to fill voids that had developed in the emergency medical services within their borders. In some cases, they turned ambulance

service over to the police or fire department. At this time, no laws are known to have existed in the United States that defined any training standard for ambulance personnel, specified any minimum criteria for ambulance design or construction, or mandated any ongoing medical oversight. The only noteworthy training program at all that existed was the American Red Cross's basic first aid course.[60] Until the 1960s, little else would change regarding civilian EMS, few advances would be made, and virtually no further systemization would occur in America.

---

[60]This standard course of instruction was released in 1910 by the ARC under the supervision of Major Charles Lynch. Dr. Mathew J. Shields, recognized as "the father of first aid" in the United States, was hired by the ARC to assist in its development. The course was largely based on Dr. Shields's work with miners in Jermyn, Pennsylvania. Initially, physicians were the only ones permitted to instruct the course, but by 1925 lay personnel were added to the trainers' ranks.

World War II, the Korean Conflict, and the Vietnam War all brought advances in trauma medicine to the military, and those changes eventually made their way into the civilian sector. Many improvements in military EMS organization and operations occurred, including the use of helicopters to rapidly retrieve critically injured patients from the battlefield and transport them to field hospitals (MASH units). This was a most noteworthy advancement because it reduced the time from injury to surgical intervention. By providing on-scene advanced medical treatment, such as intravenous fluids, nonphysician personnel marked a milestone in the progression of clinical care. However, these system attributes were slow to find their way into the civilian sector, which had stagnated since the great steps forward gained a century earlier during the Civil War.

THE IMPACT OF THE AUTOMOBILE

The invention of the automobile and its subsequent proliferation would ultimately provide the impetus for the development of modern-day EMS in the United States. Ever since it appeared in 1769,[61] the automobile wreaked havoc on pedestrian and occupant alike. The first automobile, the *Fardier à vapeur*, a steam-powered apparatus designed and built by French Military engineer Nicholas-Joseph Cugnot, actually crashed against a garden wall. Soon after the first motorized automobile was built and routinely operated

in 1885,[62] it caused the first related fatality, a pedestrian in Croydon, England.[63] Then, 18 months later, on February 12, 1898, in Surrey—a borough of London—the first fatal car accident occurred.[64]

In America, the first recorded automobile fatality occurred in New York City on

---

[61]The Fardier was a large, three-wheeled vehicle that moved slowly, at a walking gait, and was built to haul cannon for the French Military. Even though earlier self-propelled vehicles using springs, compressed air, and even windmills had been invented, Cugnot's device is widely accepted as the first true automobile. The Fardier's accident along with budget problems ended the French Army's experimentation of mechanical vehicles for the time being.

[62]Carl Benz is usually accorded this honor. His motorized automobile was the first to attain commercial success. He is credited with championing the concept of a vehicle powered by the internal-combustion engine and driven by one person. His first model was a little three-wheeled vehicle produced in 1885. In 1890, Benz manufactured a four-wheeled model. However, the French inventor de Rochas built a motorized automobile in 1862. Two years later, despite his earlier statement that automobiles were "a senseless waste of time and effort," an Austrian Jew named Siegfried Markus built a car, the existence of which was covered up by the Nazis. Records indicate, however, that the earliest internal-combustion-driven auto was developed in England in 1826. Samuel Brown, an engineer, adapted an old Newcomen steam engine to burn gas and used it to power his car up Shooter's Hill in London.
[63]The accident occurred on August 17, 1896, in the Croydon borough of London, England. The victim's name was Bridget Driscoll, age 44, who was visiting with one of her two children and a friend to watch a dancing program. The accident occurred on the terraced grounds of Crystal Palace. She was hit as she stepped off a curb by a car traveling 4 miles per hour. Witnesses described the car as moving at "tremendous speed." She died of head injuries within minutes. The car was owned by the Anglo-French Motor Car (Roger-Benz) Company and driven by Arthur Edsell, an employee, who was giving public demonstration rides on behalf of the company. He had learned how to drive only 3 weeks earlier (no driving tests or licenses existed at that time). It was purported that he tampered with the vehicle, causing it to double its speed. Some witnesses said he was distracted by conversation with one of the passengers. After a 6-hour coroner's inquest, the jury returned an accidental death verdict. Neither the driver nor the company was prosecuted. The coroner, William Percy Morrison, remarked, "I trust that this sort of nonsense will never happen again." He is credited with being the first coroner to apply the term *accident* to violence caused by speed.
[64]The victim's name was Henry Lindfield, a Brighton businessman, who crashed his auto into a tree on Russell Hill Road in the Purely section of London, England. He was 42 years old, thrown from his auto and trapped underneath the tree. His leg was subsequently amputated at Croydon General Hospital, where he died the following morning. His teenage son, Bernard, who had been traveling with him, escaped unhurt.

September 13, 1899.[65] The victim was Henry Bliss, age 68, who was stepping off a streetcar at the time and was struck by a taxi at West 74th Street and Central Park West. The driver of the electric-powered automobile, Arthur Smith, was charged with manslaughter but later acquitted because his actions were deemed unintentional. Bliss's chest and head were crushed by the accident, and he died the next day at Roosevelt Hospital.

As the morbidity and mortality associated with traffic accidents compounded each year, a series of **National Street and Highway Safety Conferences**[66] were organized. They focused on the planning and design of roadways and the creation and implementation of uniform codes of vehicle rules. The conferences explored vehicle-related injury and deaths, but limited the discussion to prevention, with little attention to any aspect of medical treatment or emergency medical services.

By the 1950s, fatalities resulting from accidents involving automobiles had reached epidemic proportions, more than 36,000 a year. Even though the rate of mortality had declined steadily since records were initiated in 1922,[67] which was mostly attributable to the overall general advancement of medicine in

society, the aggregate death toll was staggering. As a result, and in spite of his reluctance to interject the federal government into areas traditionally under state authority, President Dwight D. Eisenhower created the President's Committee on Traffic Safety.[68] Its purpose was to bring together previous recommendations of the National Street and Highway Conferences, augment them with new analysis targeted on safety, and push forward in developing remedial plans.

While car design and construction were improving and safety devices were beginning to make their appearance,[69] the nation continued to enhance its traffic laws and enforce its regulations more stringently. Engineers were building roadways better, and educational safety programs, aimed at both the youth and the general public, made their way into the mainstream. Despite advances in military medicine, civilian prehospital emergency medical care was not even a topic for consideration, even at this late stage. There was practically no cohesive system of EMS anywhere in the civilian sector of American society—certainly nothing compared to what was available in the military (National Research Council, 1966).

Significant advances in medicine and the lack of a prehospital treatment philosophy promoting aggressive intervention at the scene, led to a default model of rapid recovery and transport of the injured to the nearest facility. The primary providers of this service at the beginning of the 1960s included municipally based operations, such as police or fire departments and some private companies, but mostly funeral homes (National Research Council, 1966). The latter was well suited for the time to supply ambulance service since they had large,

---

[65]This was also the first fatal car accident in the Western Hemisphere. A plaque was dedicated at the site on September 13, 1999, to commemorate the event. It reads, "Here at West 74th Street and Central Park West, Henry H. Bliss dismounted from a streetcar and was struck and knocked unconscious by an automobile on the evening of September 13, 1899. When Mr. Bliss, a New York real estate man, died the next morning from his injuries, he became the first recorded motor vehicle fatality in the Western Hemisphere. This sign was erected to remember Mr. Bliss on the centennial of his untimely death and to promote safety on our streets and highways."

[66]Held in 1924, 1926, 1930, 1934, 1946, and 1954, these conferences were first inaugurated by President Calvin Coolidge, through his then Secretary of Commerce, Herbert Hoover, and continued through to the Dwight D. Eisenhower administration.

[67]In 1922, 14,859 people were recorded as killed by automobile accidents, a rate of 24.08 per 100 million vehicle miles traveled (VMT). By 1959 the rate had fallen to 5.17 per 100 million VMT.

[68]Informally established on April 13, 1954, Eisenhower provided the committee with formal status through Executive Order 10858 on January 13, 1960, with the charge to "advance the cause of street and highway safety."

[69]First patented in the United States in 1885 by Edward J. Claghorn, seatbelts didn't appear in American cars until the Tucker in 1947. Ford began supplying seatbelts in its general production models as early as 1956.

fast vehicles capable of transporting bodies in a supine position, were prolifically located in or near virtually every community, and were readily available at almost any time.

MODERN-DAY AMERICAN EMS IS BORN

A convergence of several landmark events occurred in the mid 1960s that altered the very foundations of EMS in the United States, commencing a new era of modernity and organization. For decades, a crescendo had been building regarding the carnage experienced from automobile accidents on the nation's highways. Finally, in 1961 President John F. Kennedy declared, "Traffic accidents constitute one of the greatest, perhaps the greatest, of the nation's public health problems" (West Virginia Department of Education, n.d.). Instantly, a new focus was established on the need for emergency medical aid for traffic accident victims in the United States.

Then, during President Lyndon Johnson's administration several crucial events took place. First, in 1965, **Medicare** was created by an act of Congress.[70] In the original legislation, ambulance transportation was recognized as a covered beneficiary service. With this legislation the federal government had established a long-term funding mechanism for EMS and medical transportation.

Next, in 1966, the **President's Commission on Highway Safety** in its final report, "Health, Medical Care and Transportation of the Injured," listed emergency care and transportation of the accident victim as one of its community action programs. This recognized that more than just better road design, preventative programs and safety education were needed to curb the death toll accumulating on the highways.

President Johnson championed the cause, declaring support for passage of the federal **National Highway Safety Act** of 1966 (Public Law 89-564) and signing it into law that year. It highlighted, for the first time, emergency medical care[71] as a necessary element to reducing death and disability associated with traffic accidents. Expanding considerably from the letter of the law, extensive regulations promulgated pursuant to the act created the first comprehensive description of an EMS system, components, and standards,[72] defining a system far from one associated only with trauma injuries on highways.[73]

---

[70]Medicare was passed by Congress and signed into law by President Johnson in July 1965. Officially part of the Social Security Amendments of 1965, Medicare established a two-part insurance program for older Americans. The first part was a program of hospital and related benefits, financed by Social Security taxes. Key benefits included 90 days of hospital care, 100 days of nursing-home care, 100 home-nursing "visits" in each "spell" of illness, and hospital outpatient service. All benefits were subject to deductibles and coinsurance. The second part, a voluntary program of supplementary benefits, covered 80 percent of physicians' fees, additional home-nursing services, in-hospital diagnostic and laboratory work, certain kinds of therapy, ambulance services, surgical dressings, and more. This supplementary plan would be financed initially through a $3 monthly premium from each beneficiary, matched by the federal government out of general revenues. In addition, the act provided for a substantially expanded Kerr-Mills program extending "medical indigent" benefits to other age groups besides those over age 65.

[71]Neither the term *emergency medical services* nor *EMS* appeared in the legislation. The terms *emergency services*, *emergency medical care*, *emergency service plans*, and *transportation of the injured* were used, but very sparingly. Although many authors attribute great detail to what the law mandated, it was essentially void of any specific language regarding EMS features. It was the regulations issued in 1969, pursuant to the act, that formally identified EMS and its characteristics.

[72]Standard 11 of the "Highway Safety Program Manual" is the definitive text that first defined an EMS system and delineated its elements. It was published on January 17, 1969, and appeared in Appendix A of the manual under the title "Implementation Guidelines."

[73]It is most probable that this deviated expansion from the automobile trauma–related intent of the 1966 Traffic and Motor Vehicle Safety Act was the result of the personalities involved at the time, both in and out of government (Leo Schwartz of the Department of Transportation's NHTSA EMS division and David Boyd, then of Baltimore's Shock Trauma Center), and the tandem explosion of cardiac related medical research and cardiac/medical oriented paramedic units surfacing around the country in the late 60s and early 70s.

The Highway Safety Program Manual included nineteen volumes[74] ranging from "Periodic Motor Vehicle Inspection" to "Accident Investigation and Reporting." Volume 11 was titled *Emergency Medical Services* and incorporated eight chapters (with several appendices) that provided the guidelines and descriptions of an EMS system's elements as well as technical assistance for their implementation. For the first time, America had a national resource tome that created a standard guide for the structure of an EMS system.

With a suddenly burgeoning bureaucracy, initial steps were taken to control, through consolidation, the several new and existing agencies that incorporated roadway safety and EMS as a part of their missions. On November 9, 1966, the National Traffic Safety Agency[75] (authorized by the National Traffic and Motor Vehicle Safety Act of 1966, P.L. 89-563) and the National Highway Safety Advisory Committee[76] (authorized by the Highway Safety Act of 1966, P.L. 89-564), both in the Department of Commerce, were merged[77] and commenced operations under the direction of Dr. William J. Haddon, Jr. They would ultimately be moved to a newly created Department of Transportation (DOT) on April 1, 1967, as part of the transfer of the Federal Highway Administration (FHWA).[78]

It is important to note that a competing government program surfaced shortly after EMS was first inaugurated into the modern era. In 1972, President Richard M. Nixon refocused the mission of the Department of Health, Education, and Welfare's (DHEW, predecessor of today's Department of Health and Human

Services) EMS division,[79] operated within the Public Health Service, toward EMS. Congress subsequently expanded its mission even further in 1973 when it passed the EMS Systems Act of 1973 (P.L. 93-154). DEMS's newfound assignment would last only 7 years, under the leadership of Dr. David R. Boyd, but would have profound impact on the expansion and medical orientation of EMS systems across the country. By virtue of its significant grant appropriations,[80] DEMS would provide funds for more than three hundred experimental, demonstration EMS systems throughout the nation.

Coincidentally in the 1960s, monumental research would be completed and published, creating a vanguard for the advancement of multispecialty EMS. Two watershed investigative papers, **"Accidental Death and Disability: The Neglected Disease of Modern Society"** by the National Research Council of the National Academy of Sciences (National Research Council, 1966) and "A Mobile Intensive Care Unit [MICU] in the Management of Myocardial Infarction" by **J. Frank Pantridge, M.D.** (1916–2004) and John S. Geddes (Pantridge and Geddes, 1967) scientifically established both the need and the efficacy of prehospital emergency medical services for both trauma and cardiac cases. More research would follow, expanding even further the types of medical conditions that would benefit from prehospital care, but these two documents were the first definitively empirical evidence that America's

---

[74]It is often misreported that 18 volumes existed. This is because the first volume was number "0."

[75]Which would become commonly known as the National Traffic Safety Bureau.

[76]Which would become commonly known as the National Highway Safety Bureau.

[77]By Presidential Executive Order 11357.

[78]Originally established as the Office of Road Inquiry (ORI) in 1893, the FHWA attained its current name on April 1, 1967.

[79]Although it existed before 1974, DEMS was originally formed to prepare United States medical services for nuclear attack. Its mission was drastically changed by President Nixon in his January 1972 State of the Union address when he directed the DHEW "to develop new ways of organizing emergency medical services and providing care to accident victims."

[80]A total of almost $8 million was awarded to five "pilot" EMS programs in Florida, Illinois, California, Ohio, and Arkansas. Also, nearly $11 million was authorized by Congress between 1970 and 1972 for the national regional medical program (RMP) initiative.

lack of a cogent EMS system needed to, and was capable of, change.

The introduction and propagation of prehospital medical care, especially advanced clinical treatment, would not wait for government bureaucracy. Oftentimes with no legislation regarding their activities, physicians around the country were spearheading in the field, at the scene of incipient need, the use of medications, defibrillators, and other advanced medical modalities. Most of these services started with almost a single-minded focus on cardiac emergencies, but rapidly expanded into treating many other medically urgent conditions. The emphasis was shifting from the rapid recovery and transport of victims, to the rapid response of specialized personnel and apparatus and the stabilization of patients before movement to a hospital.

It was during this time, and within this context of excited academic camaraderie, that the first advanced life support ambulance in the United States was launched. Credited to St. Vincent's Hospital in Manhattan, New York, and the brainchild of Dr. William J. Grace, this unit was staffed by physicians and responded to the scene of suspected cardiac emergencies. Dr. Grace published his findings with his colleague Dr. John Chadbourne, documenting a reduction in mortality from 21 percent to 8 percent with prehospital intervention of advanced cardiac treatment. Their Mobile Coronary Care Unit (MCCU) was operational by the late 1960s (Page, 1979).

The first nonphysician, mobile, advanced medical treatment service in America was initiated in Miami, Florida, in 1968.[81] **Eugene Nagel, M.D.** was the visionary who blended the training of surrogate quasi-physicians with radio technology to invent the paramedic using telemetry communication to receive real-time medical command from a doctor at a hospital. This service was followed shortly thereafter by similar programs in Columbus, Ohio; Jacksonville, Florida; Seattle, Washington; and Los Angeles, California.

The legislative impetus for the birth of modern American EMS was centered almost exclusively on trauma associated with motor vehicle accidents. The simultaneous, and serendipitous, medical research thrust revolutionary, prehospital, nonphysician clinical care on cardiac emergencies (essentially myocardial infarctions and cardiac arrests). Despite this disparity, these two distinct versions of the new EMS paradigm would eventually amalgamate into a single, comprehensive construct. With the passage of the EMS Systems Act of 1973, the two divergent themes of prehospital emergency care would be reconciled and formally recognized as a single, medically broad-based, ideology. Language from the act officially defined EMS as the provision of "health care services under emergency conditions," a substantial expansion of the vague reference in the 1966 Highway Safety Act, whose title and entire context set the parameter for the term it used, *emergency medical care*, as related solely to injuries sustained from auto accidents.

In 1979, **Mickey Eisenberg, M.D.**, published the results of a study he conducted on the effects of rapidly instituted cardiopulmonary resuscitation (CPR) and definitive medical care provided to patients suffering sudden cardiac arrest in the field, prior to arrival at a hospital. This landmark research demonstrated that the elapsed time from the onset of sudden cardiac arrest to the initiation of CPR, as well as definitive medical care, were critical determinants in the outcome of the patient. His study has been widely cited to support the need for training the public in CPR and has

---

[81]It was organized by Dr. Eugene Nagel in collaboration with Drs. J. Miller and Jim Hirchman. The University of Miami Medical School sponsored the first paramedic training classes at the University of Miami and called its graduates "Physician Extenders." By March, 1967, these paramedics were operational, transmitting heart rhythms to Jackson Memorial Hospital, with a medical-radio telemetry contraption that weighed 54 pounds, administering medication and defibrillating patients.

been used to help design the delivery component and structure of EMS systems around the country. However, Dr. Eisenberg's paper has been erroneously referred to as identifying 8 minutes and 59 seconds as a preferred maximum response time standard. This mistake emanates from the statistical segregation of time periods he used in reporting his findings.

By the close of the 1970s, EMS was firmly established in the medical infrastructure of the United States as its own discipline with its own science. During the next several decades it would become more sophisticated, evolving into an industry within its own right. As a result, unique business and economic models would arise to govern its administration, operation, and financing. While the clinical and operational natures of EMS have matured substantially in a common direction since 1965, no predominant business scheme has surfaced as the most appropriate or the most widely accepted.

From embryonic afterthoughts to well-refined, and sometimes complex, integrated organizations, the provision of EMS at the beginning of the twenty-first century is vastly different from the EMS of our ancestors. The types and extent of medical care treatments provided in prehospital emergencies has expanded significantly over the years. The scope of clinical interventions that EMS caregivers provide today is far advanced from what was initially permitted, or even envisioned, at their inception in the late 1960s. However, the maturity and sophistication of how this care is delivered and how EMS systems are operated today, has developed in a varied and diversified fashion. No single theme or predominant system schema is considered premier in the United States.

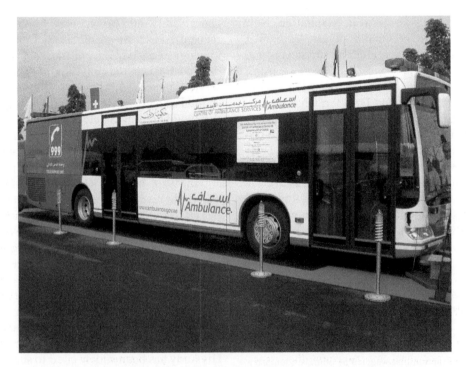

FIGURE 1.8 ■ Dubai field support mobile hospital. *Source: Courtesy of MONOC, by permission.*

As prehospital care has become more advanced, **delivery models** have become stratified in many parts of the country, with more than one entity responsible for different components of the EMS system. These variously layered configurations of EMS provision have generated a multitude of business structures, differing by participant, that are discussed later in this text (Figure 1.8). *Source: Reprinted by permission from MONOC Mobile Health Services.*

CHAPTER REVIEW

Summary

The development of EMS in the United States spans several centuries and matured in tandem with the growth of general medicine throughout the country. It was heavily influenced by the needs of the military and by developments in other countries. As EMS entered the twentieth century in America, the publication of several investigative and medical research papers, as well as the passage of key legislation that enabled both a stable funding source and a federally standardized programmatic structure, allowed EMS to blossom rapidly and become recognized as a specialized public health and medical service. EMS now exists in many forms around the country with no single delivery model preferred over another.

WHAT WOULD YOU DO? Reflection

XYZ Ambulance Service's orientation presentation reviewed the inception and evolution of EMS in America as follows:

1. *What is an EMS system?*

An EMS system is a network of prehospital emergency medical care that is coordinated to provide medical treatment of the suddenly ill or injured from primary response to definitive care. It includes personnel trained in the rescue, stabilization, transportation, and advanced treatment of traumatic or medical emergencies. It is linked by a communication system that functions on both a local and a regional level. It is often tiered to include first responder, basic life support, and advanced life support components. It also includes stages of activation, response, treatment, and transportation. These stages include emergency medical dispatch, medical response, ambulance personnel and apparatus (basic life support), medium and heavy rescue equipment, and paramedic (advanced life support) units.

2. *What landmark events helped shape our modern perception of an EMS system?*

+ The National Research Council's Accidental Death & Disability white paper.
+ The Highway Safety Act
+ The National EMS Systems Act
+ The enactment of Medicare, specifically its medical transportation eligibility section
+ Dr. Mickey Eisenberg's studies on prehospital definitive care and rapid CPR
+ Drs. Pantridge and Geddes's study on prehospital definitive care of myocardial infarction patients
+ Dr. Eugene Nagel's design and implementation of mobile intensive care units using telemetry and paramedics

3. *How did the American Revolution, the Civil War, and American Military conflicts of the later twentieth century influence EMS in the United States?*

These military events influenced American EMS in the following ways;

- The American Revolution introduced the concept of emergency medical care being provided at the scene of injury with evacuation capability to tiered levels of definitive care.
- The Civil War introduced specialized apparatus for the transportation of wounded persons from the site of injury and the training of dedicated personnel for the treatment of injured persons at the scene and during transportation to definitive care.
- American Military conflicts of the later twentieth century introduced advances in trauma medicine and improvements in EMS organization and operations, most noteworthy of which were the use of helicopters to rapidly retrieve critically injured patients from the battlefield and the rapid intervention of advanced medical care by nonphysicians as quickly after injury as possible.

Review Questions

1. Name three seminal events that helped initiate modern EMS in the United States.
2. Where did the word *ambulance* originate, and what was its meaning?
3. What impact did the enactment of Medicare have on EMS in America?
4. What was the National Research Council's white paper on accidental death and disability, and how did it influence the development of EMS in the United States?
5. What is the modern meaning of an EMS system?
6. What were the main contributions derived from the Civil War regarding modern American EMS?
7. What were Larrey's "flying ambulances"?
8. What was the impact of Pantridge and Geddes's research on the management of myocardial infarctions on the U.S. EMS system?
9. What did Dr. Mickey Eisenberg's 1979 study reveal?

References

Air University. (n.d.). "Military Medicine During the Eighteenth and Nineteenth Centuries." See the organization website.

American Red Cross. (2013). "A Brief History of the American Red Cross." See the organization website.

Answers.com. (n.d.). "Travois." See the organization website.

Cavallo, G. (1997). "The Byzantines." In G. Cavallo, *The Byzantines* (pp. 19, 25). Chicago: University of Chicago Press.

Dammann, G., and A. J. Bollet. (2008). "Images of Civil War Medicine." In G. Dammann and A. J. Bollet, eds., *Images of Civil War Medicine* (pp. 48–63). New York: Demos Medical Publishing.

Encyclopædia Britannica. (n.d.–a). "Hospital." See the organization website.

Encyclopædia Britannica. (n.d.–b). "History of Medicine." See the organization website.

Encyclopædia Britannica. (n.d.–c). "Travois." See the organization website.

Free Dictionary. (n.d.). "Dooly." See the organization website.

Garrison, F. H. (1966). *History of Medicine.* Philadelphia: W. B. Saunders Company.

Gillett, M. (1981). "The Army Medical Department, 1775–1818. *Army Historical*

Series, Maurice Matloff, General Editor. See the organization website.

Homer. (2004). *The Iliad, Book IV.* Trans., Samuel Butler. See The Literature Network website.

Major, R. H. (1954). *A History of Medicine.* Springfield, MA: Charles C. Thomas.

Munson, E. L., H. Thompson, and R. J. Deering. (1911). "The Photographic History of the Civil War." In E. L. Munson, H. Thompson, and R. J. Deering, eds., *The Photographic History of the Civil War*, vol. IV (pp. 297–344). New York: The Review of Reviews Company.

National Research Council. (1966). *Accidental Death and Disability: The Neglected Disease of Modern Society.* Washington, DC: National Academies of Science.

NewYorkCity.gov. (n.d.). "New York City Fire Department. Part 1." See the organization website.

NobelPrize.org. (n.d.). "History of Organization" [Red Cross]. See the organization website.

O'Gara-Hess. (2005, March 18). "O'Gara-Hess History." See the McLellans Automotive website.

Ortiz, J. M. (1998, October–December). "The Revolutionary Flying Ambulance of Napoleon's Surgeon." *U.S. Army Medical Department Journal* (p. 17).

Page, J. O. (1979). *The Paramedics.* Basking Ridge, NJ: Backdraft Publications.

Pantridge, J., and J. S. Geddes. (1967). "A Mobile Intensive Care Unit in the Management of Myocardial Infarction." *Lancet 2*, 271. 1967.

Sayad, A. J. (2005, February 26). *EMedicine 26.*

Science & Society Picture Library. (n.d.). "'Clarence' ambulance, c. 1897." See the organization website.

United States Library of Congress. (2011, May 12). Legislation PL 93-154 Summary. Washington, DC.

University of Pittsburgh. (2004, Fall). "Emergency Medicine Marches on at Pitt." *Facets*, 18–19.

West Virginia Department of Education. (n.d.). "A Brief History of Emergency Medical Services." See the organization website.

Whonamedit? (n.d.). "René-Théophile-Hyacinthe Laënnec." See the organization website.

Wikipedia. (n.d.–a). "Pannier." See the organization website.

Wikipedia. (n.d.–b). "Bellevue Hospital Center." See the organization website.

Key Terms

"Accidental Death & Disability: The Neglected Disease of Modern Society" Published by the National Research Council of the National Academy of Sciences in 1966, this report provided an overview of the woefully inadequate medical care given to victims of vehicle accidents. It scientifically established the need for specialized emergency medical services for patients suffering trauma from motor vehicle accidents.

ambulance A vehicle (automotive, airborne, or waterborne) used for transporting medical personnel and equipment to the location of a sick or injured person, and for transporting sick or injured individuals to a location where further care can be provided.

American Red Cross Beginning as the Sanitary Commission during the Civil War this private organization provided necessary items, such as blankets, food, medicines, and so on, and aided in the establishment of field hospitals. It also trained and provided nurses for the army. Its most important contribution may have been its codifying of criteria to be used by medical personnel for the maintenance of sanitary conditions in the treatment of soldiers and the environment of the hospitals.

Baron F. P. Percy Introduced the idea of a regular corps, specially trained in and equipped for the transport of injured, using stretchers and educated in a formal, regimented course of instruction. The corps accompanied a large medical wagon to the scene of the battle wounded, striking out in a radial fashion to rapidly retrieve the injured. Once returned to the mobile hospital wagon, the surgeons would immediately provide medical care to the wounded, treating them sufficiently until they were either ambulatory or could be transported in the wagon.

delivery models The ways in which EMS systems are designed in order to provide service to the public. Some types include fire department agencies and hospital-based and commercial services.

Dominique-Jean Larrey Chief surgeon for Emperor Napoleon Bonaparte, who conceptualized and implemented a cogent, comprehensive prehospital care system that, for the first time, triaged the injured, provided immediate, temporary medical care and transported the injured from the site of injury to medical aid stations in a formal, regulated way using special apparatus.

emergency medical services (EMS) The provision of medical care by specially trained and authorized personnel to the suddenly ill or injured prior to, and in the absence of, a hospital setting.

EMS Systems Act of 1973 Federal law that determined an EMS system provides for the arrangement of personnel, facilities, and equipment for the effective and coordinated delivery of health care services in an appropriate geographical area under emergency conditions.

Eugene Nagel, M.D. The visionary who blended the training of surrogate quasi-physicians with radio technology to invent the paramedic using telemetry communication to receive real-time medical command from a doctor at a hospital.

hospital A permanent structure that houses the appropriate facilities, equipment, and personnel necessary to provide immediate diagnostic services and emergent, definitive, and sustaining medical care for those patients who arrive, by whatever means.

J. Frank Pantridge, M.D. Researched and scientifically established both the need and the efficacy of prehospital emergency medical services for myocardial infarction cases, through a landmark study entitled "Mobile Intensive Care Unit Management of Myocardial Infarction."

Jonathan Letterman, M.D. Established an effective ambulance corps and included techniques

in the loading and unloading of patients on stretchers into and out of ambulance wagons. He ordered that all ambulances be staffed with dedicated attendants at all times and be prepared to move immediately and quickly when called upon.

medical transportation systems The movement of patients to, from, or between medical facilities of any kind, including physicians' offices, ambulatory care centers, and such specialized medical facilities as dialysis centers and hospitals.

Medicare Federal legislation that established ambulance transportation as a covered beneficiary service. In so doing the federal government had established a long-term funding mechanism for EMS and medical transportation.

Mickey Eisenberg, M.D. Published the results of a study he conducted on the effects of rapidly instituted cardiopulmonary resuscitation (CPR) and definitive medical care provided to patients suffering sudden cardiac arrest in the field, prior to arrival at a hospital.

National Highway Safety Act Federal law that highlighted emergency medical care as a necessary element to reducing death and disability associated with traffic accidents. Extensive regulations promulgated pursuant to the act created the first comprehensive description of an EMS system, components, and standards.

National Highway Traffic Safety Act (NHTSA) On November 9, 1966, the National Traffic Safety Agency (authorized by the National Traffic and Motor Vehicle Safety Act of 1966; PL 89-563) and the National Highway Safety Advisory Committee (authorized by the National Highway Safety Act of 1966; PL 89-564), both in the Department of Commerce, were merged. Because both acts included many overlapping items, many of their components were eventually merged or consolidated. Both acts are now collectively referred to as the "National Highway Safety Act."

National Street and Highway Safety Conferences A series of conferences focused on the planning and design of roadways and the creation and implementation of uniform codes of vehicle rules. They were associated with the prevention of vehicle-caused injury and deaths and did not address emergency medical services.

President's Commission on Highway Safety This commission's final report listed emergency care and transportation of the accident victim as an important community action program.

system A group of objects or subsystems interacting in an organized manner to produce an intended outcome.

U.S. Public Health Service Established on July 16, 1798, through the Act for the Relief of Sick and Disabled Seamen, creating the Marine Hospital Service, which became the U.S. Public Health Service. The act established a network of medical care, with a system of hospitals, for the aid of American merchant seamen, beginning along the northeast coast and eventually proliferating to the Great Lakes and the Gulf and Pacific coasts.

CHAPTER 2

Levels of Ambulance Service

Matt Zavadsky, MS-HSA, EMT

Objectives

After reading this chapter, the student should be able to:

2.1 Define the four levels of ambulance service.

2.2 Identify the role each of the levels of ambulance service could play in an emergency medical services system.

2.3 Explain the clinical and fiscal implications of deploying levels of care.

2.4 Explain the potential impact of current research on patient outcomes for ALS and BLS levels of care and how that may impact future deployment of ALS and BLS ambulances.

Overview

Ambulance services in the United States range in size from one ambulance operated by volunteers and managed by a community board of directors to large governmental agencies and even larger, private, for-profit corporations. This text presents information that the manager of an ambulance service, large or small, needs in order to keep the business solvent and provide clinically excellent service to the community.

Key Terms

advanced life support (ALS)

basic life support (BLS)

critical care transport (CCT)

emergency medical dispatch (EMD)

intermediate life support (ILS)

medical director

scope of practice

system deployment, or deployment

WHAT WOULD YOU DO?

You have just been named as the executive director of a large ambulance service located in an urban area covering 420 square miles and 880,000 residents. Your governing board is interested in looking at ways to improve service delivery while reducing expenses and has asked you to come up with a proposal to use a mixed ALS and BLS service delivery model.

1. What are your considerations in developing this proposal?
2. What are the advantages and disadvantages of running a mixed ALS/BLS fleet?
3. How would a mixed ALS/BLS fleet change your deployment methodology and costs?
4. What would be your final recommendation?

■ INTRODUCTION

Modern-day ambulance services evolved from humble beginnings with ambulance workers who were livery attendants with little or no training in medical care. Today's ambulance services are a hybrid of clinically sophisticated services with specialized training and technology designed to bring the right care to the right patient, at the right time, and in the right setting, and to safely and expediently transport those patients to locations where definitive care can be rendered.

Each community (municipality, county, and region) determines the level of sophistication of its ambulance service, which may require effective combination levels of care in order to meet the community's expectation. This chapter will help you understand the various levels of clinical care that ambulance services can provide.

It is important to understand that the concept of *levels of care* is a changing one. Treatment modalities that once fell clearly within the definition of *advanced life support*, such as defibrillation and medication administration, now (with improvements in technology and education) are able to be delivered by lesser-trained providers and have become incorporated into intermediate or basic life support programs.

■ SCOPE OF PRACTICE

A **scope of practice** is established by the state government to outline the medical procedures authorized through licensure by a state licensing authority (NASEMSO.org, 2012). It defines what the licensee[1] can and cannot clinically perform in the treatment of patients. Some states have very specific scope-of-practice requirements defined generally in state statute through definitions first of what constitutes advanced and basic life support care, and in the definitions of EMT and paramedic. For example, in Florida, the scope of practice for EMTs and paramedics is delineated in state statute (State of Florida, 1997). In other states, such as Texas, the scope of practice definition is very general, and is left to the discretion of the local **medical director**.

Other states have less prescriptive approaches to scope of practice, allowing greater flexibility to local EMS systems and individual medical directors to determine the

---

[1]The debate about license versus certification versus registration is endless and ongoing. For purposes of this text, a "license" is granted by governmental authority and grants the holder with a right to practice a trade, occupation, or profession, regardless of what the individual state may call it. For a detailed discussion of the issue, see www.nremt.org/nremt/about/Legal_Opinion.asp

drugs and procedures available for use by local EMS providers. Some states allow for "pilot programs" to test various proposed changes to the scope of practice subject to a variety of approvals, conditions, and limitations.

Side Bar

Definitions

(1) "Advanced life support" means treatment of life-threatening medical emergencies through the use of techniques such as endotracheal intubation, the administration of drugs or intravenous fluids, telemetry, cardiac monitoring, and cardiac defibrillation by a qualified person, pursuant to rules of the department. . . .

(7) "Basic life support" means treatment of medical emergencies by a qualified person through the use of techniques such as patient assessment, cardiopulmonary resuscitation (CPR), splinting, obstetrical assistance, bandaging, administration of oxygen, application of medical antishock trousers, administration of a subcutaneous injection using a premeasured auto injector of epinephrine to a person suffering an anaphylactic reaction, and other techniques described in the Emergency Medical Technician Basic Training Course Curriculum of the United States Department of Transportation. The term "basic life support" also includes other techniques which have been approved and are performed under conditions specified by rules of the department. . . .

(11) "Emergency medical technician" means a person who is certified by the department to perform basic life support pursuant to this part. . . .

(17) "Paramedic" means a person who is certified by the department to perform basic and advanced life support pursuant to this part. (State of Florida, 1997)

LEVELS OF CARE

In most areas of the United States, ambulance service levels of care as defined by scope of practice statutes fall into four main categories:

1. Basic Life Support (BLS)
2. Intermediate Life Support (ILS)
3. Advanced Life Support (ALS)
4. Critical Care Transport (CCT)

Basic Life Support

Basic life support (BLS) is generally accepted as the use of noninvasive medical care administered by emergency medical technicians (EMTs) who are certified by state EMS agencies after successfully completing a 110- to 200-hour EMT-Basic training program (NHTSA, n.d.).

The procedures typically authorized for EMTs to administer include basic patient assessment, auto-injector use for epinephrine, nebulized medications for treating bronchospasm, oxygen administration, spinal immobilization, splinting, bleeding control, automated external defibrillation for cardiac arrest cases, and some advanced airway techniques, such as multilumen airway management devices.

Advanced Life Support

Advanced life support (ALS) is generally accepted as *invasive* medical care administered by paramedics who are certified by state EMS agencies after successfully completing 1,000 to 1,500 hours of EMT-Paramedic training (NHTSA, 1998a).

The procedures typically authorized for paramedics to administer include advanced patient assessment; advanced airway management through the use of endotracheal intubation or even surgical airway procedures, such as surgical or needle cricothyroidotomy; medication administration for the treatment of cardiac, respiratory, or other serious medical conditions either through intravenous, intramuscular or subcutaneous administration routes; and electrocardiogram interpretation for the diagnosis of cardiac dysrhythmias.

Intermediate Life Support

Intermediate life support (ILS) is a hybrid of BLS and ALS care. ILS care is administered by EMT-Intermediates (NHTSA, 1998b).

This level of care typically includes all of the BLS care, plus nonmedicated IV placement; advanced airway management through endotracheal intubation; and limited medication administration for the treatment of cardiac, respiratory, or other serious medical conditions.

Critical Care Transport

Critical care transport (CCT) is the provision of very complex care not typically provided by paramedics. CCT may involve specially trained paramedics or other health professionals, such as registered nurses, nurse practitioners, physician assistants, or physicians. CCT is generally utilized only to transport high-risk patients undergoing specialized treatments or requiring invasive monitoring from one medical facility to another.

This level of care can include airway management through the use of ventilators, monitoring invasive arterial lines, multiple vasoactive intravenous medication infusion through intravenous pumps, administration of specialized medications that could have profound impact on the patient's hemodynamic state, and administration of blood or blood byproducts (UMBC, 2012).

ROLES OF LEVELS OF CARE IN EMS SYSTEMS

A high-level view of the roles played by ambulance services in many communities reveals distinct business units. Emergency ambulance service is an element of the community's EMS system (the way the community responds to unplanned, unscheduled requests for emergency medical assistance, usually via the 9-1-1 system). A second, sometimes separate and sometimes not, business unit provides interfacility medical transportation, ranging from nonambulance medical transportation through critical care interfacility services.

Before discussing the various ways ALS and BLS care can be utilized in a community, it is important to understand the main components of a community EMS system.

DISPATCH, CONTROL, OR COMMUNICATIONS CENTER

An ambulance communications center typically includes two primary components. The first component, often referred to as a public safety answering point, receives requests for ambulance service either through a 9-1-1 call or a private call through a ten-digit phone number. The second component is a dispatch or control center, which alerts, communicates with, and maintains awareness of the status and needs of ambulances in the field.

Most EMS communication centers provide **emergency medical dispatch (EMD)**, which encompasses two important functions: (1) determining the appropriate level and mode of response and (2) providing medical instructions over the phone to callers who are with the patient and willing to carry out the medical instructions.

Not all requests for emergency medical service require a maximal response by the EMS system. A conscious and alert patient who has suffered an ankle injury while playing soccer generally does not require the same response as an unconscious patient who was thrown out of a moving vehicle on the interstate. The soccer player may simply require a nonemergent (no lights, no siren, or "cold") response by personnel trained to the BLS level, while the ejected patient may require an emergent (lights and siren, or "hot") response by personnel trained to a higher level, along with other emergency response services. Through scripted questions (caller interrogation) and locally approved protocols, call takers certified in EMD assign the appropriate level of care and mode of response based on the information obtained from the caller.

FIRST RESPONDERS

Many EMS systems utilize *first response* agencies to place trained personnel more quickly at an emergency scene, and to augment the usual two-person staff of an ambulance. These agencies respond to medical calls in non-patient-transport-capable vehicles and are designed to arrive at the scene of an EMS call before the ambulance. In most urban and suburban communities, the local fire departments provide first response services since their static and geographic deployment model for fire protection makes them well suited for efficient EMS first response. In some communities, especially in rural areas, first response may be provided by law enforcement agencies or even volunteer first response organizations.

AMBULANCE TRANSPORT

The ambulance component of an EMS system may be provided by one of several different types of organizations. The ambulance service may be a contracted or franchised private, for-profit ambulance company; a municipal or county governmental organization; a hospital-operated ambulance service; or a volunteer ambulance service organization.

CRITICAL CARE TRANSPORT

CCT is an important component of the EMS system, although it is often not connected to the business unit that responds to 9-1-1 calls.

Most areas of the United States have developed regional systems of care, with hospitals of varying capability. Patients frequently must be moved to higher echelons of care, from local or community hospitals (often level 3 or level 4 trauma centers) to regional medical centers (level 2 trauma centers) or tertiary medical centers (level 1 trauma care and many specialist services). Often, medical care that has been initiated at the sending facility needs to be maintained during transport to the receiving facility. This may include specialized procedures, such as mechanical positive pressure ventilation, intra-aortic balloon pumps, blood administration, chest tubes, or other high-risk modalities. CCT services may be provided by specially trained personnel and specially equipped vehicles that are staffed and operated by an ambulance service. In some communities, discrete hospital-operated CCT ambulances may provide this service.

Side Bar

Special Discussion of Intermediate Life Support

Intermediate life support (ILS) care is typically found in communities that desire the benefit of some advanced life support (ALS) care but do not have the call volume or fiscal resources to support a full paramedic level of service. ILS care is generally considered ALS by state EMS governing boards since EMT-Is are able to initiate some invasive treatments beyond the scope of practice of basic EMTs. For the purposes of this chapter, we consider ALS care to mean the provision of a paramedic level of service.

■ LEVEL OF CARE AND RESPONSE CONFIGURATIONS——————

A community can configure its EMS system to incorporate BLS, ILS, and ALS emergency care in many different ways.

In considering system configuration, readers should note that within the EMS community, much discussion has arisen about the appropriateness and potential legal risks of transferring patient care from one level of provider to another. No problems have been found with the appropriate transfer of care from a provider with a lesser certification to a provider with a higher level of certification (e.g., from an EMT responder to an ambulance paramedic). However, some are concerned about a paramedic responder transferring patient care to an ambulance EMT. Done individually and ad hoc, should harm result, a claim of "abandonment" might be raised. However, done within the guidance provided by EMS system directive or protocol, such a transfer should incur no more legal risk than when an emergency physician examines a patient and transfers care to a staff nurse in the emergency department for further care and monitoring.

The following configurations are possible:

+ BLS first response and ALS ambulance
+ ALS first response and BLS ambulance
+ ALS first response and ALS ambulance
+ BLS first response and BLS ambulance
+ BLS first response and BLS ambulance with ALS intercept

BLS FIRST RESPONSE AND ALS AMBULANCE

In this model, the first responders typically arrive on scene first and provide BLS care. In many urban and suburban EMS systems, the time difference between the first responder's arrival and the ambulance arrival is about six minutes. These minutes can be crucial in serious medical cases such as cardiac or respiratory arrest. The initiation of CPR, application of an automated external defibrillator (AED), or control of serious bleeding can be life saving for these patients. Research has shown that

the fast initiation of BLS care has a more profound impact on patient outcome than ALS care at any time (OPALS, n.d.; AHA, 2010).

Under this system design, the BLS first responders initiate the BLS care and hand off care to the ALS ambulance. In serious cases, one or more first responders may accompany the patient to the hospital to assist the ambulance crew with patient care.

ALS FIRST RESPONSE AND BLS AMBULANCE

Some communities elect to have the first response agency provide ALS care and the ambulance provide BLS care. This model was used extensively in some West Coast communities in the early years of EMS. In this scheme, the first response agency arrives and initiates any needed BLS or ALS care. When the ambulance arrives on scene, the ALS provider may transfer care to the BLS ambulance, or ride with the BLS ambulance along with the patient to continue the ALS assessment and/or treatment.

ALS FIRST RESPONSE AND ALS AMBULANCE

In this model, ALS can be provided by both the first responder and the ambulance provider. Transfer of care is usually fairly easy, especially if both agencies are operating under the same protocol and the same medical director. There is a risk that this model involves more paramedics than the community can support with adequate training and exposure to critical procedures, thereby reducing the level of experience and proficiency of each individual paramedic.

BLS FIRST RESPONSE AND BLS AMBULANCE

In some regions, especially rural areas, both the first responder and the ambulance provide

BLS care. The first responders again provide the rapid initial response and then the ambulance provides the transport component. First responders may ride in the ambulance to provide assistance with patient care.

BLS FIRST RESPONSE AND BLS AMBULANCE WITH ALS INTERCEPT

In some areas, there is insufficient call volume to maintain proficiency of paramedics assigned to either the first response or the ambulance component of the EMS system. In these cases, the community may enter into an agreement with a neighboring community, hospital, or other organization to provide "ALS intercept" for certain cases. The ALS intercept may be provided in single paramedic response vehicles or, in some cases, an ALS ambulance. If an ALS ambulance is used for the intercept, a paramedic with equipment from the ALS ambulance could board the BLS ambulance and provide ALS care, or the patient could actually be transferred from the BLS ambulance to the ALS ambulance.

The latter of these two options tends to be confusing to the patient and patient's family, and, depending on environmental and geographic conditions, can be logistically challenging. For example, one EMS system in western Wisconsin used to transfer the patient from the rural BLS ambulance to the ALS ambulance. As you might imagine, this transfer was difficult on state highways in subzero weather. Today, that EMS system has one paramedic from the ALS ambulance board the BLS ambulance and accompany the patient in the BLS ambulance. This model also presents economic challenges, as most reimbursement sources (Medicare, Medicaid, and commercial insurance) will pay for only one service, leaving the interacting EMS agencies to sort out any division of fees that might be required.

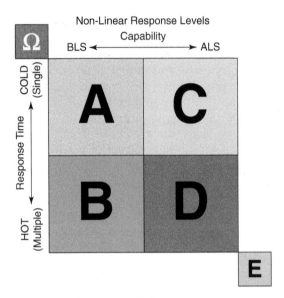

FIGURE 2.1 ■ AMPDS® suggested response configurations. *Source: Reprinted by permission from IAED © 2012 IAED. All rights reserved.*

■ DETERMINING RESPONSE CRITERIA ─────────

Within these configurations, the EMD criteria used by call takers in the control center can effectively determine the correct response level for the patient based on the caller interrogation. The National Academies of Emergency Dispatch (NAED) uses a matrix of response determinants to help local medical directors configure response criteria for medical calls. The matrix is shown in Figure 2.1. This matrix coincides with the response determinants contained in a series of 37 separate response protocols built into the Priority Dispatch Advanced Medical Priority Dispatch System (AMPDS).

As you can see in Figure 2.2, the AMPDS chest pain protocol has specific response configurations based on the patient's age and clinical presentation, as determined by the scripted caller interrogation questions asked by the NAEMD-certified call taker. The

LEVELS	#	DETERMINANT DESCRIPTORS	CODES	RESPONSES	MODES
D	1	**Not** alert	10-D-1		
	2	**Difficulty speaking between breaths**	10-D-2		
	3	**Changing color**	10-D-3		
	4	**Clammy**	10-D-4		
C	1	**Abnormal** breathing	10-C-1		
	2	**Heart attack** or **angina** history	10-C-2		
	3	**Cocaine**	10-C-3		
	4	Breathing **normally** $\geq$ **35**	10-C-4		
A	1	Breathing **normally** < **35**	10-A-1		

For use under MPDS® license agreement only. © 1979–2012 Priority Dispatch Corp. All rights reserved.   AMPDS™ v12.2, NAE-std, 120401

FIGURE 2.2 ■ AMPDS® determinants for chest pain. *Source: Reprinted by permission from IAED © 2012 IAED. All rights reserved.*

patients at greatest at risk receive an ALS "hot" response with ALS "hot" first responders, while patients at lower clinical risk receive a "lesser" response. Many EMS systems use this criterion to ensure an operationally and clinically safe response.

■ SYSTEM DEPLOYMENT

The term **system deployment,** or **deployment**, refers to the method used to distribute EMS resources throughout a service area. Deployment encompasses the number of units placed in the system, as well as the geographic distribution and level of care.

ALL ALS VS. TIERED SYSTEMS

The determination of whether to deploy all ALS resources in a community has both clinical and fiscal considerations.

Clinical Considerations
Any health care practitioner must be able to practice clinical skills regularly to maintain proficiency. This is true of cardiac surgeons as well as paramedics. Cardiac surgeons are required by their accrediting boards to perform a certain number of procedures per year to maintain credentialing. The same is true for paramedics under the supervision of progressive medical directors. Research has shown that high-risk procedures, such as endotracheal intubation, can be harmful to patients if they are not provided by paramedics proficient in the skill (Wang, Lave, Sirio, and Yealy, 2006). This same research suggests that in order to maintain proficiency, providers should perform the skill at least fifty times per year. Therefore, unless the paramedics in the EMS system are performing endotracheal intubation four times per month, they are at a great risk of not performing the skill adequately when called on to do so. The same concept can be applied to patient assessment or any complex medical procedure, including medication administration.

As a result, some medical directors, and even some state agencies, restrict the number of paramedics operating within an EMS system. In recent highly publicized media stories, the medical director in Naples, Florida, tested paramedics in his system and found that many were unable to perform critical skills or patient assessment. As a result, he de-credentialed the paramedics and limited their scope of practice to essentially BLS care (Freeman and Mills, 2009). Similarly, the State of New Jersey

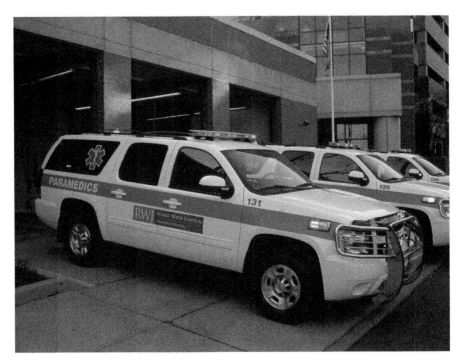

Figure 2.3 ■ A Robert Wood Johnson University Hospital EMS non-transporting mobile intensive care unit provides advanced life support services to municipal and not-for-profit basic life support transporting ambulance services. *Source: Courtesy of MONOC, used by permission.*

recognizes the need for paramedics to be highly utilized to maintain proficiency and restricts the provision of paramedic-level services to hospital-operated paramedic services, of which there is only one per region (Figure 2.3). Thus, even in dense urban areas, first responder agencies and ambulances are BLS only and the local hospitals provide paramedic intercept services.

Fiscal Considerations

Paramedics are typically paid a higher wage than EMTs, and ALS equipment is much more expensive than BLS equipment (a cardiac monitor alone can cost as much as $35,000). Further, paramedics require extensive initial training and continuing medical education compared to their EMT counterparts. Therefore, fiscal considerations in deploying paramedics in a system are significant.

In Fort Worth, Texas, the Fort Worth Fire Department provides BLS first response with forty-one fire engines and eight hundred EMT personnel (Figure 2.4). They provide high-quality BLS care for typically 4 minutes on scene prior to arrival of the ALS ambulance for high-priority cases. If Fort Worth were to decide to deploy paramedics throughout the first response component of the EMS system, the initial cost to make this change has been estimated at close to $8.5 million in equipment and training costs.

For the ambulance provider, the fiscal considerations are a little more complex. Although operating ALS ambulances is more expensive than operating BLS ambulances, efficiencies are gained by being able to send any ambulance to any type of call. If there were a mix of ALS and BLS ambulances, the provider would need to segregate the types of

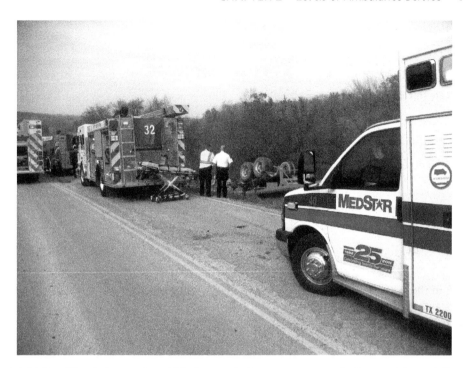

FIGURE 2.4 ■ Fort Worth fire truck and Medstar ambulance at a car wreck. *Source: Glen E. Ellman.*

calls and types of ambulances. For example, if a BLS unit were the closest unit to an ALS call, it would be passed over for an ALS ambulance that would be farther away. Depending on the geography and population density in a community, this deployment model may lead to the need for more actual ambulances on the street at a higher overall cost. For example, the two-tiered ambulance service in the City of Boston operates with great efficiency, whereas that same model in a large county would require far more ambulances to operate. Thus, in some communities it has been found to be more efficient to operate a single-tiered ambulance service utilizing all ALS (paramedic) ambulances.

IMPACT ON REVENUE

The Centers for Medicare and Medicaid Services (CMS) and most third-party payers

recognize the cost difference for the provision of ALS versus BLS care. As such, ALS service is charged and reimbursed at a higher rate than BLS service. Further, emergency service is more expensive to provide than nonemergency service since most emergency service is time sensitive and requires additional costs to deploy ambulances at the ready to meet specific response-time criteria. Nonemergency service can in many cases be prescheduled and either performed by ambulance staff between emergency calls or by personnel specifically scheduled to complete nonemergency calls on a scheduled basis (Figure 2.5).

IMPACT OF PARAMEDIC SHORTAGE ON AMBULANCE DEPLOYMENT

The shortage of available paramedics in some areas of the United States is well known. This makes the deployment of ALS ambulances a

Area Metropolitan Ambulance Authority Rate Schedule FY 2010–2011		
Base Rate (includes supplies)	**Emergency**	**Non-Emergency**
	$1,544.00	$947.00
PROCEDURE/SERVICE RATE		
SCT / CCT Base Rates	$2,640.00	
Response & Assessment (Includes Supplies)	$126.50	
*Emergency/Non-Emergency Mileage (per mile)	$10.00	
Long Distance Transfer Mileage	$10.50	

FIGURE 2.5 ■ This figure represents the charge matrix for MedStar EMS in Fort Worth, Texas.

challenge in these areas, leading to ambulance shortages and delayed responses to both ALS and BLS calls. Consequently, in some communities (e.g., San Antonio, Texas; Cincinnati, Ohio; and Philadelphia, Pennsylvania) system administrators are transitioning from an all-ALS fleet to a mixed-ALS/BLS fleet. These system leaders feel that since only 60 percent of the EMS calls require ALS care, they can safely send BLS ambulances to 40 percent of the calls. This adds to the overall ambulance deployment, thereby reducing the workload and improving response times to all types of ambulance calls.

■ CURRENT RESEARCH ON ALS VS. BLS CARE AND RESPONSE TIMES

Recently published research regarding the impact of ALS care and response times on eventual patient outcomes has been interesting. Researchers appear to be finding that on a *patient outcome* basis, relatively few patient conditions are truly impacted by ALS prehospital care or response times. In fact, even in hemodynamically unstable trauma patients, there was no statistically different change in

patient outcomes for patient delivery to a trauma center within the commonly accepted "golden hour" (Feero, Hedges, Simmons, and Irwin, 1995). Additional research on cardiac arrest patients continues to demonstrate that the single most important determinant of patient outcome is the provision of fast, effective BLS care, regardless of ALS response times or even the provision of ALS care at all.

Recent research has begun to address the concern that ALS interventions do not improve patient outcomes. "Bundles" of interventions, when properly performed, have been found to have significant patient benefit in a variety of clinical conditions, including myocardial infarction, pulmonary edema, bronchospasm, and status epilepticus (Myers, Slovis, Eckstein, Goodloe, et al.). Groups of interventions that include ALS interventions are found to reduce or limit morbidity, mortality, and the need for additional care. As more research becomes available, further EMS system design changes (ALS vs. BLS care) are likely to occur.

CONSIDERATIONS FOR THE FUTURE

EMS and the provision of ambulance service are continually evolving. Recently, several EMS systems have developed advanced practice paramedic (APP) or community paramedic programs to support community health programs and provide additional clinical resources for the high-frequency/low-acuity calls, as well as the low-frequency/high-acuity calls. The systems in Wake County, North Carolina (Wake.gov, 2012), MedStar EMS in Fort Worth, Texas (MedStar EMS, 2013), and elsewhere have demonstrated exceptional results in reducing EMS system use by frequent callers and have allowed medical directors to train a limited group of providers in the special skills needed to provide these nontraditional services.

These systems are able to deploy different resources for "typical" EMS calls, while sending expert resources along with the regular ambulance crews to the most life-threatening calls. As these systems mature, the efficacy of an expanding role for EMS to provide care to the right patient, at the right time, in the right setting with the right resources will dramatically change the EMS profession. It also could dramatically change the levels of education and training needed by paramedics of the future. Watch for this evolving trend and how it may apply to systems you manage.

CHAPTER REVIEW

Summary

It's often said that if you've seen one EMS system, you've seen one EMS system. Most EMS systems evolved without the benefit of carefully thought-out public policy with a focus on mobile health care delivery. The various scope-of-practice rules present in most state EMS regulations offer EMS leaders a myriad of options for levels of service delivery. Clinical, operational, and economic balance needs to be continually evaluated and refined to meet the needs of the local community served.

WHAT WOULD YOU DO? Reflection

What are your considerations in developing this proposal?

1. Engage all the stakeholders in any discussion regarding a transition from an all ALS to a mixed ALS/BLS fleet.
   a. Medical control
   b. First responders
   c. Elected and appointed officials
   d. Hospital leadership

2. Thoroughly identify the types of calls that the BLS units would be handling to ensure that there is sufficient volume and need for this level of service.

3. Determine if there is any impact on how BLS calls are billed and paid to evaluate if there will be any impact on revenue streams.

What are the advantages and disadvantages of running a mixed ALS/BLS fleet?

1. BLS units can safely and effectively handle nonemergency, interfacility transports that have been carefully screened by a medical director-approved call-taking process. Using BLS units for this type of service would free up ALS units for medically appropriate ALS calls and balance the workload over additional deployed ambulances.

2. It needs to be clearly communicated to the community stakeholders that the BLS units would be utilized exclusively for the basic interfacility calls, and not used for any emergency calls.

3. BLS units can serve as a training ground for bringing new employees into the agency to learn about the agency and the service area.

4. It is possible that some stakeholders would feel the system is putting patients at risk by allowing lesser trained personnel to transport patients.
   a. This concern might possibly be mitigated through strong stakeholder education and involvement in program development.

5. There is a risk that a BLS unit would be assigned to a nonemergency call that, on arrival, may need ALS care.
   a. In these cases, there may be a loss of system efficiency.

How would a mixed ALS/BLS fleet change your deployment methodology and costs?

1. The marginal unit hour cost is very similar; however, the limited availability of paramedics makes the use of dual EMT (BLS) units a desirable option for adding field resources to the deployment plan. From a pure deployment perspective, BLS units should be scheduled during times of peak demand for non-emergency BLS calls. Geographically, these units should be posted or stationed in areas close to the facilities that have a high probability of utilizing BLS resources.

What would be your final recommendation?

1. If all stakeholders agree with the deployment and utilization strategy, move forward with a limited scope pilot project prior to full implementation. This way, it is easier to make modifications if necessary and warranted.

Review Questions

1. Describe the struggle to maintain consistent definitions of levels of service over time.
2. What is one approach that states have taken to deal with restrictive scopes of practice?
3. What are the primary roles of first response personnel in EMS systems?
4. Discuss one significant quality-of-care challenge in low-volume EMS systems, or EMS systems where there are high numbers of paramedics relative to the number of patients seen.
5. What recent information has been developed regarding the value of advanced life support services?

References

AHA (American Heart Association). (2010). "AHA Guidelines for Cardiopulmonary Resuscitation and Emergency Cardiovascular Care." See the organization website.

Feero, S., J. R. Hedges, E. Simmons, and L. Irwin. (1995). "Does Out-of-Hospital EMS Time Affect Trauma Survival?" *The American Journal of Emergency Medicine 13*(2), 133–135. See the organization website.

Freeman, L., and R. Mills. (2009, October 30). "Tober Pulls Paramedic Certification for All East Naples Firefighters." See the Marco News website.

MedStar EMS. (2013). "Community Health Program." See the organization website.

Myers, J. B., C. M. Slovis, M. Eckstein, J. M. Goodloe, et al. (2008). "Evidence-Based

Performance Measures of Emergency Medical Services Systems: A Model for Expanded EMS Benchmarking." *Prehospital Emergency Care 12*(2), 141–151.

NASEO.org (National Association of State EMS Officials). (2006, September). "National EMS Scope of Practice Model." National Highway Traffic Safety Administration. See the organization website.

NHTSA (National Highway Traffic Safety Administration). (n.d.). "Emergency Medical Technician–Basic: National Standard Curriculum." U.S. Department of Transportation. See the organization website.

NHTSA (National Highway Traffic Safety Administration). (1998a). "Emergency Medical Technician–Paramedic National Standard Curriculum (EMT-P)." U.S. Department of Transportation. See the organization website.

NHTSA (National Highway Traffic Safety Administration). (1998b). "EMT-Intermediate National Standard Curriculum." U.S.

Department of Transportation. See the organization website.

OPALS (Ottawa Pre-hospital Advanced Life Support). (n.d.). "OPALS Study for Adults." See The Ottawa Hospital Research Institute website.

Philadelphia Fire Department. (2008). "Field Medic Units." See the organization website.

State of Florida. (1997). Florida Statutes, Chapter 401, Section 401.23. See the organization website.

UMBC (University of Maryland, Baltimore County). (2012, July 1). "Critical Care Emergency Medical Transport Program." See the organization website.

Wake.gov. (2012). "Advanced Practice Paramedics." See the organization website.

Wang, H. E., J. R. Lave, C. A. Sirio, and D. M. Yealy. (2006). "Paramedic Intubation Errors: Isolated Events or Symptoms of Larger Problems?" *Health Affairs 25*(2), 501–509. doi: 10.1377/hlthaff.25.2.501. See the Health Affairs website.

Key Terms

advanced life support (ALS) Enhanced assessment, invasive life support techniques provided by EMT-Paramedics who have completed a 1,000- to 1,500-hour vocational/technical certification course.

basic life support (BLS) Basic assessment and noninvasive clinical techniques provided by basic-level EMTs who have completed a 110- to 200-hour vocational/technical certification course.

critical care transport (CCT) Specialized clinical care transport provided by specially trained paramedics or registered nurses during transport from one facility to another facility.

emergency medical dispatch (EMD) The use of specific, script-based call-taking protocols to determine appropriate levels and modes of response and providing pre-EMS arrival medical instructions to callers.

intermediate life support (ILS) Assessment and limited invasive treatment provided by EMT-Intermediates who have completed a 250- to 300-hour certification course.

medical director The physician designated to authorize medical care administered by out-of-hospital EMTs and paramedics.

scope of practice The defined medical procedures authorized by state regulatory authorities to be administered by EMTs and Paramedics.

system deployment, or deployment The process by which EMS units are placed in the field for response to EMS calls.

Corporate Models for Ambulance Service Delivery

Skip Kirkwood, M.S., J.D., NREMT-P, EFO, CEMSO; Rob Luckritz, J.D., NREMT-P; Art Groux, B.S., EMT-P; Robert K. Waddell II, EMT-P (Ret.); Mike Touchstone, M.A., EMT-P, Vincent D. Robbins, FACHE

Objectives

After reading this chapter, the student should be able to:

3.1 Distinguish an emergency medical services system from an ambulance service.

3.2 List at least five different corporate models for the delivery of ambulance service to a community.

3.3 Discuss key strengths, weaknesses, and attributes of each corporate model for delivery of ambulance service to a community.

3.4 Explain the implications of federal anti-kickback regulations.

3.5 Understand the relationship between ambulance service and hospital profits.

Overview

Ambulance services in the United States range in size from one ambulance operated by volunteers and managed by a community board of directors to large governmental agencies and even larger, private, for-profit corporations. This text presents information that the manager of an ambulance service, large or small, needs in order to keep the business solvent and provide clinically excellent service to the community.

Key Terms

field EMS	**charity care**	**public utility model**
dual-role, cross-trained	**cooperative hospital**	
member	**service organization**	
	(CHSO)	

WHAT WOULD YOU DO?

You have completed your degree and worked for ten years as a field EMS provider, serving in a variety of EMS agencies and rising to the rank of shift supervisor. Seeking to advance your career, you've been watching the ads, expanding your network, and applying for positions that fit your ideal for the next step in your career ladder. Last week, you were interviewed for a most exciting position: emergency services director for Newtown, Georgia—a brand-new municipality being incorporated in an area that was previously unincorporated county territory. Newtown has been chartered using a council–manager form of government, and this morning the town manager called to offer you the job. The bad news (or maybe not so bad) is that the manager has just discovered that, under state law and the new town charter, the town is responsible for providing

emergency medical services, including ambulance service, within its town limits and according to standards set by the state EMS office. Although plans for addressing other public service requirements (police, fire, animal control, streets, parks, etc.) are well underway, no plan has been made to address the community's need for EMS and ambulance service.

Your first assignment is to develop, recommend, and justify to the manager and council the best method for providing ambulance service to your community. Just to keep it interesting, the membership of the town council includes the owner of a local ambulance service that does primarily nonemergency interfacility transports, a fire captain from a neighboring town, and the chief operating officer of the hospital located just outside the town limits.

■ INTRODUCTION

It is often said that "If you've seen one EMS system, you've seen one EMS system." This quote, first attributed in the 1980s to the well-known EMS economist Jack Stout, Ph.D., has risen in status to become the title of an article published in a peer-reviewed medical journal (O'Connor and Cone, 2009). Similarly, the options for communities to structure ambulance services for their citizens

are nearly endless—although the many options can be categorized, as we have attempted to do in this chapter.

When discussing corporate models, terminology becomes important. Many people use the terms *EMS* and *ambulance service* as interchangeable. They are not. *EMS* has been defined, by the federal government and others, so broadly that it takes in everything from prevention (before the emergency) through notification, response, prehospital care, hospital

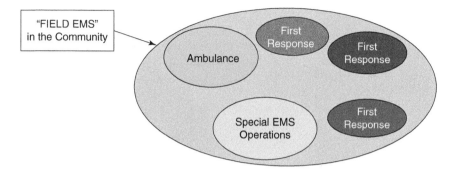

FIGURE 3.1   ▓ In this "American model," the various components may be delivered by any combination of public or private entity operating within a legally defined or informally involved arrangement, with (or often without) common medical direction.

care, and even rehabilitative care (Becknell, 2010). This breadth has become so significant that even the United States Congress now refers to the component of the larger EMS system that is provided outside of the hospital as **field EMS** (U.S. Congress, 2010).

Several conceptual models can be put forward in the design of a field EMS system.

One or more ambulance services are included within this field EMS system. An ambulance service is a service that responds to requests for ambulance service and transports patients between one point and another. A typical community in the United States has a field EMS system that looks something like Figure 3.1.

Side Bar

International EMS

* In the United Kingdom, the community is defined as the entire nation, and field EMS is provided by National Health Service (NHS) "Trusts," which is the term used in the United Kingdom for nonprofit corporations. The NHS trusts provide all elements of the field EMS system. The fire service is minimally involved or not involved at all in medical care delivery.

* The EMS system in Canada is in a state of transition. Whereas in the past ambulance service was a provincial (state) function, some provinces are today devolving EMS from the provincial level to the local or regional municipality (county) level. In some communities, the model looks much like that in the,

although in others it looks more like that in the United States.

* In Australia, field EMS is provided by large, state-operated ambulance services that are responsible for first response, ambulance transportation, and certain aspects of community and preventive health. Several of these services are responsible for technical rescue, including automobile extrication, although as EMS has expanded in to the primary care arena, technical rescue has begun to migrate to the service matrix of the fire brigades.

* Land ambulance services in New Zealand are provided primarily by two organizations: Wellington Free Ambulance and St. John Ambulance New Zealand. St. John Ambulance

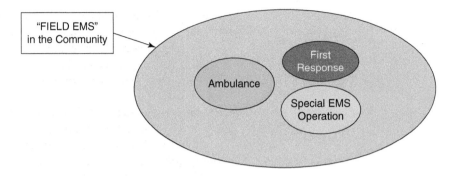

provides service to approximately 85 percent of the land mass of New Zealand, through a network of 553 ambulances and 183 ambulance stations (St. John, n.d.).

♦ In the United Kingdom and some of the Commonwealth countries (Canada, Australia, and New Zealand), the model looks as depicted above.

The United States is served by a potpourri of corporate structures that can be grouped into five large blocks:

♦ **Community-owned nonprofit organizations** may employ paid personnel, rely on volunteers, or utilize some combination of the above.[1]

♦ **Private for-profit ambulance services** typically utilize all paid personnel, sometimes operating under contract or franchise with a community, and sometimes operating in an unregulated (at the local level) economic environment.[2]

♦ **Fire-based ambulance services** operate within the local fire service organization. Generally, there are two types of fire-based ambulance services: one that utilizes dual-role, cross-trained personnel who provide both fire suppression and EMS service, and one that utilizes non-fire personnel in a separate EMS division within the fire service organization.

♦ **Municipal (including county) ambulance services** are separate departments of local government. Although the term is disfavored among municipal ambulance personnel, these services are often referred to as "third services" (with law enforcement and fire suppression being the first and second services).

♦ **Hospital-operated ambulance services** are operated as an arm of a local health care institution or system, either as a revenue center for the hospital or as a service to the community that the hospital serves.

Each of these blocks will be described separately, from the perspective of an author who is intimately familiar with the details of that model. In addition, we will describe the **public utility model**, an approach to EMS delivery in a community that reached a peak of popularity in the late 1980s but has faded somewhat due

---

[1]To avoid confusion and clarify what knowledge the student may bring to this topic, it is important to identify what difference, if any, exists between the terms *nonprofit* and *not-for-profit*, especially in the context of corporate structure and governmental taxing status. This chapter will use a meaning consistent with that of the Internal Revenue Service (IRS): *Not-for-profit* refers to activities, including hobbies such as chess or knitting. The term *nonprofit* describes an organization established for purposes other than making a profit, as codified by the IRS, and confers an exclusion from the legal obligation of paying taxes. It is important to note that *nonprofit* does not necessarily mean an organization must be "charitable" in nature or cause.

[2]Ambulance services are regulated to some degree or another at the state level in all states in the United States.

principally to changes in reimbursement for ambulance transportation on the part of the federal government, also will be described.

COMMUNITY-OWNED NONPROFIT ORGANIZATIONS, from the perspective of Art Groux, B.S., EMT-P

Community-based ambulance services have played a major role in the delivery of EMS in the United States since the first days of ambulance services. Many of these services originated from first aid and rescue squads that were developed at the turn of the twentieth century. They started with a core group of individuals identifying the need for some form of medical care and ability to transport the sick and injured from outside of a hospital to definitive care. These first squads were developed with the noble goal of filling this need, and relied primarily on volunteers.

These services were the forerunners of the modern community-owned nonprofit organizations. Although many of these modern-day services still rely entirely on volunteer staff, others have evolved into career or combination paid/volunteer departments. Many of these organizations began as individual departments serving small communities and have since merged into larger regionalized services serving multiple communities.

The makeup of these services varies greatly from community to community and state to state, in the same manner that the delivery model of EMS care varies by community. This model of service has evolved over time and has many advantages and disadvantages.

ADVANTAGES OF COMMUNITY-OWNED NONPROFIT ORGANIZATIONS

The advantages of this form of EMS organization vary from community to community. Local needs, politics, population, service area demographics, revenue and funding sources, and many other factors can influence what are considered advantages in a particular community.

Nonprofit boards, if comprised properly, can provide some level of insulation from changes in political tides; however, partisan issues often impact patient care. An appropriate nonprofit board should be focused on providing quality patient care in a manner that is fiscally responsible. When selecting board members, it is imperative for the organization to assess its needs and seek out members who can help the organization meet those needs. For example, an organization may be in need of a treasurer and will seek out a certified public accountant (CPA) in the community whose skills might be a good match for that position.

Nonprofit organizations provide some freedom from typical governmental processes. The controls that exist in governmental procurement systems can lead to lengthy purchasing and acquisition processes that may include multiple quotes, bid processes, and potential bond requirements. These processes can inadvertently drive up the overall cost of items and eliminate opportunities for negotiated deals and special offers. Nonprofit organizations also may enjoy greater flexibility in human resources matters (hiring, structuring jobs, compensation, discipline, etc.) than do governmental agencies.

CHALLENGES OF COMMUNITY-OWNED NONPROFIT ORGANIZATIONS

Although board makeup can be an advantage for nonprofit services, it can also be a challenge. The composition of a nonprofit's board of directors is one of the most important predictors of the success of the organization. Board structures that do not allow for continuity between board terms can result in snap decisions that fail to consider long-term consequences. The use of long-term strategic plans can help prevent such decisions. Utilizing staggered terms for board members also helps ensure that a portion of the board maintains support of long-term plans.

Another potential challenge includes the overall makeup of the board. In some services, boards are comprised of line members (paramedics) from within the agency. This model can lead to decisions made in the best interests of the provider rather than those of the organization. In contrast, a board comprised of all non-EMS providers can lead to a long decision-making process that requires education of board members on the tasks involved in providing services. Board members have a legal (fiduciary) duty to the organization they serve, and they may find it difficult to separate the interests of the organization from their interests as line members and employees.

As with all corporate models, funding is a challenge in a nonprofit model. Many nonprofit ambulance services receive a subsidy from a governmental body, and therefore they must be cognizant of political processes and tides. Other organizations rely heavily on fund-raising to provide operational funds. Unfortunately, fund-raising may vary significantly from year to year. "Good" years are not always good years from a fund-raising standpoint if you don't use some of those "excess" funds to plan for bad years. "Bad" years can be devastating if you have no plan or capital set aside to address to those years.

Still other organizations' funding comes almost entirely from fees for service. These structures require planning for changes in call volume. A dramatic increase in call volume can leave the agency short staffed or ill prepared, and a dramatic decrease in call volume can leave the organization with insufficient funds to meet its operational requirements.

ORGANIZATIONAL STRUCTURE OF COMMUNITY-OWNED NONPROFIT ORGANIZATIONS

The organizational structure of a nonprofit service can vary and should be defined in the articles of incorporation and bylaws of the organization. Poor planning in the creation of these documents can cause issues for the organization that may be difficult to resolve in the future. Several items must be addressed when considering the most appropriate corporate structure for a community-based nonprofit ambulance service.

As mentioned, some organizations include providers (ambulance paramedics) on their boards, although others limit membership on the board of directors to individuals not involved in daily operations. Those who choose to allow providers to be members of their board must consider the requirements for voting and recusal (abstinence from participation) in discussions related to compensation or human resources. Some organizations implement probationary periods or different classes of membership. Those that are volunteer based must consider which individuals are eligible to become full-fledged members of the organization. Organizations must consider when corporate officers are elected and how they are structured; specifically, consideration must be had with regard to term and whether officers are elected or appointed. If the board has a separate group of corporate officers (the board of directors) and another group of operational officers, the mechanics of appointment, retention, and removal from office must be carefully defined in corporate documents.

Financial practices within the organization must be addressed when considering the organizational structure. Decisions must be made regarding what accounting practices the organization is going to use, and who is responsible for maintaining financial records and reports. The use of independent auditors should be considered. Similarly, the organization must consider what will happen to the assets of the service should the service be dissolved; options include divesting the assets to another community organization, another EMS provider, or to the local municipality.

Matters that are determined by state and federal regulation should be addressed in the organization's bylaws. It is imperative that every nonprofit have its bylaws and proposed changes reviewed by an attorney who is familiar with the laws of the state and those governing nonprofit corporations.

PRIVATE FOR-PROFIT ORGANIZATIONS, from the perspective of Robert K. Waddell II, EMT-P (Ret.)

As the United States prepared to enter World War II, shortages of resources, including health care personnel, became a significant issue both domestically and abroad. The war movement led many hospitals to discontinue their ambulance services. Demands and requirements for these resources forced hospitals to keep their physicians and staff inside the facility. Prior to this time, many ambulances had been staffed by physicians and hospital interns. Aside from fire departments, funeral homes were the only other businesses that had the vehicles (hearses) capable of transporting people in a horizontal position. The profession that was ultimately responsible for providing emergency care to the living became commingled with the profession responsible for caring for the deceased.

In September 1966, the National Academy of Sciences and National Research Council produced a white paper entitled "Accidental Death and Disability: The Neglected Disease of Modern Society" (also see Chapter 1). This research stimulated discussion and action at all levels, including the United States Congress. Shortly thereafter, in the early 1970s, with the support of Congress, the ambulance service industry began its transformation from a response service to a system of prehospital care. Funeral homes continued to be a major provider of

private, and frequently for-profit, prehospital care throughout the United States. Unfortunately, this arrangement was easily perceived as a conflict of interest. This author was told by a legacy funeral home and ambulance owner, tongue firmly planted in cheek, "Three hundred dollars to treat 'em, three thousand dollars to bury 'em! Where do you think my priorities are?" Although his statement was in jest, public perception was exactly as stated.

In the early 1980s, nearly two hundred private ambulance services across the United States began merging into larger regional corporations. This led to two companies—Rural/Metro Corporation (R/M) and American Medical Response (AMR)—becoming the largest and most dominant for-profit ambulance services in the nation. R/M is the second largest (as of 2011) and considered one of the oldest ambulance providers in the United States. The largest (as of 2011) ambulance provider is AMR. AMR was the first for-profit ambulance service to become publicly owned and to be listed on the New York Stock Exchange. Although the operational functions of the nonprofit and for-profit ambulance services are the same, the underlying purposes are clearly different. The for-profit organization exists to generate income for its owners (be they individuals or corporate stockholders), whereas any excess of revenue over expenses may not accrue to the officers or directors of a nonprofit.

RELATIONSHIPS OF PRIVATE FOR-PROFIT ORGANIZATIONS WITH JURISDICTIONS

For-profit ambulance service providers conduct business according to any of numerous models. One such model is a simple contract for services, with municipalities or quasigovernmental agencies paying the company to provide a legally specified level of service.

In the fee-for-service model, the municipality provides a monetary stipend in exchange for not only the provision of ambulance service but also formal guarantees of performance, including fractional response time, minimum staffing requirements, minimum equipment, resource allocation, and the level of service (basic life support and/or advanced life support). In a third model, the municipality authorizes the corporation to provide services within its jurisdiction without any implied or guaranteed revenue (see Figure 3.2).

Another model provides services strictly to the interfacility market, rather than 9-1-1 or emergent response. The interfacility requirements may have less strenuous accountability requirements due to the fact that the patients being transported are more likely to be medically stable and lack an urgent need for acute care. These services include transporting patients to and from physician's offices, hospitals, specialized diagnostic facilities, treatment centers, or extended or dependent care facilities.

Many for-profit ambulance services function similarly to nonprofit, fire-based, and

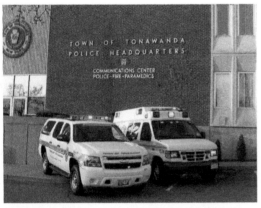

FIGURE 3.2 ■ A municipality may authorize a private corporation to provide services within its jurisdiction without any implied or guaranteed revenue. Here, a Town of Tonawanda Police Department paramedic unit is shown with an ambulance provided by Twin Cities Ambulance, Tonawanda, New York. *Source: Town of Tonawanda Emergency Medical ALS Response.*

hospital-based services in the level of customer service they provide to their staff and affiliated agencies. Training, continuing education, recertification requirements, and clinical quality assurance are all components of these services.

■ FIRE-BASED AMBULANCE SERVICE, from the perspective of Mike Touchstone, M.A., EMT-P ————

The fire service has a long history of providing protection for lives and property. This has been the role and responsibility of fire departments since the inception of fire suppression. Early in their history, in the early 1900s, fire department personnel started providing oxygen and first aid to their fellow firefighters. Transitioning to providing treatment to community members was a natural outgrowth of that practice (Eckstein and Pratt, 2002). Some fire departments "began providing first aid and medical rescue services to the public as early as the 1920s" (Carter and Rausch, 2008). Before *emergency medical services (EMS)* was a recognized term, fire departments were among the organizations providing prehospital emergency medical care. As EMS evolved, and became established as a necessary service, fire departments continued to be one of the most prevalent agencies delivering EMS. With the ongoing challenges of access to health care, issues of reimbursement, and the difficult economic situations that face EMS organizations, today's fire service is taking steps toward providing the full spectrum of EMS services, including both first response and ambulance transportation.

HISTORY OF FIRE-BASED EMS

The fire service has been part of the growth and development of EMS systems in the United States from the beginning. Part of the history of the modern fire service and fire-based EMS predates the development of EMS as a separate discipline or a distinct public safety/public health/health care function. The involvement of fire departments in providing ambulance service dates back to the 1940s. During World War II, shortages of personnel caused by the war effort led many hospitals, which had traditionally provided ambulance services, to turn over the provision ambulance transportation to local fire departments (Dyar and Evans, 2010).

One of the earliest, and common, arguments in support of fire-based EMS was articulated by Dr. Eugene Nagel in the mid-1960s: The fact that fire departments have available an established infrastructure—including personnel, equipment, stations, communications capabilities, and organizations—makes taking on the roles and responsibilities of providing EMS relatively easy and cost effective. Recognizing these advantages, Dr. Nagel initiated a partnership with the Miami Fire Department and in 1964 began training firefighters on how to perform CPR and other emergency medical techniques. He found the firefighters to be quick learners and soon began teaching even more procedures that he deemed essential for what he was calling his Cardiac Care Unit. Dr. Nagel reasoned that firefighters were the best people waiting for emergencies, and he had faith that they could learn enough to intervene with advanced life support to save lives by using these firefighters as the eyes and ears of physicians (Trebilcock, n.d.).

By the late 1960s, Dr. Nagel and colleagues at the University of Miami Medical School had conducted the first paramedic program (Heightman, 2010). Today, local fire departments are common EMS providers. The fire department may be a small rural volunteer department or a large urban municipal department. Regardless of department size, location, or pay scale, the EMS provider who responds to 9-1-1 EMS calls is often a member of a fire department. These EMS systems are commonly referred to as "fire-service-based EMS" or "fire-based EMS."

Fire-based EMS is configured in many different ways and utilizes various organizational structures to provide the resources necessary to successfully operate an EMS system. In 1999, the United States Fire Administration (USFA) reported that "fire/EMS in the United States was present in 26 different models with 52 different permutations" (McNamara, 1999). The many models and permutations of those models result from fire-based EMS systems delivering several levels of service and differing components. Depending on local needs and available resources, fire-based EMS systems may be run exclusively by the fire department or partially run by the fire department with other service components provided by private entities, third-service government agencies, or other EMS providers such as hospital-based EMS.

Fire-based EMS service levels may include basic life support (BLS), advanced life support (ALS), or a combination of both. Departments may provide first responders at the BLS or ALS level, and they may also incorporate ambulance transportation. Because reimbursement for EMS is presently based solely on patient transportation, fire departments that provide ambulance transportation can recover a significant percentage of the cost of providing EMS through billing. For this reason, more fire-based EMS systems are moving toward including ambulance transportation among the services they provide. Some are also considering providing nonemergency ambulance transportation services.

Other operational components of fire-based EMS systems can include fly cars or quick response units, field supervisors, field training officers, and a command structure. There must also be administrative staff to provide support, such as logistics, apparatus, equipment and supply, quality and performance improvement, research and planning, education and training, investigations, and communications. The support functions can be incorporated within the department or, as previously indicated, provided by other agencies. Some fire-based EMS units' members may have additional training and education to provide services such as special event coverage, dignitary protection, rescue services (vehicle, high angle, swift water, trench, etc.), tactical support, and hazardous material response.

The number of models and permutations of those models are influenced by the level of training, education, and certification that a department deploys. Members of fire-based EMS systems can be dual-role cross-trained or they may be single-role providers. A **dual-role, cross-trained member** is a firefighter who also holds an EMS certification or an EMS provider who also holds firefighter certification. Single-role members are either exclusively firefighters or exclusively EMS providers. Some systems employ both dual-role and single-role members. Regardless of the makeup of the system, the majority of fire department members in fire-based EMS systems are considered uniformed personnel, and the departments are generally operated in a paramilitary fashion.

ADVANTAGES AND CHALLENGES OF FIRE-BASED EMS

The International Association of Fire Chiefs (IAFC), the International Association of Firefighters (IAFF), and the Metropolitan Fire Chiefs Association have produced a document entitled "Fire Service-Based EMS Electronic Tool Kit: Resources for Leaders" (International Association of Fire Chiefs, n.d.). The document includes thirteen "talking points" in support of fire-based EMS. These points state that fire departments deploy resources throughout communities and already pay for personnel, apparatus, and facilities; have firefighters positioned for rapid response; train firefighters in EMS; don't have to pay as much overtime to firefighters as compared to private sector EMS paramedics; provide a seamless

service including response, treatment, and transportation; and have lower turnover.

The California Professional Firefighters' website includes an article in support of fire-based EMS titled "Fire-Based EMS . . . The Right Choice for Public Safety." This article lists three main benefits to fire-based EMS: higher survival rates, rapid response times, and quality of care (California Professional Firefighters, 2007). Both of these documents represent the opinions of fire service organizations; neither document references studies or scholarly publications to support the opinions.

A third document, "Prehospital 9-1-1 Emergency Medical Response: The Role of the United States Fire Service in Delivery and Coordination," provides additional and more complete arguments in support of fire-based EMS.

There are also challenges for fire-based EMS. Eckstein and Pratt (2002) suggest the most fundamental challenge is "whether firefighters possess the desire to provide EMS" (p. 73). They also describe the significant contrast between the traditional fire service culture; providing the physically and emotionally demanding service of fighting structure fires, and the more recent demands of providing EMS; and compassion, caring, and careful patient assessment. They conclude that "It would be shortsighted to assume that an experienced firefighter in a traditional, busy urban fire department would easily adapt to the integration of EMS" (p. 73).

Bruegman (2009) echoes the position that fire department culture presents challenges to fire-based EMS. He says:

> Today, EMS accounts for the majority of calls. Yet many metropolitan-sized organizations have resisted the incorporation of EMS into their fire service deployment package; or if they have, it is not embraced in the firehouse as an important service. In many cases, the resistance was due to the culture of the organization, which was so engrained that they were there to fight fires and provide rescue related services,

even though the number of fires and other such calls has continued to decline. The culture had created a level of arrogance that did not allow these people to see the changing context of the industry and their own environment. (p. 29)

Carter and Rausch (2008) identify conflicting forces that will impact the future of fire-based EMS. These include:

* The continuing changes in health care that require frequent training to maintain competency and new equipment
* The emergence of new for-profit and nonprofit local organizations that provide complete or partial EMS
* The cost of government-supported EMS
* Conflicts about appropriate compensation for the higher training and skill required of EMS personnel
* Conflicts with police over which agency (fire service or police) should provide the various components of EMS, especially in light of the potential for higher compensation
* Quality assurance and medical control (p. 248)

In order for fire-based EMS systems to be most effective, the challenges in the preceding list must be overcome. Changing organizational culture is possible with strong leadership, clear vision, and a consistent, disciplined effort to make changes.

There are both advantages and challenges related to fire-based EMS systems. Regardless of this fact, nearly all of the two hundred largest cities provide EMS first response, and fire departments provide transport in 35 percent of those cities.

FIRE-BASED EMS SYSTEM MODELS

Some might question the use of the term *accompany* with respect to EMS trained and certified responders. In most cases, single-role EMS responders do not "accompany" fire resources; they respond separately and have different roles and responsibilities on the emergency scene.

These roles and responsibilities vary depending on the nature of the incident. On a fire scene, single-role EMS responders most often play a support role, providing medical coverage for the incident. On an EMS response, dual-role fire personnel are often in a support role, such as a BLS first responder who initiates BLS care then turns the patient over to a paramedic who may be a single-role provider who responded separately in a quick response unit or in an ambulance.

As Dr. McNamara (1999) referred to a USFA report that found 26 models with 52 permutations; there are still many models and permutations of those models. Recognizing the fact that the three "white paper" configurations are broad generalizations, let us use them as a starting point to explore models of fire-based EMS systems in greater detail.

Dual-Role Cross-Trained Provider Models
Dual-role cross-trained firefighters can achieve several levels of training: emergency medical responder, emergency medical technician, advanced EMT, or paramedic.

Many fire departments utilize some form of the dual-role cross-trained model for their EMS system. According to the *JEMS* 2009 "200-City Survey" (Williams and Ragone, 2010), of the 56 reporting fire departments that provide transport, 49 (87.5 percent) use dual-role providers and 7 (12.5 percent) use single-role providers for transport. There are many possible applications of the dual-role cross-trained model, and fire departments use dual-role cross-trained members to staff BLS and ALS first responder fire apparatus, as well as BLS and ALS ambulances. Cross-trained firefighters can also serve in specialty units, such as hazardous material response units.

Single-Role Fire-Based EMS Models
Some fire-based EMS systems use combinations of dual-role cross-trained and single-role

personnel. Single-role fire-based models that utilize only single-role personnel are less common. These systems deploy some personnel whose training and certification are limited to fire suppression, and other personnel whose training and certification are limited to EMS. These departments staff ambulances with EMTs and paramedics who are not trained as firefighters, and these personnel do not participate directly in fire suppression activities. Fire suppression activities are the responsibility of firefighters with training limited to fire suppression.

Combined System Models

Combined system models may refer to staffing patterns or to public–private partnerships. EMS systems that use both fire-based resources and resources outside the fire department can be referred to as public–private systems, or combined systems. In this model, the fire department provides BLS or ALS first response, and another entity provides ambulance transportation.

Another combined system model uses both dual-role and single-role providers. The Philadelphia Fire Department (PFD) is an example of a fire-based EMS system that deploys both dual-role and single-role resources. The department initially trains firefighters to the EMT-B (EMT) level of certification, but not all firefighters are required to maintain the certification throughout their careers. All engine and ladder (truck) companies have at least one firefighter/EMT-B assigned to the company, and all type of fire apparatus are utilized for first response services. Each apparatus is equipped with an automated external defibrillator (AED), oxygen, and oxygen delivery systems, as well as other basic life support equipment, such as splints, dressings and bandages, cervical collars, and long spine boards. Firefighter/EMTs also staff BLS ambulances utilized for BLS transport, and they may be assigned or detailed to an ALS ambulance to work with a paramedic.

The paramedics in the PFD are single-role EMS providers who staff ALS ambulances; they do not participate directly in fire suppression activities. They do, however, provide medical support as well as rest and rehabilitation on fire incidents.

Side Bar

General Examples of Fire Service EMS Configurations

Dual-Role Cross-Trained Personnel

* Fire service engine or ladder company BLS first response staffed with firefighters holding First Responder or EMT-B certification. BLS transport provided by fire service ambulance staffed with two firefighter/EMT-Bs.
* Fire service engine or ladder company BLS first response staffed with firefighters holding First Responder or EMT-B certification. ALS transport provided by fire service ambulance staffed with firefighter/EMT-B and firefighter/ EMT-P (paramedic) or two firefighter/paramedics.
* Fire service engine or ladder company ALS first response staffed with at least one firefighter holding paramedic certification. Transport provided by fire service ambulance staffed with two firefighter/EMT-Bs, firefighter/EMT-B and firefighter/paramedic or two firefighter/paramedics. In the case of the ambulance being staffed by two EMT-Bs, ALS transports could be provided by having the paramedic from the fire company move to the ambulance to provide ALS care during transport.

Dual-Role and Single-Role Personnel

* Fire service engine or ladder company BLS first response staffed with firefighters holding First Responder or EMT-B certification. Transport provided by fire service ambulance staffed with single-role EMT-B and paramedic or two paramedics.

Combined System

- Fire service engine or ladder company BLS first response staffed with firefighters holding First Responder or EMT-B certification. Transport provided by another agency's ambulance staffed with two single-role EMT-Bs, a single-role EMT-B, and one paramedic or two paramedics.
- Fire service engine or ladder company ALS first response staffed with at least one firefighter holding paramedic certification. Transport provided by another agency's ambulance staffed with two single-role EMT-Bs, a single-role EMT-B, and one paramedic or two paramedics.

The particular fire-based EMS model used dictates the level of EMS certification required of firefighters. A system may use firefighters certified to any of the certification levels to staff fire apparatus dispatched as first responders.

FIRE-BASED AMBULANCE SERVICE: SUMMARY

The fire service in the United States has been involved in providing protection of lives and property for over three hundred years. Firefighters have been providing first aid and oxygen to their fellow firefighters since the early 1900s and to the public since the 1920s. Fire departments in some cities took on ambulance service in the 1940s during World War II. The first paramedic class was delivered to firefighters in the Miami Fire Department in the 1960s. All of this shows the long history of fire department involvement in EMS.

Today, most first responders are fire departments, and provide a portion of emergency ambulance transportation. Those models that include fire departments providing EMS service are referred to as fire-based EMS systems. As the landscape of EMS evolves and changes under financial, political, and cultural

pressures, the fire service and fire-based EMS will continue to play a part in the ambulance service industry. Fire service organizations advocate for expanding the role of the fire service in EMS and will continue to be an ongoing force influencing the future of EMS.

▓ MUNICIPAL AND COUNTY AMBULANCE SERVICES, from the perspective of Skip Kirkwood, M.S., J.D., NREMT-P, EFO, CEMSO ──────

One of the historical threads of the evolution of ambulance services in the United States, particularly in large cities, involves the transition of ambulance service provided by a city or county hospital to a separate service provided directly by the municipality or county. These so-called third services (with police and fire being the first and second services in this paradigm), serve some of the oldest and most populous U.S. cities, including Boston (MA), Pittsburgh (PA), Honolulu (HI), Austin (TX), and Denver (CO). At the other end of the spectrum, many rural communities are served by independent municipal or county governmental ambulance services (MCGAS). County-operated ambulance services are common in certain states, such as North Carolina (Figure 3.3), where state statute and regulations require counties to provide emergency medical services to all citizens (NCGS, n.d.).

Generally, MCGAS are a uniformed public safety service, although this description often conflicts with specific legal classifications in individual states.[3] These conflicts generally arise as a result of statutes that were in place long before the dawn of modern-day EMS, when ambulances

---

[3]For example, in Pennsylvania governmental EMS workers are considered a "uniformed service" by some portions of the state code, although in other sections they are not "essential service" workers.

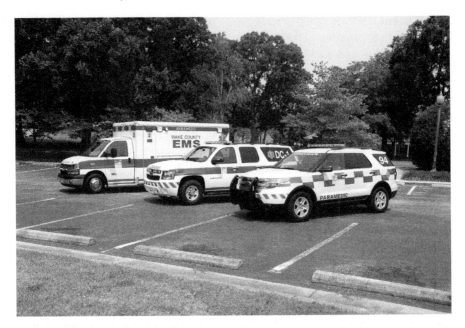

FIGURE 3.3 ■ EMS is a statutory responsibility of counties in North Carolina, thus the county is served by many county government EMS services. The Wake County EMS Division has provided EMS throughout the county since 1976, and utilizes paramedic ambulances, advanced practice paramedics, and field supervisors as part of its daily service mix. *Source: Official Wake County EMS Photo by Mike Legeros, used by permission.*

were operated by drivers with little or no clinical training. In general, these issues have not been resolved because they carry a cost associated with providing ambulance paramedics the more-generous benefit packages provided by municipalities to law enforcement officers and firefighters. In certain jurisdictions, these "distinctions without a difference" have become matters of contention between labor organizations and their political allies.

Like every other organizational option, the MCGAS model has strengths and weaknesses.

STRENGTHS OF THE MCGAS

Employees of the MCGAS are single-focus paramedics, whose only job is to provide emergency medical care and ambulance transportation. Thus recruitment, training, and personnel management can focus on matters of clinical excellence alone, as opposed to models where operating an ambulance is a secondary job responsibility of personnel in other departments. MCGAS have the ability to be more flexible and efficient than fire-based models in staffing plans since the demand for ambulance service is dynamic in both the spatial and temporal sense. A variety of flexible schedules can be utilized to more efficiently match supply (available ambulance unit hours) with demand (number of calls for service and a particular time of the day).

Elsewhere in this text, we discussed the differences between an ambulance service and emergency medical services. MCGAS usually function as a full-service EMS organization for their communities, handling EMS issues beyond ambulance-based care and transportation. Some well-known nonambulance EMS services include the mass gathering activities of Boston EMS and the Denver Paramedics; the medical rescue capabilities and expertise of Austin-Travis County (TX) EMS and Pittsburgh EMS; and the innovative advanced practice paramedic (APP) program in Wake County, North Carolina.

MCGAS are directly accountable to the citizens they serve, unlike other models where the primary accountability may be by way of a contract, a private owner, or a board of directors not selected by the community at large. The citizens, through their elected representatives, are able to directly determine the costs and performance standards for their community's ambulance service, and to make informed local decisions about structure, funding, and infrastructure. This is often cited as a weakness of the MCGAS model (Fitch, Ragone, and Griffiths, 2010); however, this is purely a matter of perspective. Accountability for the performance of a MCGAS is direct (management may be disciplined or replaced for nonperformance), although accountability for a contracted service is indirect (a financial penalty is imposed). City and county councils and commissions are free to impose and to modify response performance and clinical standards in the best interests of their constituency, unfettered by contractual limitations.

The expenditure of public tax dollars to fund the operation of the MCGAS beyond the ambulance transportation revenues that are recouped may be less controversial than the provision of subsidy payments to a private, for-profit ambulance company. As federally funded reimbursements continue to decrease while the beneficiary populations (Medicare and Medicaid) increase, the need for expenditure of local tax dollars will likely increase in order to ensure the community of the availability of EMS and ambulance service.

WEAKNESSES OF THE MCGAS

As a relative newcomer to the departmental structure of the municipality, EMS may be accorded a position in the administrative and political structure of less prominence than law enforcement and fire services. Unless questions related to the legal status of personnel are effectively resolved, employee relations issues may loom large, with EMS personnel in constant turmoil as they urge for parity with their police and fire brethren.

From a financial standpoint, the MCGAS may fall victim to poorly conceived governmental cost-control strategies, such as across-the-board budget reductions. Similarly, revenue capture may suffer if billing for ambulance transportation services is not well managed.

A high-level look at municipal and county ambulance services in the United States reveals a mixture of results. Boston, Austin-Travis County, Wake County, and several other North Carolina counties have and continue to demonstrate excellent operational performance and clinical outcomes. Some ten years ago, the MCGAS serving New York City was merged with the New York City Fire Department (FDNY) as a cost-cutting measure, and it is now managed by the fire service (although no cost savings have ever been reported). MCGAS serving Pittsburgh and Honolulu are being assessed for possible consolidation with their local fire service agencies, and Cleveland is in the process of consolidation. Past experience suggests that these consolidations will succeed or fail based on political considerations separate from issues of operational or clinical performance, while the cost savings that form the foundation of the consolidation argument remain illusory.

■ HOSPITAL-OPERATED AMBULANCE SERVICES,
from the perspective of Vincent D. Robbins, FACHE ——————————

One of several models in the delivery of ambulance services in the United States includes entities owned and operated by hospitals. This model may be further subdivided into those which are internalized departments within hospitals; wholly owned and separately incorporated subsidiaries of single hospitals; or mutually owned, shared ambulance companies, such as those operated by cooperatives. Although nonprofit hospitals may own and operate either nonprofit or for-profit ambulance services, it is practically impossible for a for-profit hospital, or group of hospitals, to own a nonprofit ambulance service.

GENERAL CRITERIA OF NONPROFIT AND FOR-PROFIT COMPANIES

Companies organized as tax-exempt nonprofit entities under the federal Internal Revenue Code are required to demonstrate their tax-exempt purpose,[4] as specified in regulation, and are forbidden to inure financial benefit to individuals (i.e., stockholders) (IRS, 2012). Thus, nonprofit organizations do not have "owners" that receive a share of profits. As such, it is not possible to design a corporate structure that would legally permit a for-profit organization to own a nonprofit. However, a for-profit company could establish a nonprofit and appoint a controlling number of board members to govern the organization. Again, though, no fiscal benefit would be permitted to flow from the nonprofit to the board members, and therefore to the for-profit.

---

[4]Exempt purposes set forth in section 501(c)(3) of the Internal Revenue Code are "charitable, religious, educational, scientific, literary, testing for public safety, fostering national or international amateur sports competition, and preventing cruelty to children or animals." The IRS defines *charitable* as the term is used in its generally accepted legal sense and includes relief of the poor, the distressed, or the underprivileged; advancement of religion, education, or science; erecting or maintaining public buildings, monuments, or works; lessening the burdens of government; lessening neighborhood tensions; eliminating prejudice and discrimination; defending human and civil rights secured by law; and combating community deterioration and juvenile delinquency.

In the reverse, when nonprofits own for-profits, care must be taken to avoid jeopardizing the tax-exempt status of the former. Because nonprofits must demonstrate a purpose that supports their tax-exempt status, such as charitable programs, becoming involved in business lines or services which generate profits that do not further their tax-exempt mission would be of serious concern. Regardless, whatever profit is generated by the owned for-profit organization is taxable, even though it is flowing back to a nonprofit.

It is important to understand that state laws governing for-profit and nonprofit corporations may further limit and restrict ownership relationships and structure. In addition, local, regional, and state rules may also control how ambulance services are corporately designed and what tax statuses are permissible.

AMBULANCE SERVICES AS HOSPITAL DEPARTMENTS

When for-profit or nonprofit hospitals internalize ambulance services and operate them as a department within the organization, they function as do other divisions of the institution (Figure 3.4). Departments in the modern-day bureaucracy of the U.S. hospital are typically separate silos with different managers operating toward their own, often independent, goals. Although they frequently strive to cooperate, following the overall mission of the hospital, they act as segregated services, usually placing their immediate department needs and objectives above others within the organization. This frequently causes competition and conflict among departments within a hospital. Significant managerial energy must be expended to maintain the many departments of a hospital functioning in a mutually supportive and symbiotic style (Campbell, 2010).

Internal hospital ambulance services may be considered to be a clinical, support, or operations department, depending on the philosophy

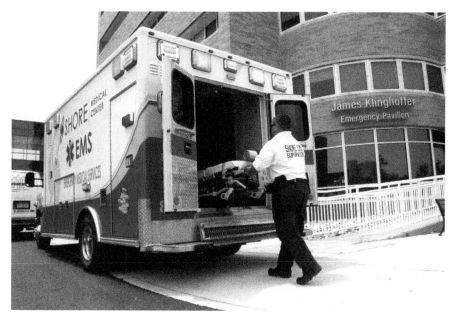

FIGURE 3.4 ■ Part of the mission of a hospital-operated ambulance service may be the promotion of the hospital name and brand in the community. *Source: Shore Medical Center.*

of the organization. They fall within the table of organization of the hospital with a managerial reporting structure that emulates other departments. The perceived importance of the service typically drives its hierarchical position on the organizational chart and the authority given its department head.

If considered a clinical department, the ambulance service is likely to be integrated closely with the departments of the hospital that actually provide health care to patients, such as nursing, and is also likely to receive significant medical oversight, including a strong physician liaison along with quality improvement review. The service is apt in this alignment to bill for its operations and be more fiscally accountable; to be assigned goals for expenses and income, as are other revenue-generating hospital departments; and to be judged more closely for fiscal success. This arrangement is more akin to the emergency department or the same day surgery center when delineated as a clinical program.

However, some hospitals view their ambulance service as simply a support function, similar to inside patient transport or materials management. In this approach, ambulance service is a department whose responsibility is to efficiently move individuals from one place to another, not necessarily focused on clinical care. Such operations are less likely to be scrutinized for quality of patient care, more likely for customer service and the timely movement of patients. Their primary goal is to enhance the productivity of other departments, usually those that produce revenue, such as the operating rooms (OR) and ambulatory care centers.[5] They are also less likely to bill or generate

---

[5]Ambulatory care is health care service delivered on an outpatient basis and not requiring the individual to be admitted to the hospital. Examples of ambulatory care centers include same day surgery, many radiology tests, a number of cardiac catheterization diagnostics, and a wide array of medical treatments.

revenue for their operation and more likely to be viewed as a cost center within the budgetary structure of the organization.

Some hospitals that maintain their ambulance service as departments within their overall organization choose to outsource[6] its management. They do this through management agreements with other companies based on the assumption that expertise for this function lies outside the hospital's management acumen. These management contracts can be based on fixed compensation paid to the outside company; they might also include performance-based reimbursement criteria, even bonuses based on attainment of predetermined goals associated with cost containment and efficiency of operation. When hospitals engage an outside entity to operate their ambulance department, they rely on the outside firm's specialized capabilities and expect better performance when compared to what they anticipate from a traditional internally managed department. Hospitals will typically analyze the expected benefits and disadvantages, including projected expenses and revenues, between internal and outsourced management scenarios before making a determination regarding this issue.

Larger hospitals or hospital systems often maintain management firms within their overall corporate umbrella. These entities act to concentrate a pool of individuals with special management skill sets within a separate group. Some health care organizations do this to centralize managers who possess more of a profit-oriented outlook on management of operations or those who are more entrepreneurial in business attitude. Such a management company can economize overhead if the group's resources are shared among several departments or operating companies throughout the hospital. It is also a mechanism used to allocate fixed costs to multiple components of a hospital or health care system and avoid duplication of costly management resources. It can serve as a way that large organizations drive compliance of varied and disparate sections within the overarching corporate vision or strategic plan. This also provides a method to set apart certain individuals for the purpose of providing substantially different salary, benefits, and performance packages than those available to other employees.

It is important to note that when hospitals internalize their ambulance service they are almost always included in their managed care contracting process and reimbursement rates.[7] Typically, the hospital and insurance plan consider the ambulance operation as just another ancillary or support function and rarely carve it out for separate or additional compensation. It is also not unusual for insurance companies to exclude or negotiate deeply discounted rates in their traditional fee-for-service plans for a hospital's ambulance service when that service is part of the facility's organizational structure.[8] Hospitals need to consider whether

---

[6]There remains inconsistent use of the term *outsourcing* in business academia. For the purposes of this chapter, *outsourcing* refers to the contracting with a third party for the performance of a delineated service or function, which may include management of a specific hospital internal operation.

[7]Managed care contracts, in the context of this book, refers to agreements made between hospitals and insurance companies which establish rates of reimbursement that are inclusive of all services provided by the health care institution for a covered patient. They are typically fixed rates of compensation for a particular diagnosis or group of diagnoses of a single patient. This type of reimbursement mechanism places significant burden on the hospital to provide cost-efficient care to the covered patient.

[8]Fee-for-service reimbursement is the traditional way health care providers have been paid by insurance companies for the care they render to patients. Essentially, it calls for the health care institution to be compensated for each service it performs and all supplies used to care for a patient. Although the individual rates for each item of care or supply are negotiated, fee-for-service does not normally limit total reimbursement.

including an ambulance service as an internal department is justified financially as it relates to their managed care and traditional insurance contracts. When an ambulance service is separated from the hospital corporation and functions as an independent entity, it is free to negotiate its own reimbursement rates from insurers.

Such arrangements usually apply to federal and state reimbursement programs as well. If the ambulance service is part of the hospital organization, Medicare considers it as such and reimburses the facility through Part A as part of the overall patient's bill; in many cases, this will result in less total revenue when compared to a separate bill and reimbursement from Medicare for ambulance service if submitted under Part B.[9] The determining factor is whether the ambulance service is part of the hospital corporation and, therefore, part of its business cost structure (considered a Medicare Provider[10]), or is a separate company recognized as an individual Medicare Supplier.[11]

However, it may work to the financial advantage of the hospital to internalize its ambulance operations. In some states, health care institutions are provided tax subsidies for the **charity care** they provide.[12] In charity cases, it is usually required that the hospital document the services it provides for which it is not compensated. Depending on the cost and revenue ratios involved, it may benefit the hospital to provide ambulance service at a financial loss through an internalized department in order to gain these state subsidies. Careful analysis is required to calculate the impact of the hospital's ambulance department's provision of charity care on the overall formula for the hospital's total uncompensated service and the amount in state subsidies that result. Medicare rules also provide for the consideration of charity care in the calculation of reimbursement rates for individual hospitals and must be assessed when deciding on internalizing or outsourcing the ambulance service function.

AMBULANCE SERVICES AS SEPARATE CORPORATIONS, WHOLLY OWNED

Many U.S. hospitals have decided to form their own ambulance companies. In these cases, the ambulance company is a separate corporation; almost always bills for its services to attain operating revenue; and typically acts, at least in part, to benefit the hospital in some fashion. Caution is needed to ensure that the services provided by the ambulance company do not illegally benefit the hospital, especially regarding anti-kickback statutes and regulations. Inappropriate remuneration may occur when the hospital receives compensation from federal reimbursement programs that is associated with a benefit of value derived by the patient and provided for the purpose of inducing use of a hospital's service or program. In other words, inappropriate remuneration means to cause financial benefit to inure to the hospital by inducing the patient with a benefit of value. This benefit of value could be a deeply discounted or free ambulance trip, or forgiving the patient a normally obligated co-payment or deductible. Since federal reimbursement is

---

[9]Medicare reimbursement related to ambulance service is divided into Part A and Part B. Part A is generally considered compensation provided by hospitals and Part B that provided by nonhospitals. Hospitals cannot normally choose under which part to submit its bill. This is regulated by Medicare, which provides detailed requirements regarding which claims for which services must be submitted under which part.

[10]*Medicare Provider* is the term used to describe a health care entity permitted to submit claims for reimbursement under Part A.

[11]*Medicare Supplier* is the term used to describe a health care entity permitted to submit claims for reimbursement under Part B.

[12]*Charity care* refers to medical services provided by health care entities to patients who are financially unable to pay for said services. These persons are frequently referred to as "financially indigent."

almost always involved in health care services, hospital-owned ambulance companies must be careful to avoid providing services in any way that results in prohibited recompense to the hospital.

In this wholly owned submodel, the ambulance company often exists primarily to improve efficiency for the rest of the hospital's operations regarding patient care. In today's reimbursement methodologies for both inpatients and outpatients, the faster the individual is treated and released, the better the net revenue margin for the hospital (Smith and Werthem, 2010). Since both federal payment systems and managed care contracts reimburse hospitals based on diagnosis, not on length of patient stay or resources consumed, the health care facility is incentivized to care for its patients as quickly as possible. Throughput has become a paramount concern for hospitals.[13] Today's insurance payment schemes reward rapid treat of patients since that makes the hospital's resources, such as inpatient beds or outpatient surgical suites, available faster for the next case. Increasing admissions or the number of procedures performed within a given time frame increases revenue with only marginal, commensurate increases in expense. Fixed costs remain virtually the same. Therefore, net revenue per case increases.

In addition, hospitals that suffer longer inpatient stays will have fewer beds available for new admissions when needed. In addition, if the hospital's emergency department (ED) is overcrowded and placed on divert, it will turn away even more admissions (Scalise, 2010). Each admission of an inpatient represents

revenue for the hospital. Therefore, each lost admission is lost revenue. If a hospital's longer length of stays or overcrowded ED is due to inefficient ambulance service, there is an opportunity to increase revenue by improving patient movement. Hospitals that recognize this factor will be seen to focus on how best to secure ambulance service that is timely, efficient, and inexpensive.

Many hospitals believe that by owning and operating an ambulance company they will have better control over the ability to direct the movement of their patients, and thereby prioritizing which individuals need to be moved for the benefit of economizing their operations. These institutions surmise that exercising day-to-day authority over medical transportation provides them with a mechanism to improve their efficiency in reducing the cost-per-case for those revenue-producing services acutely, depending on volume. These institutions see ambulance services as a way to enhance throughput and therefore net revenue.

AMBULANCE SERVICES AS A COOPERATIVE

Another way health care facilities have chosen to closely control ambulance services is through the shared hospital services cooperative concept. This structure brings several advantages to bear that are only available through the cooperative (Figure 3.5). First, a true **cooperative hospital service organization (CHSO)** would be designated by the IRS as a nonprofit, specifically under the 501(e) section of the regulatory code.[14] As such, the hospitals that participate in the cooperative can only be nonprofits themselves. They would be members, not owners, and would be bound by the associated, normal restrictions of a nonprofit

---

[13]*Throughput* is the quantity of product or service that is made or provided in a specified period of time. It is a measure of productivity and, by extrapolation, of efficiency. An example of throughput in the hospital setting would be the number of surgical cases completed in one operating theater in a day. For ambulance operations, a well-known throughput measure is Transport UHU (unit hour utilization for completed transports).

[14]The term *CHSO* is specifically used by the IRS and Office of Inspector General of the federal government in referring to hospital cooperative companies.

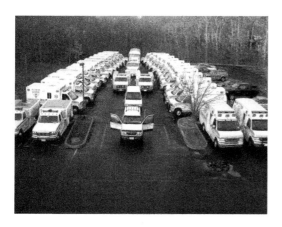

FIGURE 3.5 ▪ MONOC is a large ambulance service operated by a hospital service corporation in New Jersey. Its extensive fleet provides emergency and nonemergency ambulance transportation, helicopter EMS, and related services. *Source: MONOC Mobile Health Services.*

company. However, a main advantage of the hospital cooperative is its ability to reward members for the level of participation they refer to the company. The IRS actually requires a cooperative to distribute back to its members proportional net revenue, either through accumulation in a fund balance or via direct payment. Without what is called the "Stark safe harbor"[15] (U.S. Code, n.d.) such remuneration for referred business would violate existing federal anti-kickback regulations.

Second, by sharing membership in a cooperative, hospitals spread the financial risk associated with the ambulance service itself. Although member hospitals may pay dues to support the cooperative, they are not necessarily obligated to fund the company. Even though it is a nonprofit entity, a CHSO is free to bill for

its services, including Medicare, Medicaid, insurance plans, and patients, and it is not mandated to be funded either wholly or partially by membership contributions. In fact, if well managed and fiscally sound, CHSO ambulance companies pose virtually no concern to their members regarding fiscal matters since they are separate corporations and can be financially independent from their members.

Members maintain control through the CHSO's board of trustees and provide both management and financial oversight. Through a cooperative, however, members do not have unilateral control but must share authority over the organization. However, since the incentives of all members would theoretically be aligned on the efficient and economical movement of all their individual patients, shared control should not present a problem.

CHSOs present a structure that member hospitals can use to advance their common needs while enjoying the advantages of an economy of scale larger than themselves. These cooperatives also represent a unique model that can legally reward its members for the business each refers to the company.

SUBSIDIARY VERSUS COOPERATIVE

Whether a wholly owned separately incorporated affiliate or a CHSO, an ambulance company differs from a hospital department that provides medical transportation in some important fundamental ways. In a structure in which an ambulance service exists as a separate corporation, the entity operates more in line with typical business principles than when it functions as a department within a larger company, such as a hospital. As its own company, even if owned by only one parent organization, the ambulance service will usually have a keener focus and accountability for fiscal issues as well as administrative and operational management. Generally speaking, it will approach daily management of operations

---

[15]A portion of this safe harbor protects CHSOs from anti-kickback regulations. The safe harbor exempts payments from a member to its CHSO that support the cooperative's operational costs as well as all payments from the CHSO to its members that are required by IRS rules.

with a more targeted sense of economic survivability and will view its corporate administration as more important to long-term planning and strategic outlook.

Because it is a company itself, it will have a broader array of management responsibilities, including human resource administration, compliance with labor laws, risk management issues, financial obligations, strategic planning, medical-legal topics, and so forth. As a company, its management will be directly concerned with cash flow, billing and collections, debt service, auditing requirements, and legal and regulatory duties—particular Sarbanes/Oxley[16] mandates incumbent upon for-profit ambulance companies, as well as Medicare and HIPAA[17] compliance matters.

THE PUBLIC UTILITY MODEL, from the perspective of Skip Kirkwood, M.S., J.D., EMT-P, EFO, CEMSO

The **public utility model (PUM)**, is often discussed as a model for the delivery of ambulance services. In fact, it is not a different type of ambulance service, as much as it is a different model of governance for an ambulance service that is delivered by a separate entity. The PUM gained in popularity from its inception in 1979 and remained a stable, if strong, influence until the late 1990s, when a variety of factors—including the implementation of the National Medicare Fee Schedule and the national consolidation of private for-profit ambulance services—changed the dynamics of the environment in which the model operated.

Historically, private sector ambulance services operated, if there was any oversight at all, under the oversight of a unit of municipal or county government. Often, this involved a multitude of poorly supervised ambulance services, little or no public accountability, and poor operational and clinical performance. Competition within the market provided unwanted distractions, perverse performance incentives, and poor service to economically disadvantaged areas.

To bring greater order, efficiency, and accountability to ambulance service markets, EMS system innovator Jack Stout developed the concept of the PUM. Jay Fitch and associates also embraced and implemented this approach in a number of communities, in which a separate governmental regulatory agency, often known as the authority, provides a regulatory and oversight framework, develops a detailed performance-based contract, and utilizes a competitive procurement process to select an operations contractor (competition "for" the market rather than "in" the market). In its purest form, a PUM will also own the capital assets (ambulances, communications, dispatch systems, cardiac monitors, etc.) of the system, so that in the event of default on the contract, a contractor can be replaced without a lengthy capital procurement cycle. The operations contractor is awarded an exclusive franchise for both emergency and nonemergency ambulance work in the authority's jurisdiction, and is responsible for staffing, operating, supervising,

---

[16]The Sarbanes-Oxley Act (Public Law 107-204, 116 Stat. 745, enacted July 30, 2002), commonly referred to as Sarbanes-Oxley or Sarbox, is a federal law that established new accountability and attestation standards for all U.S. companies and their boards, management, and auditing firms. It is named after its original sponsors: U.S. Senator Paul Sarbanes (D-MD) and U.S. Representative Michael G. Oxley (R-OH).

[17]Health Insurance Portability and Accountability Act (HIPAA) (Public Law 104-191) was enacted by the U.S. Congress in 1996. It was originally sponsored by Senator Edward Kennedy (D-MA) and Senator Nancy Kassebaum (R-KS). It protects workers' health insurance coverage when there is a change or loss of jobs. It also establishes national standards for electronic health care record transactions and national identifiers for providers, health insurance companies, and employers. In addition, it mandates the security and privacy of health data.

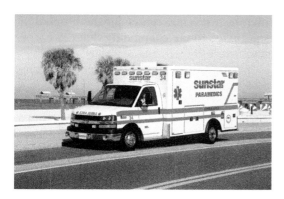

FIGURE 3.6 ■ Shown here is a paramedic ambulance of Sunstar EMS. Ambulances in Pinellas County, Florida, are operated by a private contractor, whose identity remains hidden. The county owns the brand name of this well-known public utility model EMS organization. *Source: Pinellas County Government, by permission.*

and dispatching the ambulances, gathering documentation, and providing information to the authority. The contractor is often unknown to the community, with the authority providing the brand name and brand identity for ambulance service in the community.

A variety of factors arose in the late 1990s and early in the twenty-first century that decreased the viability of the PUM. Multilevel consolidations of private ambulance companies left few organizations that were qualified to bid for major metropolitan ambulance contracts. Changes in reimbursement for ambulance transportation required the authorities to look to public tax dollars in increasing amounts to offset the losses from ambulance billing.

Competitive procurements for exclusive market share became increasingly litigious. Labor organizations became more involved with governance, procurement, and operational issues. Faced with these challenges, several well-known PUMs decided to "self operate," effectively ceasing to be PUMs at all and transitioning to freestanding municipal or county government ambulance services (MCGAS). Well-known PUMs, including MAST (Kansas City, MO), Fort Worth's MedStar, and the Richmond Ambulance Authority have gone the self-operated route. MAST has since undergone further transition, and ambulance service in Kansas City is now provided by the Kansas City Fire Department. REMSA (Washoe County [Reno], NV) operates by a separate but wholly owned nonprofit contractor. Often thought of as a PUM, the Mecklenburg EMS Agency (MEDIC), serving Charlotte, North Carolina, is actually an independent governmental agency that incorporates a unique partnership with the community's hospitals. Several PUMs continue to operate successfully in the pure form, including Sunstar EMS (Pinellas County, FL), EMSA (Oklahoma City and Tulsa, OK), and TRAA (Fort Wayne, IN).

CHAPTER REVIEW

Summary

The majority of ambulance services in the United States operate under five primary structures. Community-owned nonprofit organizations are independent nonprofit organizations that work closely with the communities they serve. These organizations originated out of volunteer organizations but have evolved to include career and hybrid paid/volunteer models. Private for-profit ambulance services typically utilize paid paramedics and often operate under contract or franchise with a community. Fire-based ambulance services operate within a fire service organization. These services may operate utilizing dual-role, cross-trained personnel who provide both fire suppression and EMS service, or single-role paramedics situated in a separate EMS division within the fire service organization. Municipal ambulance services are separate departments within local government. These services are generally uniformed services and often referred to as third services. Hospital-based ambulance services are operated as an arm of a local health care institution or system either as a revenue center for the hospital or as a service to the community that the hospital serves.

In addition to the five corporate structures, the public utility model represents a method of public/private partnership that provides for contracted EMS services within a public authority. This model has fallen out of favor in recent years due to the evolution of health care reimbursement models.

WHAT WOULD YOU DO? Reflection

As you explore these issues with your manager and various community leaders, you realize that the community is unaware of any of the many issues involved in selecting a model for your community's ambulance service. Your boss, after listening to you, recognizes that this is a potential political hot potato in the community. You recommend, and your boss agrees, to hold a series of community forum meetings on the issue, facilitated by a well-respected public administration professor from a local university.

At these sessions, you will present the strengths and weaknesses of each possible organization and the demographics of EMS needs in the community, and you will take questions from the audience. Other interested parties, including the members of the town council with expertise in the area, will have an opportunity to present their views. After the forum series is complete, the local school of government will conduct a poll of the citizens, which will be presented to the town council for consideration.

Review Questions

1. What are the most important considerations when structuring a board of directors for a community-based nonprofit ambulance service?
2. Why is the number of fire-based EMS systems growing rapidly?
3. Who were the predecessors to the modern for-profit ambulance services?
4. What are the two largest for-profit ambulance services today?
5. What is the difference between a single-role and dual-role EMS provider in the fire service?
6. What is a cooperative hospital service organization?
7. Explain why a hospital might elect to outsource the management of its ambulance service.
8. Why would a hospital want to own an ambulance service?

References

Becknell, J. (2010, April). "EMS Is Everything and Everybody: The Curse of a Big Name." *Best Practices in Emergency Services 13*(4).

Bruegman, R. (2009). *Fire Administration I.* Upper Saddle River, NJ: Pearson Prentice Hall.

California Professional Firefighters. (2007). "Fire-Based EMS ... The right choice for Public Safety." See the organization website.

Campbell, G. (2010). "7 Tips for Creating the New American Hospital." Second Curve Healthcare. See the organization website.

Carter, H., and E. Rausch. (2008). *Management in the Fire Service*, 4th ed. Sudbury, MA: Jones and Bartlett, p. 248.

Dyar, J., and B. Evans. (2010). *Management of EMS.* Upper Saddle River, NJ: Pearson.

Eckstein, M., and F. Pratt. (2002). "Fire." In A. E. Kuehl, ed., *Prehospital Systems and Medical Oversight* (pp. 68–74). Dubuque, IA: Kendall/ Hunt.

Fitch, J. J., M. Ragone, and K. Griffiths. (2010). "Executive Summary: Making Smart Choices about Fire and Emergency Medical Services in a Difficult Economy." *Strategies and Solutions for Local Government Managers* 42(5). See the Fitch & Associates website.

Heightman, A. J. (2010). "Pioneers of Paramedicine Honored in L.A." See the JEMS Emergency Medical Services website.

International Association of Fire Chiefs. (n.d.). "Fire Service-Based EMS Electronic Toolkit: Resources for Leaders." See the organization website.

IRS (Internal Revenue Service). (2012). "Exemption Requirements: 501(c)(3) Organizations." See the organization website.

McNamara, M. (1999). "The Evidence For/Against Fire Service EMS and Private Sector EMS."

NCGS (North Carolina General Statutes). (n.d.). North Carolina Administrative Code, Chapter 10P. See the Office of Administrative Hearings website.

O'Connor, R. E., and D. C. Cone. (2009, December). "If You've Seen One EMS System, You've Seen One EMS System ..." Academic Emergency Medicine *16*(12),1331–1332.

Pratt, F., P. Pepe, S. Katz, and D. Persse. (2007). "Prehospital 9-1-1 Emergency Medical Response: The Role of the United States Fire Service in Delivery and Coordination." FireCompanies.com. See the organization website.

Scalise, D. (2010). "Improving Patient Throughput." Hospitals & Health Networks (online magazine). See the organization website.

Smith, J., and S. Werthem. (2010). "Improving Revenue and Profit by Expediting Patient Throughput." Society for Health Systems. See the Institute of Industrial Engineers website.

St. John. (n.d.). "St. John Ambulance National Performance Statistics." See the organization website.

Trebilcock, M. (n.d.). "About Us: Our History." City of Miami Department of Fire-Rescue. See the organization website.

U.S. Code (USC). (n.d.). Title 42, Chapter 7, Subchapter XI, Part A § 1320a–7b: Criminal penalties for acts involving Federal health care programs.

U.S. Congress. (2010). House. *Field EMS Quality, Innovation, and Cost Effectiveness Improvements Act of 2010.* HR 6528.

Williams, D. M., and Ragone, M. (2010, February). "2009 JEMS 200-City Survey: Zeroing in on What Matters. *JEMS: A Journal of Emergency Medical Services.* See the organization website.

Key Terms

field EMS Those components of the EMS system that concern the direct provision of care to patients, beginning with the dispatch of first responders and ambulance services through the transport of the patient to the hospital, or other appropriate disposition of the patient.

dual-role, cross-trained member A firefighter/paramedic who is trained, licensed, and authorized to provide both firefighting services and emergency medical care.

charity care Care provided to individuals who do not have sufficient insurance or financial means to pay for their care, which accounted for as a loss (written off) by the organization providing care.

cooperative hospital service organization (CHSO) A nonprofit organization owned by two or more nonprofit hospitals, designed to provide shared services to participating hospitals.

public utility model (PUM) A model of EMS system design popularized in the 1980s, utilizing a governmental authority, which contracts with an operations contractor to actually operate ambulances on behalf of the authority. A typical PUM has exclusive operating rights for all emergency and nonemergency ambulance activity in the area it serves.

The Ambulance Market

4 **CHAPTER**

DAVID A. SHRADER

Objectives

After reading this chapter, the student should be able to:

4.1 Describe the ambulance and medical transportation market in the United States in economic terms.

4.2 Explain related and overlapping markets that interact with the ambulance market.

4.3 Understand the approximate demand for ambulance and related services and factors that affect that demand.

4.4 Clarify the utility nature of the economics of the ambulance market, including economies of scale.

4.5 Describe the effects of market exclusivity, and discuss horizontal and vertical consolidation within the market.

4.6 Discuss the use of competition and the antitrust implications of creating exclusive markets.

4.7 Explain various common methods used for the allocation of market rights.

4.8 Identify the effects of federal government intervention in the ambulance market, including a description of cost shifting and its predictable results on pricing.

4.9 Identify a major reason that the ambulance market is likely to grow significantly over the next twenty years.

4.10 Discuss strategies that ambulance service providers may pursue to expand the market and access new sources of revenue.

Overview

Ambulance services in the United States range in size from one ambulance operated by volunteers and managed by a community board of directors to large governmental agencies and even larger, private, for-profit corporations. This text presents information that the manager of an ambulance service, large or small, needs in order to keep the business solvent and provide clinically excellent service to the community.

Key Terms

average cost curve
average cost per call
cost shifting

economic market
horizontal
   consolidation

marginal cost per call
public utility
   economics

submarket
vertical consolidation
wholesale competition

WHAT WOULD YOU DO?

During your first week in management, the EMS chief calls a special management meeting for later in the day. He announces that projected increases in costs will cause an average loss of $30 per transport during the next budget year. City hall has said that increased subsidies are not an option and that a plan is needed to make up for this projected loss in the budget or expenses will be cut through layoffs. The chief says he wants to brainstorm some ideas in 30 minutes and has asked all members of the management team to be prepared to offer possible solutions to be investigated.

1. Is it possible to increase revenue to offset the projected loss?
2. Would changes in your current production methods improve efficiency?
3. Would an expansion of service area or services provided produce economies of scale?
4. Are other sources of revenue available by changing the services provided?

■ INTRODUCTION

Emergency medical service (EMS) systems and ambulance services are highly complex businesses. Successful management of EMS requires a broad variety of skills and competencies. In addition to clinical and human resources experience, the successful manager must understand such disparate concepts as utility economics, health care reimbursement, logistics management, and antitrust and contract law. Many experienced executives with successful experience in the airline, ground transportation, security, and technology industries have failed in EMS as a result of unintended consequences resulting from an underestimation of the complexity of the industry. Understanding the economics of the ambulance market is one of the keys to long-term success.

ECONOMIC MARKETS

In a broad economic sense, the market is the foundation of the overall economy. The exchange of all goods and services for other goods and services and for money defines commerce within the market. Noted economist Faustino Ballvé (1963) observed, "Everything…from the exchange of meat for eggs between neighboring families to international trade, constitutes the *market*, the pivot around which all economic life revolves" (p. xx).

The broad **economic market** is composed of a complex, worldwide network of smaller components. Due to its scale and intricacy, the global economic market is difficult to comprehend. For this reason, the term *market* is usually used to refer to specific subsets of the broader economic market.

The term *market* was derived from the familiar concept of a place where people met to exchange goods and services. Although markets originally described physical locations, it is now common to use the term to describe any one of a variety of systems, institutions, procedures, social relationships, or infrastructures that describe or facilitate parties in commerce. As a result, we may describe the housing market, the market for luxury cars, for health care services, or for ambulance services.

When describing a particular market, care must be taken to accurately define the types of commerce that are included and to exclude those that are unrelated to the economic activities that are to be examined. Depending on the issues to be investigated, ambulance services could be described as a subset of the broader health care market, the market for public safety services, or a portion of the transportation market. In addition, related and overlapping markets must be identified and included or excluded, depending on the particular purpose for which the market is defined.

Markets that are related and, to some extent, overlap the ambulance market include the following:

- Nonambulance medical transportation
- Paratransit operations
- Call-center operations
- Rotary and fixed wing air ambulance response and transportation
- Physician house call services
- Home health agencies
- Urgent care facilities
- Fire department (nonambulance) response systems

For the purposes of this chapter, the ambulance market is defined as the aggregate of all responses to emergency and nonemergency requests for ambulance services by one or more transport-capable ground ambulances, whether or not the response resulted in a transport. This definition includes advanced life support, basic life support, critical care transports, neonatal transfers, other specialized ground transports, and standby services.

Not included in this definition are non-transport-capable first response, extrication and technical rescue services, rotary and fixed wing air ambulance services, nonambulance nonemergency medical transportation, paratransit, urgent care facilities, and physician house call services.

Some overlapping services, including home health care, may be included in information related to the ambulance market. New initiatives among some ambulance providers have moved into this market during the past few years. Although programs, such as advanced practice paramedics and community health paramedics, represent a substantial growth opportunity for ambulance and EMS providers and are increasing in popularity, they currently represent a negligible amount of economic activity in the ambulance market.

THE AMBULANCE MARKET ———

Expenditures for ambulance services in the United States in 2010 are reported to have been approximately $14,000,000,000 (Bain & Company, 2011). Due to the difficulty in assessing local tax subsidies and shared expenses within government providers, this number is probably grossly understated in terms of the total cost of services. This figure for expenditures also does not include charges that are written off as contractual allowances for Medicare and Medicaid cases. It does, however, serve as a useful indicator of the amount of sales revenue generally available within the competitive market.

MARKET SHARE DISTRIBUTION

In 2010, government providers of all types represented approximately 54 percent of the total expenditures for ambulance services, or $7,560,000,000 (Figure 4.1). Private providers of all types accounted for 34 percent of the market, or $4,800,000,000. Hospital-based systems accounted for 5 percent, public utility models for 3 percent, and other types of providers amounted to 4 percent of the market (R/MC, 2011).

Two major categories of providers represent the majority of the government segment of the market. Fire departments serve the largest portion with an estimated 42 percent to 46 percent. Municipal and county government services serve an estimated 8 percent to 12 percent of the national market. Other government providers, such as health department or police-based services, are rare and account for a negligible share of the market. Military services are not included in these estimates since their services are primarily internal and generally do not involve reimbursement through fees or local taxes.

COMPETITIVE LANDSCAPE

The ambulance and medical transportation market in the United States is a fragmented landscape of local system designs. In 2010, over 15,000 ambulance providers were actively providing emergency and nonemergency ambulance services in the United States (American Ambulance Association, 2010). Provider types included governmental agencies, hospitals, private companies, volunteer associations, nonprofit corporations, special purpose organizations, and joint ventures.

Many fire departments directly provide ambulance services to their communities. In addition, most of the 30,125 fire departments in the United States provide EMS services—including first response, rescue, forcible entry, extrication, technical rescue, and manpower—that directly affect the speed and efficiency of

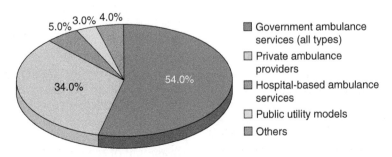

FIGURE 4.1 ■ Ambulance market share distribution.

ambulance services, even in markets in which the ambulance provider is another agency or company (National Fire Department Census, Quick Facts, 2010 Estimate)

The mix of system designs and provider configurations has been the result of independent local system evolution to meet perceived community needs with the resources that were locally available when key decisions were made. Federal grants, an action television show, hospital mission statements, opportunistic businessmen, the success of fire prevention, and charismatic personalities often influenced critical choices in the design of EMS.

No matter the structure or ownership of an ambulance provider or potential provider — whether a fire department, third-service agency, hospital or private company — each is a competitor within the ambulance market. Some providers have relatively secure market rights, although others compete daily in a retail environment for calls. Nevertheless, any provider may lose or expand its market rights and, as a result, all are involved to some degree in market competition.

SUBMARKETS

A **submarket** is a geographic, economic, or specialized subdivision of a market. Within the ambulance market, several submarkets are identifiable. These include the following:

* Geographic islands or exclusions
* Emergency (9-1-1) responses
* Interfacility responses
* Critical care transport responses
* Standby services
* Basic life support responses
* Advanced life support responses

In the United States, since no state is currently served by a single provider of ambulance services, each geographically established EMS system represents one level of submarket.

Within each EMS system, a single provider, a network of providers, or multiple specialized and/or competing providers may serve the various submarkets.

In many parts of the country, advanced life support and basic life support or emergency (9-1-1) responses and interfacility responses are thought of as separate markets or businesses. This distinction is usually the result of regulatory limitations, local practice, provider preferences, or tradition.

These submarkets, sometimes referred to as market components, generally require the same types of resources (such as ambulances), require personnel from a similar labor pool, function under similar regulations, are paid for by the same sources of revenue, and share other economic and operational similarities. In this respect, they describe submarkets or components of the total ambulance market, and thus it is difficult to draw any meaningful economic distinctions among them. Clinical distinctions are similarly difficult to make as the most critical patients may be transported between facilities, and it is nearly certain that the least clinically acute patient on any given day in most EMS systems will be encountered on an emergency (9-1-1) response.

PUBLIC UTILITY ECONOMICS IN EMS

In 1980, Jack Stout (Figure 4.2) published the first in a series of articles describing a specialized EMS system design known as a public utility model (PUM) (Stout, 1980). The PUM was developed in 1976 by a team of economists and organizational scientists at the University of Oklahoma's Center for Economic Management and Research, funded by the Kerr Foundation. The term *public utility model* was chosen because EMS is an essential public service that shares many economic

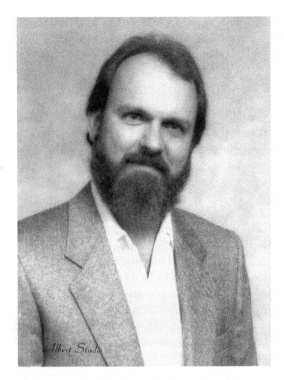

FIGURE 4.2 ■ Jack Stout, Ph.D., an economist, made great contributions to the understanding of the economics of ambulance service operation, and was one of the cornerstones of the development of the public utility model approach to ambulance service delivery. *Source: Photo provided courtesy of Jack Stout, Ph.D.*

properties of other utilities, such as water systems and electrical power distribution.

In public utilities, the majority of the cost of producing the product or service is incurred in the development of the distribution system required to deliver it to the consumer. In the case of power utilities, for example, the largest portion of the cost of the service covers the construction of power generation plants, the building and maintenance of the distribution grid, and meeting regulatory requirements. In the ambulance market, generally more than half of the cost of providing ambulance service is generated by developing the network of staffed ambulances required to cover the service area as well as essential support functions including dispatch, billing, and management.

Once the network is established, the incremental cost of handling each call is relatively small. Increases in fixed costs grow more slowly than overall growth in call volume. This results in a marginal cost for incremental business that is less than the **average cost per call**. Unless sufficient volume is added to require substantial capital investment and other fixed costs, each marginal increase in call volume decreases the overall average cost per call.

THE AVERAGE COST CURVE

As call volume increases, the **marginal cost per call** initially decreases due to the more efficient use of the network and increased productivity. If call volume growth requires the addition of ambulance unit hours and other resources, the marginal cost will increase. As long as the marginal cost per call is less than the average cost per call, additional volume will lower the overall average cost per call.

Economists refer to this as the **average cost curve** (Figure 4.3). It describes economies of scale as increasing call volume lowers the average cost per call. If the average cost per call is reduced to the point that it is equal to the marginal cost per call, economies of scale can no longer be obtained through call volume growth. If the marginal cost per call exceeds the average cost per call, increased volume causes diseconomies of scale and causes a rising average cost per call.

NETWORK DUPLICATION VERSUS EXCLUSIVITY

The infrastructure costs of public utilities, including ambulance services, make duplication of networks in the same geographic area very expensive. It is generally less expensive to serve the demand for service at marginal

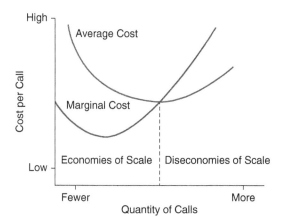

FIGURE 4.3 ■ The average cost curve.

costs of a single provider than to establish multiple providers delivering the same level of service while serving the same geographic submarket. Duplication of fixed expenses, overlapping deployment plans, inefficiencies in selecting the closest appropriate ambulance, and loss of economies of scale force the average cost per call upward.

The establishment of exclusive operating areas in which a single ambulance provider provides ambulance service is a common method of capturing the economies of scale that reduce the average cost per call. Often, political bodies and the public voice concerns that a loss of competition will lead to higher costs. These concerns are based on the economic principle that competition leads to competitive pricing as consumers choose the best deal when purchasing goods or services. Economists refer to this self-regulation of the market as "the invisible hand."

Stout explained it well when he wrote, "For the 'invisible hand' of micro-economics to work effectively, the 'consumer' must have motive opportunity and the ability to quality/ price shop for goods and services. For obvious reasons, the emergency victim makes a poor shopper, and with the advent of 9-1-1 systems, the vendor selection process is largely in the hands of local government" (Stout, JEMS, February 1985, p. 56).

HORIZONTAL AND VERTICAL MARKET CONSOLIDATION

The geographic consolidation of ambulance services is sometimes described as **horizontal consolidation**. This refers to serving a larger submarket, usually through the inclusion of contiguous geographic areas. Examples include countywide EMS systems, multijurisdictional joint powers authorities, and city services that expand outside of city limits. Horizontal market consolidation is a very common tool used to achieve increased call volume and the resulting economies of scale.

Horizontal consolidation is such a powerful tool that even large cities can achieve significant economies by combining EMS services with small neighboring communities, provided that the marginal cost of serving the new areas remains less than the overall average cost per call for the base system. Limitations in implementing horizontal consolidation include physical or transportation barriers to efficient travel, population density of contiguous areas, and political considerations.

Vertical consolidation is the combination of types or levels of service to achieve increased efficiency. The combination of emergency (9-1-1) ambulance services and interfacility transports is a common vertical consolidation strategy. By using the same vehicles and infrastructure to handle more call volume at marginal cost, the provider can lower the overall average cost per call.

In some cases, vertical consolidation can reduce costs or make resources available at a lower cost by combining ambulance resources and staff with nonambulance activities. This effectively shares the costs with the other activity, thereby reducing marginal costs to both groups.

Side Bar

Financially Viable

A study of thirteen EMS systems was designed to measure the economic viability of tiered (ALS/ BLS) versus single-tier (ALS only) ambulance deployment strategies. The study, which was presented to the National Association of EMS Physicians in 2000, involved a combination of tiered and single-tier high-performance providers. Each engaged in deployment and budgeting exercises for both strategies based on known EMS emergency and nonemergency demand. Every system reported that the single-tier strategy was more cost effective, with savings ranging from 4.9 percent to 19.82 percent with a median of 12.9 percent. Every system that participated in the study subsequently changed to a single-tier, all-ALS deployment strategy (Overton, 2000).

Other examples of vertical consolidation include providing critical care transports, paramedics working in rural emergency departments when not on calls, using existing firefighters to staff ambulances, sharing crews with an air ambulance program, and assigning EMS crews to community health programs and patient house calls. Each is a strategy to use the marginal capacity of the existing resources to capture more business, providing more service at a lower price.

■ SYSTEM OVERSIGHT AND REGULATION————————

Throughout most of the United States, state and local government share the responsibility for oversight and regulation of ambulance services. Generally, the state handles issues of service licensure and personnel certification or licensure, and sets minimum requirements for various components of EMS systems. In most states, the responsibility for the design and implementation of the local EMS system is delegated to a unit of local government. Meaningful oversight of EMS and ambulance services by a unit of local government is designed to make the level and price of service accountable to the public.

The establishment of 9-1-1 centers has positioned local government to select the ambulance service on behalf of the patient. In submarkets that employ both horizontal and vertical consolidation to achieve better service at a lower cost, local government often chooses to have a single exclusive provider of either emergency (9-1-1) or all ambulance services. The exclusive provider may be any sort of organization that provides ambulance services. Examples include public third service, private, fire department, hospital-based, law enforcement, volunteer, and joint powers authorities.

ANTITRUST

Antitrust laws were established to prevent organizations from conspiring to establish monopolies. Presumably, once all competition has been eliminated, the monopoly is expected to drastically raise prices to the detriment of the public interest. Thus, when establishing exclusivity in a submarket, care must be taken to avoid anticompetitive activities that violate state and federal antitrust laws.

EMS submarkets, due to the economic advantages of market consolidation, actually reduce costs to the public when exclusivity is achieved. When most people think of market competition, they think of retail competition in which multiple vendors openly compete for each sale. Multiple ambulance providers engaged in retail competition within the same geographic submarket usually produce lower quality and/or higher prices.

Wholesale competition is a viable alternative to retail competition in which periodic competition *for* the market is substituted for retail competition *within* the market. A local government may decide to conduct a competitive process to choose an exclusive ambulance provider for a specific period of time. Because it offers the maximum tax benefit in the depreciation of capital costs, the most common initial contract term is 5 years.

A community may therefore select an exclusive ambulance provider without displacing competition. Using a wholesale procurement process simply changes the form of the competition while gaining the economies of scale that result from exclusivity.

State laws are particularly important when establishing exclusivity in ambulance submarkets. Because they are sovereign, states cannot commit antitrust violations. By extension, any anticompetitive practice that can be shown to be a reasonably foreseeable consequence of the action of the state legislature can be defended from antitrust charges under the legal doctrine of sovereign immunity.

Laws vary greatly from state to state. For instance, in California the state provides detailed requirements for competitive processes used to establish exclusivity, whereas Oregon authorizes counties to use any method they choose with or without competition. Some states, such as Arizona, limit the pool of potential providers that local governments may consider through certificate of need (CON) requirements.

GOVERNMENT PROVIDERS

Much of the United States is served by government agencies that provide ambulance services. The most common configuration is a fire-department-based ambulance service (42 percent–46 percent). Public third services are the next most common (8 percent–12 percent). Communities decide to directly provide ambulance services through government agencies for a variety reasons.

The history of EMS systems development significantly influenced the types of providers that prevail in different parts of the United States. In some cases, federal demonstration projects, grants, the success of fire prevention, media portrayal of providers, and charismatic individuals have led to regional trends in the types of ambulance providers that serve various communities.

In 1973, Congress passed the EMS Systems Act (Public Law 93-154), which provided funding for the development of regional EMS demonstration projects. A number of the regional EMS projects were located in the mid-Atlantic and Southeast areas. In many cases, the regional EMS councils served as conduits for federal grants funding to establish county third-service EMS systems. As a result, third-service EMS systems became the prevailing model in several states.

A federal demonstration project in Jacksonville, Florida, funded a fire-based EMS model. The engaging efforts of then Captain John Waters in describing the successes of the project encouraged the development of many fire-based EMS systems in Florida. The television portrayal of fire-based EMS in the television show *Emergency!* influenced people throughout the United States to expect EMS services from fire departments.

Public-hospital- and health-department-based services were once common in large cities. New York City, San Francisco, Atlanta, and Denver were once all served by such systems. Grady EMS in Atlanta and the Denver Health Paramedic Division survive, while San Francisco has transitioned to a fire-based system for emergency (9-1-1) responses and New York employs a combination of fire department and private hospital ambulances.

VOLUNTEERS

Volunteers represent a form of subsidy to an EMS system. Since labor accounts for 70 percent to 80 percent of the cost of providing ambulance services, free or nearly free labor substantially reduces the cost of providing service to the community. Volunteer ambulance services are generally associated with rural communities and often are the only affordable method of providing ambulance services in areas with low population density.

The City of Virginia Beach, Virginia, is unusual in that it employs a network of volunteer rescue squads to serve a community of 440,000 residents. The 900 volunteers respond to over 39,000 ambulance calls each year. The Virginia Beach Rescue Squad Foundation claims that the use of volunteers saves the City over $22 million each year (Virginia Beach Rescue Squad Foundation, 2010).

PRIVATE PROVIDERS

Throughout much of the history of EMS, private providers were usually local companies established by local entrepreneurs. Beginning in 1976, Medevac, a California company, began expanding with multiple operations in several communities. As larger and more sophisticated contracting opportunities were developed in communities across the United States, new competitors—including Hartson/MedTrans and the HCA Medical Transportation Company—quickly developed to meet the need for larger, better-funded, and more sophisticated ambulance companies.

A first wave of industry consolidation began in 1988 when Secom Company Ltd. of Tokyo purchased several midsize ambulance companies. Shortly afterward, a group of investors joined with four ambulance companies to form American Medical Response (AMR) and completed an initial public offering to establish the first publicly traded ambulance company. Several other large providers, including Rural/Metro Corporation (R/MC), followed AMR into publicly traded stock markets.

To meet the financial expectations of shareholders, the publicly traded ambulance companies needed to demonstrate substantial growth. They accomplished this by acquiring many smaller companies and through aggressive pursuit of contracting opportunities. By the summer of 2011, both AMR and R/MC were no longer publicly traded, having been purchased by private equity groups.

The majority of private ambulance providers continue to be local or regional operations. They range in size from very small, deploying one or two ambulances, to large-scale regional providers with hundreds of ambulances and hundreds of millions in revenue.

HOSPITAL-BASED EMS

Hospitals and hospital networks provide various ambulance services in a number of communities. In some cases, these hospital-based ambulance services are the primary emergency (9-1-1) provider for the community. In other cases, the ambulance service provides for the transportation needs of the parent hospital organization.

The transition to the Medicare Ambulance Fee Schedule established new accounting rules that make the operation of an ambulance company less financially attractive for hospitals, spurring many hospitals to exit the ambulance market. Nevertheless, many hospitals continue to provide ambulance and medical transportation services, often due to a sense that these services are a part of the hospital's core mission.

■ ALLOCATION OF MARKET RIGHTS

Local governments often find that they must make decisions regarding how ambulance services will be provided within their jurisdictions. In some cases, state law mandates that counties or cities organize and arrange for emergency

(9-1-1) ambulance service. In many cases, the need arises as a practical matter of determining what service will be responsible for emergency (9-1-1) calls. The decision to establish an organized system of ambulance service is described as the allocation of market rights.

Market rights may be allocated in a number of ways. The local government may choose to retain some or all of the market rights for itself and establish a public EMS system through its fire department, law enforcement agency, or a third-service ambulance department. State laws may limit the ability of local governments to assume exclusive rights to ambulance services. For instance, California law requires that, with very limited exceptions, any exclusive arrangement for ambulance services must be accomplished through the use of periodic competitive processes.

LAISSEZ FAIRE

In some cases, the local government avoids making a decision regarding market rights by taking a laissez faire (deliberate abstention) approach to EMS. This is most common in communities that have been served by local ambulance providers for a long period of time. From time to time, if a local provider has been successful in an unregulated submarket, one or more new competitors may enter the market in an attempt to take business away from the successful company. As the new competitor takes away call volume that the incumbent had served at marginal cost, costs for both competitors increase. Often the result is increased cost and deterioration of performance.

Additional problems arise in unregulated markets when new providers demand access to emergency (9-1-1) calls. The common methods of distributing these calls among multiple ambulance providers are problematic.

Some communities use a system of call rotation in which each ambulance provider takes a sequential turn answering emergency calls. Rotation systems cannot ensure that the closest appropriate ambulance is sent to each call, thereby wasting resources. To avoid antitrust problems, any rotation system must be expanded to include any new competitors that choose to enter the market in the future. Each time a new competitor joins the rotation, the existing providers lose call volume and overall system costs increase.

Another common scheme for the distribution of emergency (9-1-1) calls is to divide the service area geographically. This approach is problematic for several reasons. The fair division of a service area is difficult, and each provider is at risk for being assigned a socioeconomically unattractive portion of the jurisdiction. In addition, antitrust law prohibits conspiring to divide a market.

Some communities have tried to accommodate multiple ambulance providers by assigning emergency (9-1-1) calls using a "closest unit" system. Automatic vehicle location (AVL) technology makes it possible for the 9-1-1 center to see the location and status of each ambulance in the service area and to assign calls to the closest appropriate ambulance. Unfortunately, in many instances, this approach leads to economic cherry-picking as some providers intentionally deploy their ambulances to socioeconomically attractive areas while avoiding unattractive parts of town. Often this practice leads to unequal levels of service based on socioeconomic status.

Very many communities have tried for years to cope with laissez-faire approaches to providing ambulance services. Often, when ambulance providers engage in retail competition for emergency and nonemergency calls, the cost of providing ambulance services rises and each competitor makes less money. In some cases, this eventually leads to service failures as none of the providers can maintain sufficient resources to provide reliable service. Local governments frequently respond to high-profile failures of ambulance services with increased regulation, contracting, or a public takeover of ambulance responsibilities.

FRANCHISE

One method of arranging for ambulance service is for a local government to grant a franchise to a single ambulance provider. Franchises are most commonly granted through the use of a wholesale competitive process. When designing the procurement process, the local government must make a number of decisions about the desired level of service and cost of the resulting contract. Key decisions include which services are to be included in the franchise, whether to specify a level of effort or performance standards, whether to provide tax subsidy or require that the contractor rely solely on patient revenues, and how to establish fees for service. Additional considerations include penalties for failure to perform, contract termination for breaches, and performance security.

PUBLIC UTILITY MODEL

One variation of the franchise approach to market allocation is the public utility model system design. In this model, the local government assigns the ambulance market rights to itself, a joint powers authority, or a not-for-profit organization to serve as the exclusive ambulance provider. The provider, often referred to as the "Authority," then competitively establishes an operations contract with a firm to manage the deployment of people and resources to achieve specific performance goals. The authority owns the accounts receivable and all revenue streams and pays the operations contractor based on conditions usually established through a competitive process.

USE OF COMPETITION

Communities that have established exclusive market rights for some or all ambulance services periodically consider if they should test the market by using a competitive process to determine if they are getting the best deal. Frequently, public opinion, the local media, or lobbying activity from competitive ambulance services leads the local governing body to consider a competitive process.

Well-designed competitive processes are not simple tasks. In most midsize to large EMS systems, a request for proposals (RFP) process requires 12 to 24 months to complete. Uncertainty for the incumbent contractor and the possibility of a disruptive transition of providers may affect system operational and financial performance. Local authorities must balance the risks of a competitive process against potential improvements.

In some states, the law requires periodic competition. California requires that exclusive markets undergo periodic competition. The state EMS authority interprets "periodic" as at least once every 10 years. In other states, local authorities are specifically empowered to establish exclusive market rights without the use of any competitive process at all. A legal requirement is an unavoidable reason for local authorities to resort to a competitive process.

Absent a legal requirement to conduct a competitive process, local authorities should carefully consider what they might gain by issuing an RFP or bid. If they believe that there is an opportunity to substantially improve either the quality or cost of ambulance services, then a competitive process is worth the associated risks and expense. However, if a thorough investigation of the current service indicates that it is unlikely that a procurement process will yield substantial improvements, the cost and disruption of an RFP should be avoided. Small incremental improvements can be realized more quickly and less expensively through negotiation with the incumbent contractor.

EFFECTS OF GOVERNMENT INTERVENTION

The federal government began paying for ambulance services with the establishment of Medicare and Medicaid in 1966. Growth in the number of beneficiaries for both programs has resulted in Medicare and Medicaid beneficiaries representing approximately half of ambulance patients nationwide.

Medicare payments for ambulance services nationally average approximately 6 percent to 8 percent below the cost of providing those services (U.S. Government Accountability Office, 2007; American Ambulance Association, 2006). In most states, Medicaid payments are a fraction of the Medicare fee schedule and in some states, payments have decreased in recent years.

Medicare and Medicaid payments are established by government-mandated fee schedules. Each establishes an allowable charge above which the ambulance provider must write off any additional charges as a "contractual allowance." In the case of Medicare, the provider is required to bill 20 percent of the allowable charge to the patient. Providers are prohibited from billing Medicaid patients for any portion of charges associated with ambulance transports.

ECONOMIC DISTORTION

Since approximately half of all ambulance charges are paid below cost and because increases in prices do not affect Medicare and Medicaid payments, ambulance providers must increase prices so that other payers will cover the shortfall from Medicare and Medicaid. This practice is known as **cost shifting**. Another significant contributor to cost shifting is uncompensated care provided to patients who do not have health insurance and are unable or unwilling to pay their bills.

In some markets, these "private pay" patients account for 15 percent to 20 percent of patients transported.

Another revenue-side issue is the increasing percentage of Medicare beneficiaries utilizing ambulance services. It is well documented that the Medicare-eligible population is growing, and that this demographic utilizes ambulance services with greater frequency than younger population groups (American College of Emergency Physicians, 2010).

The practical market implications of cost shifting are enormous. For example, in 2011 one large urban EMS system documented an actual, fully loaded average cost of providing ambulance services of $384 per transport. To compensate for the cost shifting caused by Medicare, Medicaid, and uncompensated care, the provider was required to charge an average patient fee of $1,505.

This economic distortion often causes confusion when ambulance providers attempt to increase fees for service to compensate for increased costs. If a provider requires an additional $10 per transport to cover increased costs, it first needs to adjust for the inability to increase Medicare and Medicaid reimbursement and then adjust for the marginal collection rate for other payers. If half of the business is Medicare and Medicaid, with a typical marginal collection rate of 20 percent, the provider must increase the average fee for service by approximately $100 in order to collect $10.

In some regards, cost shifting functions much like a hidden tax on insured patient accounts in order to pay a portion of the cost of Medicare, Medicaid, and uncompensated care.

SUBSIDIES

Some form of tax subsidy supports many ambulance services of all system designs. In some cases, due to geographic, demographic,

Best Practices

Price Subsidy Tradeoff Matrix

MedStar, a public utility model EMS system serving fifteen cities surrounding Fort Worth, Texas, publishes an annual Price Subsidy Tradeoff Matrix. This allows each member city to select any level of subsidy and its corresponding patient fees. A city may chose to fully subsidize ambulance services with patient fees set at zero, to provide no subsidy with fees set to recover full costs, or to do anything in between. When the City of Fort Worth chose to eliminate tax subsidies that it had been paying for more than 25 years, user fees were adjusted to ensure that the loss of tax money did not require reductions in the level of service provided.

Source: Area Metropolitan Ambulance Authority, Uniform EMS Ordinance and Interlocal Operating Agreement.

---

or economic conditions, some level of subsidy is required to support reliable service. In other cases, communities choose to provide subsidies to offset user fees or to compensate for lower productivity related to deliberate choices in deployment methods.

Nationally, subsidy levels range from nothing to 100 percent and are often higher in governmentally operated systems. Some system designs and contracts are designed not only to eliminate subsidies but also to recapture government costs associated with oversight and regulation.

Many urban EMS systems with a typical payer mix and better than average productivity collect all of their revenue from patient fees and operate without subsidy. A price-subsidy trade-off curve can be plotted for any EMS system that demonstrates what prices are required to fund the operation at different levels of subsidy.

Because of cost shifting, every dollar of subsidy may offset as much as $10 in patient fees. As a result, when comparing rates for ambulance services, it is necessary to adjust for the impact of subsidies before making a comparison. In the previous example, the provider with a cost of $384 per transport would be fully funded at a subsidy of $384 per transport and could provide ambulance services at no charge.

However, with charges averaging $1,505 per transport, no subsidy would be required.

Communities make decisions about ambulance subsidies for a variety of reasons. When subsidies are used to enhance service, increase the availability of ambulances, or overcome market and reimbursement inefficiencies, they may contribute to the reliability and performance of the EMS system. When unnecessary subsidies simply offset user fees, they essentially subsidize insurance companies that have already been paid to provide a benefit to the patients.

■ COST INCREASES ───────────

A number of factors combine to increase the cost of providing ambulance services throughout the market. In addition to the obvious issues such as increased fuel costs, some less obvious factors continue to push the cost and therefore the charges for service higher, year after year.

Federal regulations contribute significantly to increased costs as billing and confidentiality (HIPAA) compliance become more complicated. Ambulance providers must hire people, develop systems, and educate their employees in order to avoid civil and criminal liability. Environmental and transportation regulations have increased the cost of ambulances and affect their reliability and maintenance costs.

Technology has the potential to greatly improve productivity and accuracy in deployment and billing. However, many of the new technologies require significant up-front investments long before any economic advantages are realized. Often, the adoption of new technology is done to provide a competitive advantage in the acquisition or protection of market rights. In some cases, new technology adds more cost than it offsets.

Clinical advances continuously change the scope of practice and types of equipment required. New standards for the treatment of S-T elevation myocardial infarctions (STEMI), for instance, have required EMS systems to adopt new equipment, provide additional training, and change transport protocols, in some cases including longer transports and increased ambulance task times. Many systems are still in the planning or implementation phase of these changes and can look forward to new expenses and decreased productivity as the process is completed. Similar advances in the treatment of strokes and post-resuscitation cases will require new equipment and protocols, pushing the cost per transport higher.

In some communities, lack of emergency department capacity and increased utilization of emergency departments for primary care have resulted in situations where the transfer of the patient from the ambulance crew to the hospital ED crew is delayed. This delay results in a loss of productive time for that ambulance crew, making it unavailable for a subsequent call. Cumulatively, these delays result in increased costs to the ambulance service. Similarly, diversion of an ambulance to a more distant hospital increases the time for the total ambulance transport, again cumulatively resulting in increased costs.

Inflation, including energy costs and food, will have two effects on ambulance costs. First, when fuel and other items normally omitted from federal calculations of inflation are considered, ambulance providers are experiencing higher prices for many of their day-to-day expenses. Second, as employees are affected by increasing costs, increased pressure for higher wages is likely.

As the cost of providing ambulance services increases, ambulance providers may respond in several ways. Ambulance providers in densely populated areas may be able to compensate in whole or in part by improving the productivity of their operations, thereby reducing the marginal cost per transport. It seems likely that the majority of ambulance providers will pass along the increased costs through rate increases. Some of the more advanced and creative ambulance providers may seek new sources of revenue through the development of new lines of business, such as call-center operations, house-call services, post-discharge wellness visits, or similar ventures that can utilize some of the infrastructure that has been developed to support the ambulance service.

As costs increase, ambulance providers that cannot for some reason pursue marginal cost reduction, price increases, and/or new revenue sources are likely to require increased local tax subsidy. In 2011, economic conditions in most parts of the United States are such that additional subsidies may be difficult to obtain. As a result, competitive pressure may increase within the market and new opportunities may arise.

The exact form of competition will be dependent on the conditions in each submarket. In some cases, competition will come from fire departments seeking incremental revenue to help support their existing workforce. Alternatively, private contractors and regional EMS systems may offer to replace highly subsidized government-operated

5

ambulance operations at lower levels of subsidy. In other cases, more efficient providers will replace existing contractors through competitive processes. Some providers may not be able to adjust adequately and may simply go out of business.

It is impossible to precisely predict how the ambulance market will respond to increasing costs except to say that changes in the way the market is served are very likely.

■ PROSPECTS FOR MARKET
   GROWTH

The ambulance market is poised for substantial growth due to an aging population and health care reform. Currently, 40 million people over the age of 65 reside in the United States. That population is expected to nearly double during the next 20 years. In 2006, the Centers for Disease Control reported that patients age 65 and older arrived at hospital emergency departments at the rate of 17.5 per 100 people. That is approximately three times the rate for people under 65 and could result in an additional 7 million emergency (9-1-1) transports per year in 2030. Those over age 65 also account for an estimated two-thirds of nonemergency ambulance transports. As the population ages, call volume is expected to increase substantially (Burt and McCaig, 2006).

The Congressional Budget Office projects that health care reform through the Affordable Care Act will increase the percentage of the nonelderly population with insurance from 83 percent in 2010 to 95 percent by 2016. Whether or not the current health care reform bill is modified, it is likely that some degree of increased coverage will survive to the benefit of all health care providers.

The Medicare Ambulance Access Preservation Act of 2011 has been introduced in both houses of the U.S. Congress. Although it is impossible to know if the bill will pass and eventually be signed into law, it would provide a 6 percent increase in the ambulance fees schedule to correct the under-reimbursement of ambulance services by Medicare as determined by the Congressional Budget Office. Every dollar of increased Medicare payment has the potential to offset approximately $10 in patient fees, as a result of cost shifting.

■ EXPANSION OF THE MARKET

In addition to organic growth in call volume of the existing ambulance market, some progressive providers are exploring expansion into related and overlapping markets. Advanced practice paramedics and community health paramedics have the potential to bring new revenue into the ambulance market through the addition of new services. Managed care organizations and hospitals have powerful financial incentives to try new methods of preventing readmission of patients following discharge under various Medicare and managed care payment arrangements.

House calls made by paramedics have the potential to generate significant savings worth many multiples of the cost of providing the service. Pilot projects in several communities are meeting with success and are completely paid for by the savings they generate.

Some ambulance providers have expanded into other related markets including, among others, nonambulance medical transportation, Medicaid brokerage services, call-center operations, air medical transportation, travel assistance, and repatriation and contract dispatch and billing services for other providers. Each new source of revenue that can be accessed utilizing some of the resources required to serve the ambulance market can marginally reduce the cost of providing ambulance services by sharing the cost of common infrastructure.

CHAPTER REVIEW

Summary

The ambulance service market currently generates approximately $14 billion in net fees for service. Over 15,000 ambulance services and 25,000 fire departments—as well as third services, hospitals, and many other types of providers—compete for portions of the market.

The economic features of the industry have similarities to those of public utilities. The marginal cost of completing each additional ambulance call is usually significantly lower than the overall average cost per call. As a result, as more calls are run at marginal cost, the average cost per call is reduced. These economies of scale make the horizontal and vertical consolidation of submarkets financially very attractive.

Local governments often assign market rights using a variety of methods, including simple assignment to a government department and the use of competitive processes. Antitrust considerations are crucial when establishing exclusive market rights, and state laws often provide direction and authority for appropriate action.

Unregulated submarkets often disintegrate due to diseconomies of scale as competitors enter the market, forcing local government to act to establish reliable service. Franchises are one common strategy for the award of market rights. Competitive processes have advantages and disadvantages and should only be employed if there is a legal requirement to use them or the local governing body has reason to believe that sufficient improvements can be secured in either quality or cost to warrant their use.

Federal intervention in the market produces economic distortions because Medicare and Medicaid, on a national average, pay less than the cost of delivering ambulance services. This causes cost shifting that relies on a minority of insured patients to pay for the underfunded and uncompensated patients served by the ambulance provider. Cost shifting grossly distorts the fees charged for ambulance services.

Tax subsidies of ambulance services are frequently used for a variety of reasonable purposes. When they simply offset the fees charged for service, they in effect use local tax money to subsidize insurance companies that have already been paid to cover the service.

A variety of factors are likely to increase costs for all providers serving the ambulance market. Providers will use various strategies to respond to increasing costs, and new opportunities for providers to grow will likely arise as some providers achieve better results than others in adjusting to new costs.

The aging of the population will significantly drive growth in the number of ambulance transports, at least through 2030. Legislated relief from Medicare underpayments is a possibility, and health care reform may increase the number of insured patients, improving the financial outlook for providers.

Expansion of the ambulance market to serve related and overlapping markets holds promise for attracting new streams of revenue. In addition, by sharing key infrastructure, new markets and products may help lower the marginal cost of ambulance services, which in turn will lower the average cost of each transport.

WHAT WOULD YOU DO? Reflection

Depending on the particular circumstances of your EMS system, a number of options may be available to you. During the brainstorming session, you may suggest an increase in patient fees to offset the increase in costs. Other strategies may include improvements in productivity through vertical consolidation of tiered services or horizontal consolidation by taking over neighboring geographic submarkets, using marginal unit hour capacity. Additional possibilities, such as contracting with local hospitals or the health department for out-of-hospital wellness checks or contracting to use your EMS infrastructure to support other services such as dispatching for neighboring fire departments, may provide diversified revenue streams to offset the projected loss.

Review Questions

1. Define the ambulance market and identify related or overlapping submarkets.
2. Describe the relationship between the average cost per call and the marginal cost per call and how this relationship produces economies of scale.
3. Discuss horizontal and vertical market consolidation and the potential opportunities this may provide for your EMS organization.
4. Discuss the use of competition in assigning market rights for EMS, including the antitrust implications and the use of competitive processes.
5. Define cost shifting, and describe its effect on user fees.
6. Discuss the probable future of the ambulance market and EMS industry, including prospects for growth and potential strategies that providers may use to respond to changes within the market.

References

American Ambulance Association. (2007, May). "2006 Ambulance Cost Study." McLean, VA: American Ambulance Association.

American College of Emergency Physicians. (2010, June 14). "Elderly Patients Most Likely to Use Ambulances for Transport to ERs, Critically Ill Latinos Least Likely to Arrive by Ambulance." See the organization website.

Bain & Company. (2011, January). "Rural/Metro Corporation Investor Presentation," p. 7.

Ballvé, F. (1963). *Essentials of Economics.* New York: Van Nostrand.

Burt, C.W., and L. F. McCaig. (2006). "Staffing, Capacity, and Ambulance Diversion in Emergency Departments: United States,

2003–04." *Advance Data (376)*, 1–23. See the National Center for Biotechnology Information website.

Overton, J. (2000, January). "ALS and BLS: A Cost Effectiveness Study." Presentation to National Association of EMS Physicians, Fort Meyers, FL.

R/MC (Rural/Metro Corporation. (2011). Investor Presentation, Second Quarter 2011.

Stout, J. (1980, May). "The Public Utility Model, Part I: Measuring Your System. *Journal of Emergency Medical Services 5(3)*, 22–25.

Stout, J. (1985, February). *Journal of Emergency Medical Services,* The Public Utility Model Revisited, Part 1, Page 56.

U.S. Fire Administration. (2013). "National Fire Department Census Quick Facts." See the organization website.

U.S. Government Accountability Office. (2007, May). Report to Congressional Committees, Ambulance Providers, Costs and Expected Medicare Margins Vary Greatly, GAO-07-383

Virginia Beach Rescue Squad Foundation. (2010). "About Us." See the organization website.

Key Terms

average cost curve A graph of the average cost per call as volume increases. This accounts for the effect of variable or marginal costs decreasing the average cost per call as volume increases up to a limit.

average cost per call The total fully loaded expense for the service for a period of time divided by the number of calls run during the same time period. This accounts for both fixed and variable costs per unit of service.

cost shifting The practice of raising prices in reaction to underpayment of fees charged to government payers and bad debts from patients without insurance or the means to pay their bills.

economic market Describes any one of a variety of systems, institutions, procedures, social relationships, or infrastructures that describe or facilitate parties in commerce.

horizontal consolidation The expansion of service geographically under a single provider or network.

marginal cost per call Represents the direct additional average cost per call of running additional volume. This represents variable costs, but does not include fixed costs.

public utility economics Describes the interaction of market forces in a public service in which the majority of the cost of producing the product or service is incurred in the development of the distribution system required to deliver it to the consumer and the marginal cost of delivering each individual product or service is relatively low.

submarket A geographic, economic, or specialized subdivision of a market.

vertical consolidation The consolidation of services under a single production strategy. For example, the same ALS ambulances respond to all ALS and BLS emergency and nonemergency calls.

wholesale competition Periodic competition *for* the market rather than constant retail competition *within* the market.

CHAPTER 5

Medical Transportation– Scheduled

MATT ZAVADSKY, MS-HSA, EMT

Objectives

After reading this chapter, the student should be able to:

5.1 Explain the difference between medical and nonmedical transportation.

5.2 Explain the difference between scheduled and unscheduled services.

5.3 Identify the role each of the different service levels plays in an ambulance service.

5.4 List the three main decision points used by facilities in choosing an ambulance provider.

5.5 Identify the billing implications for interfacility and intrafacility ambulance services.

Overview

Ambulance services in the United States range in size from one ambulance operated by volunteers and managed by a community board of directors to large governmental agencies and even larger, private, for-profit corporations. This text presents information that the manager of an ambulance service, large or small, needs in order to keep the business solvent and provide clinically excellent service to the community.

Key Terms

interfacility	medical necessity	nonmedical	Physician
intrafacility	medical	transportation	Certification
kickback	transportation	patient	Statement (PCS)

WHAT WOULD YOU DO?

You are the marketing manager for a family-owned ambulance service that primarily offers nonemergency, interfacility ambulance service in a metropolitan area. The owner explains that the service needs to gain call volume in order to remain profitable and asks you to pursue an aggressive marketing campaign for additional interfacility work. A large hospital system in your service area has a stand-alone emergency department in a suburban area that is licensed under the same license as the main campus. The hospital system is looking for a good deal for ambulance transportation between the stand-alone emergency department and the main campus. It would prefer that you bill third-party insurance for all transports.

1. Based on current Centers for Medicare & Medicaid Services (CMS) regulations, who is responsible for the cost of ambulance service between the stand-alone facility and the hospital's main campus?
2. What are the implications if you bill third-party payers for this type of intrafacility transport?
3. What are your considerations when pricing transports under this arrangement?
4. If you agree to bill less than your cost of providing this service, what are the potential risks?
5. If you agree to bill less than the Medicare allowable rates for providing this service, what are the potential risks?

▪ INTRODUCTION

The provision of nonemergency, interfacility **patient** transport service is extremely complex, depending on the types of service offered and the manner of service delivery. Typically, ambulance services offer basic life support, advanced life support, or critical care transport services. Some ambulance services also offer wheelchair and/or stretcher van services. Wheelchair and stretcher van services can also be provided by nonambulance, patient transport services such as taxi companies or other private providers. Before delving into the intricacies of this service provision, let's define some of the key terms necessary to understand how these services can be provided.

▪ TYPES OF SCHEDULED MEDICAL TRANSPORTATION

Service provision can be categorized in terms of transport: interfacility, intrafacility, or transport to or from home.

INTERFACILITY TRANSPORTS

Interfacility transport implies taking a patient from one health care facility to another. For example, a patient may be transported from a long-term acute care (LTAC) facility to a hospital, from one hospital to another hospital, or from a skilled nursing facility (SNF) to a dialysis center, doctor's office, or community clinic. The key to determining whether a transport is interfacility is the recognition that both facilities are licensed health care facilities under separate state operating licenses. Interfacility transfers fall under specific guidelines for reimbursement by CMS and most third-party payers.

INTRAFACILITY TRANSPORTS

Occasionally, a licensed health care facility may have a main campus with buildings spread over a large area, or might have remote locations elsewhere in the community (Figure 5.1), which would require **intrafacility** transport. Such transports are typically not eligible for reimbursement by third-party payers but, rather, must be paid for by the facility. CMS and most third-party payers consider the transfer of patients within the same licensed facility the same as moving a patient from the emergency department to another floor of the hospital for admission. The transportation cost for the employees moving the patient in this scenario is not a separately reimbursable cost under CMS rules as it is considered part of the bundled payment for the patient's overall hospital stay under Medicare Part A coverage. Intrafacility transportation must be paid by the facility arranging for the transport. The introduction of a separate freestanding emergency department (ED) that is licensed as part of a hospital in the community has heightened this distinction: Transportation of the patient from the freestanding ED to the main campus is considered an intrafacility transport and the hospital is responsible for that cost.

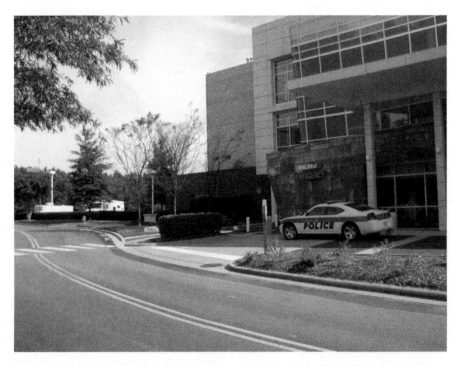

FIGURE 5.1 ■ Transportation from a freestanding emergency department to the parent hospital is considered an inpatient transfer and is the responsibility of the parent hospital. Here, a WakeMed Mobile ambulance stands by to transport a patient from the North Healthplex freestanding ED to the main campus for further treatment. *Source: Official Wake County EMS Photo. Used by permission.*

TRANSPORTS TO OR FROM HOME

Patients may also require transportation home from the hospital or from home to a medical facility. In these cases, the issue of **medical necessity** and covered locations become very important to the agency's ability to seek third-party reimbursement for the transport.

Transports from Home

In most cases, coverage is provided for medically necessary transports from a patient's home to a covered medical facility. Examples of this type of service could include trips for dialysis for bed-bound patients and outpatient treatments at hospitals or surgery centers. Sometimes patients require **medical transportation** from home to a physician's office for procedures or follow-up that may not require a hospital setting. It is rare that a third-party payer will cover ambulance transport to a physician's office, and it is specifically not included as a covered destination by Medicare. If the patient needs to be transported to locations such as a physician's office or other noncovered destination, it may still be permissible to provide the service; however, the patient must be informed that the services will not be covered by insurance and the patient may become responsible for the full cost of the transport. The mechanism for this "advanced beneficiary notice" is specified by Medicare, and is discussed by a leading EMS and medical transportation law firm on its website (Page, Wolfberg, & Wirth, 2013).

Transports to Home

Should the patient meet the medical necessity test for ambulance transportation, most trips from a hospital to the patient's home on discharge from the hospital constitute a covered service by most insurers, including Medicare. The key to determining medical necessity is evidenced by the documentation provided by the crew on the patient care record (PCR) as well as other supporting documentation such as a **physician certification statement (PCS)** of medical necessity. For many years, CMS has instructed ambulance providers and suppliers that they are not allowed to rely on the PCS for determination of medical necessity for the ambulance transport. The ambulance chart was required to independently document the medical necessity for the transport, and, if the documentation was lacking, the claim would not be paid (see Carrido, 2011). Recently, a decision of a federal court in the Middle District of Tennessee has held to the contrary, so the certainty of earlier CMS declarations remains in doubt (Justia.com, 2012).

■ DEFINING *PATIENT*

In order to be eligible for *medical* transportation, the person being transported must meet the definition of *patient*. Generally speaking, a person who is in need of medical care or medical monitoring during transport can be considered a patient. Some local or state laws specifically define *patient* in order to differentiate ambulance service from other forms of **nonmedical transportation**. For example, the Uniform EMS Ordinance that governs the MedStar EMS system in Fort Worth, Texas, defines patient as "an individual who is ill, sick, injured, wounded, or otherwise incapacitated and is in need of or is at risk of needing medical care during transport to or from a health care facility" (American Legal Publishing Company, 1998).

Understanding that a patient is someone in need of medical care or medical monitoring is important because many companies and agencies provide interfacility transport for nonpatients (people who *do not* require medical treatment or medical monitoring). Patients must be transported by medical transportation—that is, by ambulance.

MEDICAL NECESSITY

The term *medical necessity* is used by CMS and other third-party payers to ensure that a patient can only be safely transported using medical transportation (ambulance). The CMS guidelines for determining medical necessity are very specific and contained in the *Medicare Benefit Policy Manual*, Chapter 10: Ambulance Services:

> Medical necessity is established when the patient's condition is such that use of any other method of transportation is contraindicated. In any case in which some means of transportation other than an ambulance could be used without endangering the individual's health, whether or not such other transportation is actually available, no payment may be made for ambulance services. In all cases, the appropriate documentation must be kept on file and, upon request, presented to the carrier/intermediary. It is important to note that the presence (or absence) of a physician's order for a transport by ambulance does not necessarily prove (or disprove) whether the transport was medically necessary. The ambulance service must meet all program coverage criteria in order for payment to be made.
>
> In addition, the reason for the ambulance transport must be medically necessary. That is, the transport must be to obtain a Medicare covered service, or to return from such a service.
>
> As stated above, medical necessity is established when the patient's condition is such that the use of any other method of transportation is contraindicated. Contractors may presume this requirement is met under certain circumstances, including when the beneficiary was bed-confined before and after the ambulance trip (see §20 for the complete list of circumstances).
>
> A beneficiary is bed-confined if he/she is unable to get up from bed without assistance; unable to ambulate; and unable to sit in a chair or wheelchair.
>
> The term "bed confined" is not synonymous with "bed rest" or "non-ambulatory." Bed-confinement, by itself, is neither sufficient nor is it necessary to determine the coverage for Medicare ambulance benefits. It is simply one element of the beneficiary's condition that may be taken into account in the intermediary's/carrier's determination of whether means

> of transport other than an ambulance were contraindicated. (Centers for Medicare & Medicaid Services, 2010)

The specific determination of medical necessity for a medical claim in most cases will be made by a review of the statements made in the patient care record completed by the ambulance crew at the time of transport. The field providers need to provide detailed and extemporaneous explanations in their PCR supporting the medical necessity of ambulance transport as opposed to nonmedical transport. Ambulance service managers should invest a great deal of time working with their staff to ensure adequate documentation to verify medical necessity at the time of service. This is often a delicate balance for field providers as they may have difficulty understanding the significant impact their documentation plays in the agency's ability to recover fees for the service provided. Departmental rotations through the billing office for employees new to an agency, but also as a refresher for existing employees, is invaluable education and will help field providers understand the impact good documentation has on the agency's revenue stream.

PHYSICIAN CERTIFICATION STATEMENT

The PCS is required documentation for CMS for most nonemergency ambulance transportation. The PCS will assist the ambulance service with seeking reimbursement for the service, but it does not guarantee reimbursement.

NONMEDICAL TRANSPORTATION

Nonmedical transportation for people for whom medical necessity for medical transportation cannot be established are generally not considered patients (Figure 5.2). Transportation for nonpatients can be provided by public transit, wheelchair van services, and even stretcher van services. Even though the nonpatient may

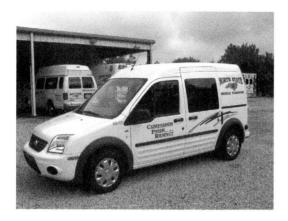

FIGURE 5.2 A nonmedical transport unit.
Source: Official Wake County EMS photo by Mike Legeros. Used by permission.

not meet the strict determinant of medical necessity for medical transportation and is therefore eligible for alternative modes, some health care facilities may desire to have the person transported by ambulance. In such situations, the facility arranging for ambulance transport for a potential nonmedical necessity case should be advised that the cost of the transport may not be eligible for insurance payment and, as such, the patient or the facility may be required to pay for the transport.

NONEMERGENCY AMBULANCE TRANSPORTATION

Nonemergency ambulance transportation can be either scheduled or unscheduled.

SCHEDULED NONEMERGENCY AMBULANCE TRANSPORTATION

In a nonemergency setting, ambulance service can be scheduled to take the patient from one location to another. Most ambulance providers consider a scheduled transportation request one that is made at least 24 hours in advance. The most common example of this type of service is repetitive dialysis patients. People undergoing dialysis generally require transport to the dialysis center three or more times per week, and transportation can be scheduled for a month or more at a time.

When a sending facility, or the patient, makes the effort to schedule ambulance transportation for a specific time, it is incumbent on the ambulance provider to arrive at the time requested for the transport. It is also important to note that the determination of on time means *at the patient's side*. In most cases, to arrive at the patient' side on time, the ambulance should arrive at a facility 10 to 15 minutes before the scheduled pickup time. This allows the ambulance crew to retrieve the required equipment (such as stretcher, oxygen, monitor, etc.), travel through the facility, and arrive at the patient's side at the requested pick-up time.

UNSCHEDULED NONEMERGENCY AMBULANCE TRANSPORTATION

When the patient requires nonemergency ambulance transportation that has not been scheduled at least 24 hours in advance, it is considered "unscheduled." Most ambulance services should be able to arrive at the patient within 1 to 2 hours for unscheduled, nonemergency service. The requestor may have some flexibility with the scheduled time and be willing to wait longer for the unscheduled service if necessary.

COST AND PRICING CONSIDERATIONS

Providing nonemergency ambulance service is typically less costly than providing emergency ambulance service. The primary reason for this difference is the cost of readiness. Most emergency ambulance service requires adherence to a response time standard, such as arriving at the scene of the emergency within 9 minutes, 90 percent of the time. Depending on the coverage area and call volume, this requires ambulances to be positioned throughout a service area "in the ready" to respond to these emergency requests. The time invested in having ambulances on standby awaiting a call adds to the cost. Conversely, calls that are scheduled do not typically require this cost of readiness, and paramedics can even be scheduled to work to coincide with the scheduled call.

As a result, most third-party payers, including CMS, allow for a higher reimbursement rate for emergency service compared to nonemergency (scheduled) service. Current CMS guidelines allow for a relative value unit (RVU) factor. RVUs set a numeric value for ambulance services relative to the value of a base-level ambulance service. Since there are marked differences in resources necessary to furnish the various levels of ground ambulance services, different levels of payment are appropriate for the various levels of service. The different payment amounts are based on level of service. An RVU expresses the constant multiplier for a particular type of service (including, where appropriate, an emergency response). An RVU of 1.00 is assigned to the basic life support (BLS) level of ground service (i.e., BLS has an RVU of 1). Higher RVU values are assigned to the other types of ground ambulance services, which require a higher level of service than BLS (Centers for Medicare & Medicaid Services, n.d.). The RVUs for various levels of ground ambulance services are listed in Figure 5.3.

As you can see, the RVU enhancement for BLS emergency service is 1.60, meaning that CMS considers it 60 percent more expensive to provide emergency service than nonemergency service. For this reason, most ambulance providers will charge less for nonemergency, scheduled service than they do for emergency service.

It is common for facilities and ambulance services to enter into a contractual relationship

Service Level	RVU
BLS	1.00
BLS - Emergency	1.60
ALS1	1.20
ALS1 - Emergency	1.90
ALS2	2.75
SCT	3.25
Paramedic Intercept	1.75

FIGURE 5.3 ■ RVUs for Various Levels of Ground Ambulance Services

for nonemergency service. Most contracts will have a provision for on-time arrival and for price. In some cases, ambulance providers will offer a discount for prompt payment of ambulance bills for which the facility is responsible for payment. Typically a 10 percent to 25 percent discount for payment within 30 days is offered. Use caution when entering into these agreements to prevent underpricing that could lead to a kickback or discounting violation through CMS.

■ CUSTOMER SERVICE AND MARKETING

In most markets, nonemergency ambulance service can be provided by any willing provider authorized by local government. This means that, unlike emergency services, the customer has a choice of providers for this type of service. In making the determination of which provider to select for their service, facilities will consider three main service delivery issues: on-time performance, price, and overall customer service.

ON-TIME PERFORMANCE

It is very frustrating for both sending and receiving facilities for ambulances to arrive late for nonemergency service. Late arrivals may not only be inconvenient for the facility and the patient but also may result in a missed appointment for a procedure leading to the potential detriment of the patient, wasted capacity for diagnostic service providers, and other losses. Therefore, it is important to meet, or better yet, exceed the customers' expectations regarding on-time performance. Chronic late performance will mean the facility will call another provider for its business.

PRICE

For some interfacility and all intrafacility transports, the sending facility is the payer for the service. This means that price is a competitive advantage. It is incumbent on ambulance providers to know their cost of delivering the service and to price their service in such a way as to not lose money on the transfer. For example, if your cost per unit hour is $140 with a mileage cost of $9 and the typical interfacility takes 90 minutes, it would be fiscally irresponsible for you to charge a base rate of $90 with a mileage rate of $5 per mile. This would result in a loss for every transport you provide. Further, CMS has very specific rules against underpricing services provided to non-CMS-funded patients as an enticement to get CMS-funded patients. Violation of these anti-**kickback** laws can result in severe civil and criminal penalties (Federal Register, 2003).

The fee charged by the ambulance provider is important for the facility regardless of whether or not it is actually paying the bill. If patients in their facility chronically complain about high charges, the facility will be encouraged to seek a different provider.

CUSTOMER SERVICE

Customer service, based on the general courtesy and professionalism of the ambulance and communications personnel, is paramount for maintaining good customer relations. Some EMTs and paramedics may view nonemergency service as an interruption of their primary mission: providing emergency medical services to 9-1-1 callers. Management should undertake great effort to demonstrate the value of nonemergency service to the organization and set the expectation that customers are to be treated with the utmost respect.

A friendly customer service approach starts with an easy service request process into the call center. Caller's phone calls should be answered professionally and courteously, and a genuine attempt should be made to meet or exceed the caller's expectations. For example, when the caller asks what time the ambulance can arrive to transport the patient, the call taker's response should be "When would you like us to be there?" If it appears that the ambulance may arrive late to the transport, it is crucial that the call center notify the caller, explain the reason for the anticipated late arrival, and offer either an alternative time or, if necessary to keep the appointment time, call another ambulance service. Although it may seem odd to call another provider, the perspective of the customers is that you went above and beyond to meet their needs, and as a result they will be more apt to call you next time.

CHAPTER REVIEW

Summary

Customer and community expectations for emergency and nonemergency transportation are vastly different. Agencies must be able to exceed the expectations of the nonemergency customers just as they do for the emergency customers. Balancing the expectations of the customer, patient, and payer communities, along with the regulatory requirements for nonemergency ambulance services, requires a careful strategy and well-thought-out service delivery model. Applying the principles outlined in this chapter will help you find the strategy and balance that works best for your community and your agency.

WHAT WOULD YOU DO? Reflection

1. Based on current CMS regulations, who is responsible for the cost of ambulance service between the stand-alone facility and the hospital's main campus?
   a. Transportation between two facilities licensed under the same Medicare license is covered by the facility's Part A payments from Medicare. Therefore, this service provision must be billed to the facility, not the patient or a third-party payer.

2. What are the implications if you bill third-party payers for this type of intrafacility transport?
   a. Knowingly submitting bills to Medicare or Medicaid for services you know are not a covered benefit could lead to potential determinations of Medicare fraud. Further, CMS routinely conducts audits of providers to determine if claims have been paid in error. CMS will review a sample of claims paid to the provider, and if it is determined that some percentage of the claims has been paid in error, CMS will require a repayment of some percentage of *all* claims paid during the period being audited. If these intrafacility claims are discovered during an audit of a representative number of claims, it may result in a higher percentage of claims paid in error, leading to potentially higher amounts being repaid to CMS and higher fines.

3. What are your considerations when pricing transports under this arrangement?
   a. Be sure that you are not pricing under the Medicare allowable rates.
   b. Be sure that you are not pricing under your cost of providing the service.

4. If you agree to bill less than your cost of providing this service, what are the potential risks?
   a. Risk of losing money on each transfer

5. If you agree to bill less than the Medicare allowable rates for providing this service, what are the potential risks?
   a. Risk of violating CMS regulations and federal law

Review Questions

1. What is the difference between interfacility transport and intrafacility transport?
2. Under what circumstances will Medicare pay for ambulance transportation from a hospital to the patient's home?
3. When is medical necessity for transportation by ambulance established?
4. What are three factors that are important to customer satisfaction in the nonemergency transport market?

References

American Legal Publishing Company. (1998). "Fort Worth Code of Municipal Ordinances, Article III, Sec 5–Area Metropolitan Ambulance Authority." See the organization website.

Carrido, N. (2011, October 14). "Non-emergent Ambulance Services: The Ambiguous Physician Certification Statement." Big Web Daily. See the organization website.

Centers for Medicare & Medicaid Services. (n.d.). 42 CFR Ch. IV § 410.40. See the organization website.

Centers for Medicare & Medicaid Services. (2010). "Chapter 10: Ambulance Services." *Medicare Benefit Policy Manual*. See the organization website.

Federal Register. (2003). 68 FR 14245 – OIG Compliance Program Guidance for Ambulance Supplier. See the U.S. Government Printing Office website.

Justia.com. (2012). *First Call Ambulance Service, Inc. v. Department of Health and Human Services et al.* See the organization website.

Page, Wolfberg, & Wirth. (2013). "Medicare Advance Notice Rules." See the organization website.

Key Terms

interfacility The transportation of a patient between two independently licensed health care facilities.

intrafacility The transportation of a patient between two facilities licensed under the same license.

kickback Offering anything of value in return for services that can be billed to Medicare or Medicaid.

medical necessity The determination of a patient's need for medical transportation services.

medical transportation The provision of medical care or medical monitoring during transport of a patient.

nonmedical transportation Transportation provided without medical care or medical monitoring.

patient A person in need of medical care or medical monitoring during transportation.

Physician Certification Statement A written statement from a physician attesting to the need for medical care or medical monitoring during transportation.

CHAPTER 6

Air Ambulance and Air Medical Transportation

EDWARD R. MARASCO, M.P.M., CMTE, EMT-P (RET.)

Objectives

After reading this chapter, the student should be able to:

6.1 Define air medical services.

6.2 Explain the common service delivery models found in air medical services.

6.3 List the most common organizational models found in air medical services and describe the key attributes of each.

6.4 Describe the regulatory agencies involved in overseeing air medical service operations.

6.5 Discuss the various staffing models commonly found in air medical services response.

6.6 Discuss the key considerations in vehicle selection and their impact on operations.

6.7 Explain the unique considerations associated with a communication center that supports air medical services.

6.8 Describe the unique aspects of a comprehensive safety program within an air medical service operation.

6.9 List some of the unique technology considerations associated with an air medical service operation.

6.10 Describe some of the educational offerings and professional certifications available to air medical services personnel.

6.11 Discuss some of the key attributes of a successful air medical service marketing program.

Overview

Ambulance services in the United States range in size from one ambulance operated by volunteers and managed by a community board of directors to large governmental agencies and even larger, private, for-profit corporations. This text presents information that the manager of an ambulance service, large or small, needs in order to keep the business solvent and provide clinically excellent service to the community.

Key Terms

air medical services (AMS)

Air and Surface Transport Nurses Association (ASTNA)

Association of Air Medical Services (AAMS)

aviation maintenance technician

Board for Critical Care Transport Paramedic Certification (BCCTPC)

Certified Flight Paramedic (FP-C)

Certified Flight Registered Nurse (CFRN)

Certified Medical Transport Executive (CMTE)

Federal Aviation Administration (FAA)

fixed wing

International Association of Flight Paramedics (IAFP)

rotary wing

WHAT WOULD YOU DO?

The county commissioners have informed emergency medical services (EMS) leadership that the county will be pursuing a joint venture to add **air medical services (AMS)** capability to the operation. The agreement calls for a specific liaison to work with the new aviation management partner to set up the AMS division and integrate it with the existing EMS operation. You have been selected to serve in that capacity and must answer the following questions at a county commission meeting in 30 days:

- What type of air medical transports would be needed in the county?
- What are the implications of the structure of the relationship forged by the county?
- What regulatory agencies will have jurisdiction over this new aspect of the operation?
- How should the operation be staffed, and what credentials will be required?
- What safety enhancements will be necessary to support the operation?
- What additional training will the leadership liaison require?

■ INTRODUCTION

In the global sense, air medical services (AMS) encompass all levels of medical transportation that are accomplished through the use of aircraft. There are more than 300 AMS operations in the United States today (Center for Transportation Injury Research, 2009, p. 8). More than 1,100 aircraft are used for AMS, and these assets can be categorized as **fixed wing** (airplanes) or **rotary wing** (helicopters) (Center for Transportation

Injury Research, 2009, p. 9). However, the earliest documented use of aircraft for medical transportation involved hot air balloons (Bock, 1988). Although this definition is fairly simple, the practical reality is that AMS operations are as diverse and complex as it gets in the out-of-hospital universe.

A typical AMS program operates as an integrated element of the regional medical transportation system. Although not always the case, AMS operations offer both scene response and interfacility transportation. For scene responses, an AMS operation is summoned directly to the site of an accident or incident and serves as the primary means of transportation to evacuate the patient to a higher level of care. It is typical for the AMS team to respond secondary to the arrival of public-safety and/or EMS personnel; however, in some systems AMS operations may serve as the first responder. Interfacility AMS include transports from one health care institution to another. The most common interfacility transport scenario involves transporting a patient from one hospital to another in order to provide access to a higher level of care. An interfacility transport will frequently originate from the emergency department; however, it is also common for the transport to originate from an inpatient setting.

■ SERVICE MODELS FOR AMS DELIVERY————

The service models found in AMS are typically differentiated by the level of care provided, the type and number of vehicles deployed as a part of the system, and the geographic area that is covered. The utilization of AMS resources is generally desired in circumstances characterized by the need for rapid evacuation of the patient, inaccessibility of the patient by ground, and/or the need for a higher level of care during transport than

what is available in other aspects of the out-of-hospital care system.

LEVEL OF CARE

Although rapid evacuation of critically ill or injured patients was the hallmark of the military model of AMS, the civilian application has included the ability to deliver a higher level of care during transport. With this in mind, the preponderance of AMS operations provides care at the critical care level. The clinical staff, medical equipment, patient care regimen, and medical direction are geared toward providing a higher level of care than is typically found in ground medical transportation resources. In relatively limited circumstances, AMS may be offered at the advanced life support (ALS) level. An ALS level of service may be found in AMS operations that serve more rural areas or in situations where the program handles scene responses almost exclusively, including some services operated by governmental entities.

FIXED WING AIRCRAFT

Fixed wing aircraft are used most often for situations that require longer-range transport (Figure 6.1) than rotary wing aircraft can accommodate. In general, fixed wing aircraft can operate

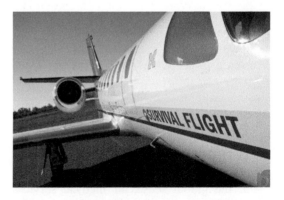

FIGURE 6.1 ■ Survival Flight, the University of Michigan Health System's fixed wing air ambulance. *Source: Courtesy of Survival Flight.*

at higher speeds, covering greater distances in a shorter period of time than can rotary wing aircraft. Although not always the case, it is most common for fixed wing resources to be used for interfacility transports. Because fixed wing work is done between airports, some other form of medical transport, most commonly by ground, is required to complete the transport between the pickup or destination and the airport. Within the scope of fixed wing capability, there are three distinct mission profiles:

- Regional transports (150 to 500 loaded miles)
- Long-range domestic transports (500 to 3,000 loaded miles)
- Long-range international transports (1,000+ loaded miles)

In the case of regional transports, fixed wing aircraft and rotary wing aircraft can be used interchangeably for certain missions. As discussed in subsequent sections of this chapter, the aircraft selection and operation relate directly to this mission profile.

ROTARY WING AIRCRAFT

Rotary wing aircraft (i.e., helicopters) are used most often to complete patient transports that are time sensitive and require less transport range than fixed wing aircraft. The ability of rotary wing aircraft to land in confined, non-airport spaces allows the team to fly directly to the scene of an accident or hospital point of origin (Figure 6.2). Likewise, rotary wing aircraft can typically transport directly to a specialty care hospital, reducing the amount of time the patient spends outside of the hospital. It is common for rotary wing resources to be used for scene responses as well as for interfacility transports. As discussed in subsequent sections of this chapter, aircraft selection and operation relate directly to this mission profile. In addition, the size and capacity of the aircraft have a direct impact on the mission the aircraft will allow.

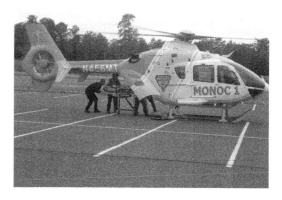

FIGURE 6.2 ■ MONOC 1, serving central New Jersey, loads a patient aboard. *Source: MONOC Mobile Health Services.*

SPECIALTY CARE TRANSPORT

It is quite common for AMS operations to either provide directly, or participate cooperatively, in an operation that offers specialty care transport by ground. Specialty care transport is difficult to describe definitively because the definition may vary from system to system; however, the Centers for Medicare and Medicaid Services (CMS) definition recognizes specialty care as a level of capability beyond the scope of a typical paramedic (Centers for Medicare and Medicaid Services, 2002). This approach acknowledges that aircraft may be unavailable from time to time due to weather, maintenance or other factors, and the need remains to complete the patient transport (Figure 6.3). In this circumstance, the clinical staff assigned to the aircraft may be used to complete a specialty care transport by ground.

INTEGRATED DELIVERY SYSTEM

The AMS program profile has changed over time from the single hospital-based helicopter operation to a more regionally focused multimodal transport profile. Although some

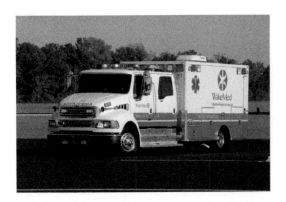

FIGURE 6.3 ■ WakeMed Mobile operates terrestrial specialty-care transport vehicles in conjunction with helicopter EMS units. *Source: Courtesy of the Author.*

single-mode (i.e., fixed wing only) operations still exist, it is quite common for an AMS program to include fixed wing, rotary wing, and specialty care transport ground capability. The combination of highly trained clinical staff with access to a variety of transport vehicles is viewed in many markets as extremely efficient and responsive to the needs of the community. The integrated delivery system allows the requesting entity to access different modes of transport by making one call.

■ ORGANIZATIONAL MODELS FOR AMS DELIVERY————————

The structure of AMS organizations has become more complex and dynamic in recent years as the health care delivery system has changed. Program structures have been transformed as the demands for service and the level of competition have evolved over time. Although the most common structural models will be described in more detail in subsequent paragraphs, it should be noted that the variations and permutations are infinite.

HOSPITAL-BASED MODEL

This approach to program structure, often referred to as the traditional model, is one of the most long-standing found in the civilian AMS community. In the hospital-based model, the AMS program is sponsored by a hospital or health system that has primary responsibility for the operation. It is common for the sponsoring organization to maintain control of the factors of production associated with providing the service with one exception. Because the aviation aspect of AMS is so heavily regulated, it has been customary for a sponsoring health care organization to seek the services of a professional aviation management company to provide aviation support. The clinical services, medical oversight, communication center services, marketing, billing services, and program management are provided by the hospital, and the pilots, **aviation maintenance technicians**, and aircraft are provided, under contract, by the aviation management company. Many hospital-based services are nonprofit entities, organized either as a part of a nonprofit hospital or as a separate corporation.

It is common for the hospital-based program to be oriented around the air medical transport needs of the sponsoring organization (Figure 6.4). This singular focus allows the transport team to be integrated efficiently as a part of the continuum of care for a specific health care system. It is also common to find integration between the AMS organization and the tertiary hospital in the areas of clinical protocols, medical devices, medical supplies, medication, medical oversight, and quality improvement frameworks within a hospital-based model. This model allows for the AMS clinical staff to take advantage of education, training, and clinical experiences offered by the sponsoring hospital. Some hospital-based services may have a particular affinity for, and/or loyalty to, the sponsoring institution.

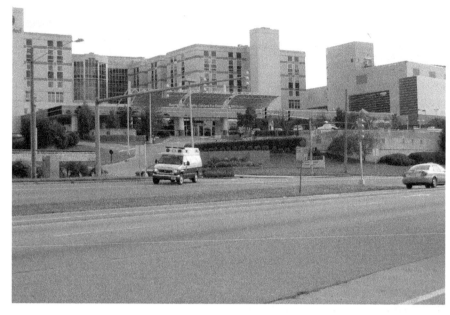

FIGURE 6.4 ▪ Integration of air transport, ground transport, and health care facilities can provide closely integrated, continuous care, while enhancing the identity of each provider. *Source: Official Wake County EMS Photo by Mike Legeros, used by permission.*

COMMUNITY-BASED MODEL

This approach to program structure is the fastest-growing approach in civilian AMS operations. The community-based model is distinct from the hospital-based model most notably because the sponsoring organization is not usually a hospital or health system. The sponsoring organization is typically some other entity that provides the service in a defined geographical area. The sponsoring organization might be an ambulance service, a nonhospital health care organization, or an aviation management company offering turnkey services, and these entities are typically organized as for-profit corporations. This phenomenon evolved during a period when hospital-based programs were being evaluated by their ownership for financial performance,

resulting in services being sold or closed. As some sponsoring hospitals elected to depart the AMS service line, a void was created for nonhospital entities to fill.

It is more common for a community-based AMS operation to serve competing health care organizations that operate in the same geographic area. It is a bit more challenging for the transport organization to be well integrated into the continuum of care because the approach used by each health care organization may be quite different. For example, the health care organizations may use different medical supplies, medications, treatment protocols, and/or patient preparation guidelines. To maintain the continuum of care, it may be necessary for the AMS clinical staff to be familiar with and make accommodation for these different standards. In this scenario, the

AMS staff may not have an affinity for one particular health care provider.

ALTERNATE-DELIVERY MODEL

This approach to program structure represents a creative strategy for shifting risk for AMS operations, including operational, financial, and public relations risks. It has been widely used as a transitional strategy as programs evolve from being hospital-based operations. The alternate-delivery model, or hybrid approach, is generally characterized by operating the AMS program as a joint venture of sorts. The parties to the transaction may include hospitals, aviation management companies, ground ambulance providers, government agencies, and/or other entities. At the most basic level, each of the sponsoring organizations contributes something to the partnership. The contribution may be determined based on the core competencies of each sponsor (i.e., clinical organization provides clinical staff, aviation operation provides aviation staff, etc.). The distribution of responsibility may also be done along the lines of control (i.e., hospital wants to retain authority over the clinical aspect of the operation). In any event, the clear delineation of authority and responsibility is one of the critical elements of success with this type of structure. Alternate-delivery models may be organized as either for-profit or nonprofit corporations.

The alternate-delivery model approach may provide more opportunity for the transport operation to be integrated into the regional system; however, it may also present substantial challenges from a leadership perspective. With multiple entities involved in the operation, it is common for such a program to have more regional buy-in. In many cases, this structure provides a mechanism for hospitals, government agencies, private corporations, and other interested parties to have a role in providing the service. Although these organizations

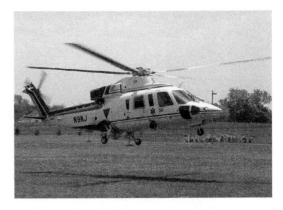

FIGURE 6.5 ■ The New Jersey State Police operates dual-role law enforcement and EMS helicopters throughout the state, in partnership with ground EMS agencies. *Source: Photo courtesy New Jersey Office of Emergency Medical Services.*

may have divergent interests, they often have enough common ground to make AMS operations successful.

PUBLIC-SAFETY MODEL

This approach to program structure also dates back to the early days of civilian AMS in the United States. A number of AMS operations are still provided by public-safety organizations (Figure 6.5). The organizations involved may be fire departments, law enforcement agencies, geopolitical government authorities, or some combination of each. Within the realm of public-safety model operations, one finds a number of diverse approaches. Some of these entities operate independently as an arm of the sponsoring government agency. In some cases, the public-safety entity will partner with a private company to provide clinical services.

A number of different funding strategies are used in the public-safety model. Some operations are set up solely as tax-funded services. Some operations are funded by user fees collected (e.g., surcharge on motor vehicle code violations). Some operations are set up as a fee-for-service provider, making them subject to Federal Aviation Regulations (FARs). Some use a combination of methods for financing the operation.

AMS organizational structure has a significant impact on the operation, financing, and regulatory considerations for an AMS program. It is a parameter that should be carefully evaluated when setting up, operating, and/or interacting with an AMS program.

Side Bar

Compliance with Part 135

In order for any AMS operation, including public safety model operations, to bill patients for services, the organization must comply with all regulations in Part 135 of the FARs.

REGULATORY AUTHORITY AND CONSIDERATIONS

One of the most complex aspects of managing AMS is the level and diversity of regulatory oversight. Out-of-hospital operations have traditionally attracted a greater level of attention by regulators because the environment is considered more complicated than the hospital setting. The clinical aspect of AMS tends to draw considerable attention because many of the procedures are considered high risk. The clinical aspect is typically regulated by state and regional medical oversight authorities. The use of aviation vehicles for transports creates yet another layer of scrutiny and oversight, particularly at the federal level.

FEDERAL AVIATION ADMINISTRATION (FAA)

A defining aspect of AMS programs is the aviation component of the operation. This creates operational and regulatory considerations that are distinct from ground medical transport programs. The **Federal Aviation Administration (FAA)** is a division of the U.S. Department of Transportation. The FAA is charged with oversight of civilian aviation operations. The mission of the FAA is "to provide the safest, most efficient aerospace system in the world" (Federal Aviation Administration, 2010). In particular, the FAA has an interest in regulating operations that involve the "flying public." The FAA sets minimum standards for the operation and maintenance of the aircraft involved in AMS. These standards may be found in 14 CFR Part 91 and 14 CFR Part 135 (James, 2004, p. 36). The subparts of the FARs that apply depend on the type and structure of the aviation operation. There are general standards that apply to all types of operations; however, some standards apply exclusively to AMS operations. The entity that is licensed to operate and maintain the aircraft is referred to as the certificated air carrier, or air operator, and is the entity that is accountable to the FAA.

NATIONAL TRANSPORTATION SAFETY BOARD

The National Transportation Safety Board (NTSB) is an independent nonregulatory federal agency that investigates every civil aviation accident in the United States and significant accidents involving other modes of transportation (National Transportation Safety Board, 2006, p. vii). The NTSB has a great deal of influence on aviation activities, due in large part to the function that it serves as a data resource. The data include a comprehensive aviation accident database and the proceedings from completed special investigations. The NTSB also conducts safety studies and issues safety recommendations that are advisory in nature. As a result of studying a series of 55 accidents that occurred between 2002 and 2005, the NTSB issued a special report in 2006 with a series of recommendations for improving AMS operations (National Transportation Safety Board, 2006). Although NTSB recommendations for aviation are typically issued to the FAA, a series of NTSB recommendations relating to AMS in 2009 included recommendations to other federal agencies as well.

STATE DEPARTMENT OF HEALTH/DIVISION OF EMS

As is the case with most medical transportation organizations, some agency within state government has oversight authority for EMS. Most frequently the state department of health has charged some agency within its confines to handle such matters as licensure of the transport organization, credentialing of its clinical personnel, and licensing of its vehicles. These state regulations cover the amount and type of equipment required aboard the aircraft. In addition, some states may regulate the crew configuration required to operate as an air ambulance. AMS operations have the unique position of needing to meet both state and federal regulations with regard to vehicle and personnel certification. Because of the distances covered by AMS programs and the regional nature of the operations, many AMS programs interface with agencies in more than one state.

REGIONAL EMS AUTHORITY

In most localities, regional authorities govern some aspect of medical transportation. In some cases the authority is delegated from statewide agencies, and in other cases the source of the authority is more local (e.g., county government). Because of the broad service area covered by most AMS programs, the leadership may need to interface with many regional authorities to actually operate in compliance with all applicable regulations. In some cases, the AMS program must be granted authority to operate county by county.

THIRD-PARTY PAYER REQUIREMENTS

Although third-party payers (e.g., Medicare, Medicaid, etc.) may establish specific requirements for medical transport organizations in order to receive payment for services, AMS providers often are required to comply with ground medical transport requirements and a separate set of requirements that apply to AMS. These requirements may reference and/or incorporate other standards, or they may have separate and distinct requirements that are unique to the payer. The process of monitoring these standards is quite time consuming.

■ STAFFING MODELS ──────────

The personnel utilized to operate an AMS program are determined by several factors, including mission profile, program structure, staff responsibilities, base site logistics, and regulatory requirements (Figure 6.6). For the purposes of this discussion, the description will focus exclusively on the AMS response team. However, it should be noted that the administrative staff, training staff, and communication center staff also play key roles in AMS operations.

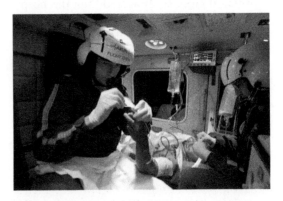

FIGURE 6.6 ■ Air medical units are often staffed with a crew composed of a flight nurse and flight paramedic. *Source: Photo courtesy of the Association of Air Medical Services.*

AVIATION STAFF

The aviation staff includes two equally important types of personnel who are integral to a successful AMS organization. Pilots are charged with the safe operation of the aircraft at all times. Aviation maintenance technicians are charged with the proper maintenance and repair of the aircraft. These staff members operate under the auspices of the FAA and any related regulations, as well as the requirements put forth by the AMS organization.

Pilot staffing in AMS is typically a function of the type of aircraft and mission profile, although some variations exist. AMS operations are widely viewed in aviation circles as some of the most demanding and complex flying done by civilian pilots. It is not uncommon for AMS pilots to fly into uncontrolled landing zones, at night, in marginal weather, with minimal prior knowledge of the surroundings. For this reason, the standards in the AMS community normally require pilots to possess more credentials, more training, and more experience than many other types of commercial pilots. Pilot staffing is done in one of two ways:

* In a single-pilot configuration, one pilot is designated as the pilot in command (PIC) and assigned to fly the aircraft. The PIC is charged with the safe and efficient operation of the aircraft at all times.
* In a dual-pilot configuration, staffing includes a PIC and a co-pilot as the standard aviation crew. The PIC would typically be the more experienced pilot with more certifications and qualifications.

The pilots are subject to flight- and duty-time requirements as published by the FAA. Unlike other personnel involved in AMS operations, the pilot is limited to a finite amount of on-duty time and is required to have a specific period of rest between duty assignments. For this reason, it is typical for the AMS pilot to be assigned to a 12-hour duty shift. In certain circumstances, the AMS pilot may be permitted to extend duty time up to 14 hours. Generally, pilots must have a minimum of 10 hours of uninterrupted (nonwork) rest between shifts.

Aviation maintenance technicians are charged with maintaining the airworthiness of the aircraft in accordance with the applicable regulations, manufacturers' requirements and recommendations, and program-specific policies. The maintenance technicians are governed by several areas of FAA regulation. In most AMS operations, a technician is assigned to care for each aircraft in the field. This technician may be supported by additional technicians with fleetwide responsibilities for certain interventions (e.g., avionics technician, engine repair specialist, etc.). Although there are some duty-time conventions, the regulations for maintenance technician duty times are less concrete than the standards for pilots.

CLINICAL STAFF

The core clinical staff for an AMS program are personnel assigned to the program or base site for the purpose of providing care to the majority of patients during transport. The most common approach is to have a team of clinical personnel dedicated to the air medical mission. In some circumstances, the clinical staff may be shared with other departments. In a hospital-based operation, a flight nurse may also provide clinical care in the hospital emergency department.

Several different crew combinations are used for clinical staff deployment. These include the following:

* One physician and one nurse
* Two nurses
* One nurse and one paramedic
* One nurse and one respiratory therapist
* Two paramedics

The most common clinical staff configuration observed in AMS operations today is one nurse and one paramedic. This configuration is recognized as one of the more versatile and cost-effective combinations to deploy. The depth and breadth of clinical knowledge typical among nurses provides advantages when caring for complicated medical cases. The field experience and technical skill capability typical among paramedics provides advantages when caring for trauma patients. It is common for only the most experienced and highly trained individuals in each profession to be employed in an AMS program.

SPECIALTY TRANSPORT TEAMS

It is quite common for AMS programs to have access to and make use of hospital-based specialty transport personnel to provide even more specialized care to patients during transport. The specialty teams are often deployed as supplemental staff to the core clinical crew; however, they will usually assume primary responsibility for patient care during the transport. The team may consistent of specially trained physicians, nurses, respiratory therapists, and/or technicians. Specialty teams can be organized around a particular patient type and/or a specific capability that is required to care for the patient. Common specialty teams include neonatal, pediatric, obstetric, and intraortic balloon pump transport teams.

Regardless of the specific discipline, it is common for members of an AMS operation to be among the most experienced, highly credentialed, and intensely trained individuals within their profession.

■ VEHICLE SELECTION AND PROCUREMENT ————————

One of the critical aspects of AMS operations includes the selection, procurement, and operation of the vehicles used to complete the mission. The choice of aircraft has a profound impact on the capability of the AMS program, the clinical staff configuration, the service area, and the marketing strategy. Certain aircraft may limit the ability to complete certain transports, whereas others may provide unique advantages for an AMS program. The typical categories of aircraft include rotary wing and fixed wing.

ROTARY WING AIRCRAFT

The selection of a helicopter for an AMS program should be based on the mission profile, the operating environment, and the economic framework of the operation. Each aircraft has a specific set of performance characteristics and operating costs that impact how the aircraft is able to meet the needs of the program. Aircraft selection is based on several parameters:

* **Single versus twin engine**

  Although the number of engines itself may not necessarily determine the ability to complete a certain mission, the number of engines may be a function of program philosophy. At the present time, no data conclude that twin-engine aircrafts are safer than single-engine aircrafts, although a portion of the community believes this to be true. On the other hand, performance data do suggest that single-engine aircraft perform better in high-altitude, high-temperature conditions. The practical consideration is that a twin-engine aircraft that loses one engine may still be able to maneuver safely with one engine engaged. A single-engine aircraft that sustains an engine failure would be forced to auto-rotate to the ground, a procedure that offers limited maneuverability.

Side Bar
Single-engine versus Twin-engine?
The debate over single-engine aircraft versus twin-engine aircraft is one of the most hotly contested issues facing the AMS community today. Making a decision in this regard should be done as objectively as possible based on the data available to the program.

+ **Cabin size and weight**

The capability of a helicopter in terms of cabin size and lift (ability to carry a certain amount of weight) has a prominent impact on patient care capability. A program with a mission profile that consists primarily of scene responses for trauma patients may be able to operate with a less capable aircraft than a program that specializes in interfacility transports requiring the use of specialized clinical equipment and/or personnel.

+ **Cost**

The cost of an aircraft for use in AMS operations can vary quite a bit depending on the aircraft selected. The cost is typically evaluated on two parameters: acquisition cost and hourly operating cost. Most AMS operations use light to midsize helicopters that range in acquisition cost from $500,000 to over $10,000,000. Likewise, the hourly operating cost of aircraft in this size range, not including fuel, can vary from $250 per hour to in excess of $1,200 per hour. Fuel cost can add another $200 to $500 per flight hour.

FIXED WING AIRCRAFT

The selection of an airplane for an AMS program should be based on the mission profile, the operating environment, and the economic framework of the operation. Each aircraft has a specific set of performance characteristics that impact how the aircraft is able to meet the needs of the program. Aircraft selection is based on several parameters:

+ **Single versus twin engine**

Fewer single-engine airplanes are acceptable for AMS operations, therefore this has not been a particularly salient issue. There is also less sensitivity around the loss of an engine in fixed wing operations. Likewise, there is a substantial difference between engine types (e.g., turboprop vs. jet). However, a substantial financial consideration is associated with one approach versus the other.

+ **Cabin size and weight**

The cabin size and configuration may be more of a consideration in fixed wing AMS operation because, on average, the patient and clinical staff will spend more time in the aircraft with the patient. The ability of the aircraft to lift a certain weight is a lesser consideration because the class of aircraft used generally has more capability than rotary wing aircrafts.

+ **Cost**

The cost of an airplane for use in AMS operations can vary quite a bit depending on the aircraft selected. The cost is typically evaluated on two parameters: acquisition cost and hourly operating cost. Most AMS operations use airplanes that range in cost for acquisition from $1,500,000 to $20,000,000. Likewise, the hourly operating cost of aircraft in this size range, excluding fuel, can vary from $500 per hour to in excess of $5,000 per hour.

The vehicle costs are usually the second-largest operating expense, behind staff costs; therefore, this is one of the most important considerations in providing a financially viable AMS program.

▧ COMMUNICATION CENTER CONSIDERATIONS ──────

Emergency medical communication centers often possess a common set of characteristics and capabilities. These core capabilities and characteristics also apply to a communication center that supports an AMS program. A number of additional capabilities must be part of an AMS communication center (Bock, Samuels, and Campbell, 1988, p. 36), including, but not limited to, scene responses, interfacility transports, fixed wing transports, and flight following and support.

SCENE RESPONSES

In facilitating AMS scene responses, communication center personnel have a more active role in coordinating the response. In most circumstances, the communication center staff is integrally involved in identifying the location of the incident and directing the aircraft to the scene. In addition, the communication center staff is typically directly involved in coordinating communication between the aircraft and the ground emergency responders.

INTERFACILITY TRANSPORTS

In coordinating interfacility transports, the communication center staff has an active role in facilitating the response. The staff is typically involved in communicating with personnel at both the sending and receiving facilities. This may involve everything from notifying security personnel to clear the helipad to coordinating the delivery of a patient care report, to facilitating physician-to-physician communication.

FIXED WING TRANSPORTS

Although fixed wing transports typically occur over longer periods of time and generally have more advanced notice, they can be more labor intensive than rotary wing transports. The communication specialist may assist the pilot with flight planning by identifying the closest airport to the patient, evaluating the resources at the airport (e.g., access to fuel after normal business hours), and arranging ground ambulance transport at both ends of the flight.

FLIGHT FOLLOWING AND SUPPORT

One of the unique aspects of AMS operations is the size of the service area and the great distances covered by the program during a single transport. It is typical for the communication center to be actively involved in tracking the progress of the aircraft from point to point

and recording the position at specific intervals. This provides a layer of safety: In the event an aircraft must make an unplanned landing, the communication specialist may be able to locate the aircraft promptly. The communication specialist will often provide other support (e.g., weather updates, patient care updates, etc.) to the staff aboard the aircraft during the mission. The communication center may also be delegated the operational control function as required under 14 CFR Part 135 of the FARs.

The AMS communication center has certain unique requirements that impact the personnel, training and equipment that are essential for success.

■ SAFETY CONSIDERATIONS———

Out-of-hospital operations present unique challenges to medical transportation providers. The environment adds a layer of special considerations that are not common in the hospital. Medical transport providers must be more aware of environmental hazards on scene, climate control, crowd control, and the media, among other matters. Many of these special considerations have a direct or indirect impact on the safety of the providers and the patient. The number of AMS accidents over the last decade and the associated fatalities has created a renewed focus on creating a safety-based culture in AMS organizations. Adopting a safety-based culture requires a commitment to safety as a value within the organization and special attention to several aspects of safety (Nelson, 2010, p. 8).

PATIENT SAFETY

In recent years, patient safety has been recognized as a high priority for patient care providers. It is the focus of performance improvement initiatives by health care providers, new performance standards by accrediting agencies, and compliance audits by government agencies. Likewise, recently it has been written about frequently in the news media.

AMS providers must manage some of the most clinically complex patients in some of the least controlled environments. The clinical needs of patients in AMS operations are frequently some of the most demanding and complicated. It is common for the most severe trauma, cardiac, neonatal, and other patients to be transported by AMS providers. The number and variety of interventions are often greater in this patient population. It is extremely important for an AMS organization to devote time, attention, and resources to the clinical aspects of patient safety.

Developing and implementing sound patient safety practices in medical transport operations is certainly a challenge. AMS providers operate in extreme aspects of the out-of-hospital setting. Patients are being cared for in uncontrolled settings in many cases, and their exposure to hazards is greatly increased. Such considerations as noise abatement, exposure to foreign objects, and complicated patient loading and unloading procedures represent an added layer of risk for AMS patients. It is extremely important for an AMS organization to devote time, attention, and resources to the environmental aspect of patient safety.

PROVIDER SAFETY

Provider safety may be discussed less often, but the operating environment for AMS poses many risks and increased hazard exposure for staff members. AMS providers operate in extreme aspects of the out-of-hospital setting and must clinically manage some of the most complex patients in some of the least controlled environments. Such considerations as noise abatement, exposure to foreign objects, and complicated patient loading and unloading procedures represent an added layer of risk for AMS providers.

It is extremely important for an AMS organization to devote time, attention, and resources to the environmental aspect of provider safety. AMS personnel are typically trained in air medical resource management (AMRM), a multidisciplinary training program that focuses on teamwork, communication, situational awareness, and fatigue effects.

AVIATION SAFETY

The unique risks associated with aviation operations makes safety an even greater consideration in AMS operations. Decision making, human error, fatigue, and equipment failure can have more drastic consequences in the aviation environment (Pickering, 2010, p. 12). For this reason, aviation safety is a major consideration for all AMS programs. Although the aviation environment presents many unique risks, the aviation environment has also produced a number of safety concepts and sound strategies for pursuing excellence in safety.

Safety management systems (SMS) are a construct developed by the aviation community to mitigate risks. It involves managing the interface between procedure and training, the equipment, the environment, and human factors. SMS embraces a convention that includes use of a formal risk assessment prior to the acceptance of each mission. Elements of risk assessment may include terrain, fatigue, weather, time of day, experience, aircraft readiness, and readiness of the crew. SMS offers a standardized approach to risk assessment and mitigation.

▨ TECHNOLOGY CONSIDERATIONS—

The complexity of the operating environment makes the application of technology even more critical than the similar technology that may be applied in the ground medical transport environment. Technology is particularly important to increase the margin of safety in operations. Based on a series of recommendations published in recent years, several evolving technologies are being embraced.

NIGHT VISION IMAGING SYSTEM

Night vision imaging system (NVIS) technology, in general, and night vision goggle (NVG) technology, specifically, have been used widely in military operations for many years; however, the value in civilian operations has only been embraced in recent years (Figure 6.7). NVIS technology provides enhanced visibility in low-light situations. The ability to see more clearly has the potential to reduce the risk of flying into obstacles, which is one of the most common causes of AMS accidents. The number of AMS operations performed in low visibility conditions makes the use of NVIS technology, most commonly NVGs, very valuable.

SATELLITE TRACKING SYSTEMS

The ability to monitor aircraft location and progress more closely can provide advanced notice of hazards, reduce the workload of the onboard staff relating to live position reports,

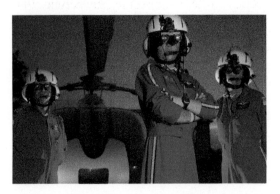

FIGURE 6.7 ■ Night vision technology adds an additional margin of safety by aiding in the avoidance of obstacles in limited light conditions. *Source: Photo courtesy of the Association of Air Medical Services.*

and reduce the workload of communication center staff. It also enables the communication center staff to locate the aircraft more quickly in the event of an emergency during transport.

TERRAIN AWARENESS WARNING SYSTEMS TECHNOLOGY

One of the deadliest risks to AMS helicopter operations is flying the aircraft into an obstacle, including towers, buildings, and the ground. Terrain awareness warning systems (TAWS) technology allows the pilot to receive active warnings when the aircraft is approaching an obstacle. Deploying this technology involves the installation of hardware and software aboard the aircraft. Although the use of this technology is not yet a regulatory requirement, many AMS programs have already installed the systems.

OTHER TECHNOLOGY OPTIONS

Other technology options that find their way into the discussions of AMS safety include the following:

> **Traffic collision avoidance systems (TCAS)** warn the pilot of a possible collision course with another aircraft.
>
> **Radar altimeters** allow the pilot to know how far they are flying above the ground, unlike regular altimeters that measure current altitude above sea level.
>
> **Live satellite weather** allows the pilot to receive current weather information for their area and their flight path.
>
> **Flight data monitoring (FDM) systems** monitor various aspects of a flight. These systems monitor the operation of aviation systems onboard the aircraft. The information can be downloaded following a flight to review how the flight was conducted.

EDUCATIONAL CONSIDERATIONS

The unique nature of AMS operations requires a number of special credentials for the staff associated with these programs. Over years, a specific body of knowledge and skills necessary for success has been identified by professionals working in the industry.

COMMUNICATION SPECIALISTS EDUCATION

The communication specialist community is diverse and challenging to categorize. The knowledge and skill sets required for success in different environments are just as diverse. The National Association of Air Medical Communication Specialists (NAACS) has assumed the leadership role in developing educational offerings for the profession. NAACS leadership developed the Certified Flight Coordinator (CFC) training and certification process. The CFC credential is valid for 4 years and can be renewed by completing 32 hours of continuing education. Additional education offerings are provided by NAACS that focus on specific functions. By requiring this credential, an AMS organization is able to ensure recruitment of staff with a core set of knowledge and skills.

FLIGHT NURSES EDUCATION

The nursing profession recognized in the early days of the AMS industry that the skill set required of nurses in the AMS environment was somewhat different from the requirements in a more traditional hospital setting. AMS programs require nurses to meet all of the licensure requirements within the jurisdiction and typically expect a significant level of experience in critical care delivery prior to employment. Most flight nurses have a background and more than 5 years of experience in an intensive care unit and/or emergency department setting. With the leadership of the **Air and Surface Transport Nurses Association (ASTNA)**, a curriculum, program, and certification process was developed to measure the attainment of a defined body of nursing knowledge pertinent to nurses operating in the AMS environment (Board Certification for Emergency Nurses, 2012). The process is currently managed by the Board Certification for Emergency Nurses (BCEN). At the completion of the program, the nurse is recognized as a **Certified Flight Registered Nurse (CFRN)** for a period of 4 years. Recertification is handled through examination and continuing education. This credential allows an AMS organization to ensure that new staff possess certain core knowledge before providing program specific education.

FLIGHT PARAMEDICS EDUCATION

The paramedic profession recognized in recent years that the level of expertise required in the AMS environment was somewhat different from the requirements in a more traditional ground EMS setting. AMS programs require paramedics to meet all of the certification/licensure requirements within the jurisdiction and typically expect a national registry certification prior to employment. Most flight paramedics have more than 5 years of experience in an active EMS setting. With the leadership of the **International Association of Flight & Critical Care Paramedics (IAFCCP)**, a specific curriculum, program, and certification process was developed as a voluntary credentialing process designed to elevate professional standards and enhance individual performance of paramedics operating in the AMS environment (**Board for Critical Care Transport Paramedic Certification**, 2009). At the completion of the program, the paramedic is recognized as a **Certified Flight Paramedic (FP-C)** for a period of four (4) years. A paramedic may recertify as an FP-C through continuing education by obtaining 100 contact hours, including completion of an approved FP-C prep class. Most AMS programs require FP-C certification as a condition of employment.

LEADERSHIP EDUCATION

Although good leadership qualities are important, the management expertise and experience required to lead an AMS organization are unique in some respects. The **Association of Air Medical Services (AAMS)** founded the Medical Transport Leadership Institute (MTLI) in 1998 to develop a specific curriculum, program, and certification process for leaders operating in the AMS environment (Association of Air Medical Services, 2010). At the completion of the program, the individual is recognized as a **Certified Medical Transport Executive (CMTE)** for a period of 3 years. An individual may recertify as a CMTE through continuing education by obtaining 30 management education units. Requiring this certification ensures that leaders have a certain set of core knowledge that is important to running an AMS organization and/or serving in a leadership role (i.e., chief flight nurse, lead pilot, etc.).

Best Practice

AMS Leadership Training

In 1995, the Association of Air Medical Services (AAMS) recognized that leadership in AMS was critically important to the success of the community. In many cases, AMS programs were operated as part of a larger organization with limited expertise and experience in some of the core competencies associated with AMS. Likewise, many of the industry leaders were experienced clinicians who had ascended to leadership positions without much formal leadership training. The complexity and demands of leading an AMS program are substantial. AAMS embarked on an initiative to develop a process to promote excellence in AMS operations by providing education and verification in certain core competencies for AMS leaders. The Medical Transport Leadership Institute (MTLI) was established as the educational program, and the Certified Medical Transport Executive (CMTE) process was established for verification.

The MTLI content was developed by a set of experienced leaders from the community. A small committee was formed to identify key areas of focus for the training. The content includes focus in the areas of clinical competency, compliance, excellence, finance, human resources, quality, service, and technology, among others. Following definition of the core competencies, a team of content area experts from within the industry were invited to become faculty members.

In order to deploy an educational program and a certification process, AAMS sought an experienced partner. In 1996 AAMS forged a relationship with the Oglebay National Training Center, in Wheeling, West Virginia, to develop and deploy the MTLI. The Oglebay National Training Center had experience developing and conducting more than a dozen leadership institutes for various professional associations. This experience and perspective proved very valuable during the early evolution of the program, and the partnership remains today as one of the strengths of the Institute.

The first MTLI course was conducted in 1997 for a capacity attendance of eighty AMS professionals. Since that time more than 700 students have successfully completed the program. The program now includes a robust graduate school offering that focuses on current challenges facing the industry. Each spring more than 200 professionals assemble in Wheeling, West Virginia, to participate in the program. Today, more than 300 CMTEs are active in the industry at some level.

MARKETING AIR MEDICAL SERVICES

Marketing AMS programs presents some challenges because the audience can be somewhat diverse and each audience segment may have different needs and expectations. Because the community is so diverse, the process of defining the four Ps of marketing (product, price, place, and promotion) is more difficult in the AMS environment (Landis and Jones, 2010, p. 12). The *product* varies, depending on the mission profile and the perspective of the requestor. The *price* may not be a substantial consideration for the requestor at the time of the request; however, it may become an issue in retrospect. The *place* is often defined by the requestor, and the AMS provider may have little to no impact on this parameter. The *promotion* aspect of marketing may be quite diverse because the *product* is so variable. Competition has many different characteristics as well. One of the real challenges is to accurately identify the decision makers who can impact the request for AMS. Often, promotion is conducted by way of air-medical educational seminars.

SCENE RESPONSES

The decision makers for scene responses are usually dictated by state law and local practice and may include a number of different public-safety professionals. The decision-making process itself is multifaceted. At the most basic level, it involves making a triage decision about whether AMS is actually indicated given the needs of the patient. Once it is determined that the patient requires air medical evacuation, the decision maker must decide which AMS provider to contact. In some systems, this decision may be done by protocol based on such factors as clinical capability, response time, and/or professional affiliation.

Ground ambulance providers are probably the most notable decision makers. In many systems the first EMS unit on the scene has the authority to make the triage decision and ultimately select the provider. In many systems, the ground ambulance provider makes the triage decision in consultation with a medical control authority.

Public-safety officials may also be involved in the decision-making process once the triage decision has been made by the clinical care provider. Law enforcement authorities on scene may be charged with making the request for AMS resources. The ranking fire officer on scene may have an impact on the choice of AMS provider because it is quite common for this individual to serve as the incident commander. In some cases, the actual decision regarding which AMS provider to request rests with the dispatcher. For these reasons, it is incumbent on the outreach personnel charged with representing the AMS provider to educate all of the audiences associated with this type of mission.

INTERFACILITY TRANSPORTS

Interfacility transports are very diverse in nature, ranging from the transport from a rural emergency department, to a tertiary care center for definitive care, to a long-range repatriation transport to return a patient home for care. The decision makers associated with these extremes and the many call types in between can be quite different. For more emergent transport requests, the target audience may be emergency physicians, critical care medicine physicians, and emergency department and intensive care unit nurses. For less emergent requests, the target audience may be social workers and discharge planners.

The hospital environment is very complex, and the AMS provider must understand these nuances to be able to reach the proper decision maker.

CHAPTER REVIEW

Summary

AMS operations are an integral part of the regional EMS system. Understanding the role and nuances of AMS programs is an important consideration for all EMS leaders. The delivery and organizational models may be very diverse. In each case, the particular model in use may impact how the program is integrated. The regulatory considerations are substantial, and this may result in additional oversight for the AMS program. The unique operating environment makes staff deployment, safety programs, communication center capability, and technology deployment special considerations.

WHAT WOULD YOU DO? Reflection

What type of air medical transports would be needed in the county?

It is likely that the county would benefit most from a helicopter capability. This solution would allow the new operation to support scene responses for trauma and other time-sensitive patient types who will require rapid access to a higher level of care. It would also allow for interfacility transports serving the health care institutions located within the county.

What are the implications of the structure of the relationship forged by the county?

The new arrangement seems to have been conceived as a joint venture between the county and the aviation management partner. Although the details of the agreement are not clear, it seems reasonable to expect that benefits and risks are shared on several elements of the operation. Both parties typically share the financial risk, the operational responsibility, and the marketing and public relations responsibility.

What regulatory agencies will have jurisdiction over this new aspect of the operation?

In this situation, multiple areas of regulatory oversight are applicable. The liaison will likely need to become familiar with requirements of the FAA, the rules of the state department of health applicable to air medical transport, and any regional guidelines that might apply. It may also be useful for the liaison to seek additional background information from applicable accrediting agencies.

How should the operation be staffed, and what credentials will be required?

Based on the mission profile and related considerations, the liaison and the medical leadership would need to evaluate various options for the clinical staff. It would seem likely that a nurse–paramedic crew composition would be suitable. The aviation staffing is prescribed by applicable FAA regulations.

What safety enhancements will be necessary to support the operation?

The air medical operation will require an expanded safety effort that incorporates some new elements of patient safety and provider safety, along with a robust aviation safety program. A number of tools are available from outside organizations, such as the FAA, AAMS, and various professional associations that should be considered to support development of an enhanced safety program.

What additional training will the leadership liaison require?

A variety of resources are available for learning more about the leadership considerations in AMS. The MTLI program sponsored by AAMS is a solid place to start. It would be logical for all members of the leadership team to become Certified Medical Transport Executives.

Review Questions

1. Define the current AMS capability in your jurisdiction, and describe how these resources are integrated into the system.
2. What are the four common organizational models found in AMS operations?
3. List three parameters that should be evaluated when selecting a rotary wing aircraft for AMS operations.
4. What segment of the Federal Aviation Regulations (FARs) is applicable to AMS?
5. Prepare an analysis of the pros and cons of each common AMS staffing model, and recommend one for the operation in your jurisdiction.
6. What are some of the unique functions that should be included in a job description for a communication specialist employed in a center that supports AMS operations?
7. List the key elements of a safety management system as defined by the FAA.
8. Investigate the cost and prepare a cost-benefit analysis for deploying an NTSB-recommended safety technology.

Chapter Review continues on p. 126

References

Association of Air Medical Services. (2010). "Medical Transport Leadership Institute." See the organization website.

Board Certification for Emergency Nurses. (2012). CFRN. Emergency Nurses Association. See the organization website.

Board for Critical Care Transport Paramedic Certification. (2009). "Frequently Ask(ed) Questions." See the organization website.

Bock, H., D. Samuels, and P. Campbell. (1988). "Air Medical Crew National Standard Curriculum." Washington, DC: National Highway Traffic Safety Administration.

Center for Transportation Injury Research. (2009). "Atlas & Database of Air Medical Services." Accessed September 15, 2010, at www.adamsairmed.org

Centers for Medicare & Medicaid Services. (2002). "Medicare Benefit Policy Manual, Chapter 10 – Ambulance Services (Rev. 133, 10-22-10)." See the organization website.

Federal Aviation Administration. (2010, April 23). "Mission." See the organization website.

James, Scott. (2004). Module 2: Industry Standards in "Guidelines for Air Medical Crew Education." Alexandria, VA: Association of Air Medical Services and National Highway Traffic Safety Administration. p 83.

Landis, D., and K. Jones. (2010). "Enhancing Your Public Image: Beyond Trinkets and Trash." Alexandria, VA: Association of Air Medical Services: Medical Transport Leadership Institute (MTLI).

National Transportation Safety Board. (2006). "Special Investigation Report on Emergency Medical Services Operations." Washington, DC: National Transportation Safety Board.

Nelson, K. (2010). *Creating A Safety Based Culture.* Alexandria, VA: Association of Air Medical Services: Medical Transport Leadership Institute (MTLI).

Pickering, T. (2010). *SMS: A Culture of Safety.* Alexandria, VA: Association of Air Medical Services: Medical Transport Leadership Institute (MTLI).

Key Terms

air medical services (AMS) Refers to the provision of medical transport services with the use of aircraft.

Air and Surface Transport Nurses Association (ASTNA) Formerly the National Flight Nurses Association (NFNA). The professional association that represents a large number of nurses involved in AMS and critical care ground transport.

Association of Air Medical Services (AAMS) An international trade association that represents a large segment of AMS providers.

aviation maintenance technician An individual with special expertise and training to maintain aircraft. The technician is required, in most cases, to maintain certification by the proper authorities to provide this service.

Board for Critical Care Transport Paramedic Certification (BCCTPC) The professional body that awards special certification to paramedics who operate in the AMS and/or critical care ground environment.

Certified Flight Paramedic (FP-C) A special certification issued to paramedics who are or seek to be involved in the AMS industry.

Certified Flight Registered Nurse (CFRN) A special certification issued to nurses who are or seek to be involved in the AMS industry.

Certified Medical Transport Executive (CMTE) A certification acknowledging satisfactory mastery of leadership materials and concepts. It is offered at the successful completion of the Medical Transport Leadership Institute.

Federal Aviation Administration (FAA) The primary arm of the U.S. government with jurisdiction over aviation-related matters. Many other countries have equivalent entities.

fixed wing Airplanes.

International Association of Flight & Critical Care Paramedics (IAFCCP) Formerly the National Flight Paramedics Association (NFPA). The professional association that represents a large number of paramedics involved in AMS and critical care ground transport.

rotary wing Helicopters.

CHAPTER **7** # Deployment and Staffing Models

STEVEN COTTER, M.B.A., NREMT-P

Objectives

After reading this chapter, the student should be able to:

7.1 Explain and demonstrate basis techniques of temporal or time series demand analysis.

7.2 Explain the differences, advantages, and disadvantages of geographic versus demand-based ambulance deployment.

7.3 Define the limitations of deterministic maximal and set-coverage geospatial modeling.

7.4 Explain the importance of appropriately managing "controllable" time segments, such as chute times, hospital drop times, and lost unit hours.

7.5 Explain the impacts of shift scheduling patterns in system efficiency as well as any potential negative impacts to patient clinical outcomes and operations safety.

Overview

Ambulance services in the United States range in size from one ambulance operated by volunteers and managed by a community board of directors to large governmental agencies and even larger, private, for-profit corporations. This text presents information that the manager of an ambulance service, large or small, needs in order to keep the business solvent and provide clinically excellent service to the community.

Key Terms

geospatial demand	**set covering model**	**temporal demand**	**unit hour utilization**
lost unit hours	**Structured Query**	**total task time**	**(UHU)**
maximal covering	**Language (SQL)**		
model			

WHAT WOULD YOU DO?

You have just been named director of an urban/suburban ambulance service that serves a population of 300,000 and responds to approximately 40,000 calls for service per year. Despite the addition of three ambulances over the past 2 years, the service's response performance to 9-1-1 calls for service continues to remain worse than expected, and in some areas it is actually increasing. When speaking to the service's staff, many people tell you that it seems like, at certain times of the day, the service does not have enough available ambulances to serve all of the incoming calls. In addition, those ambulances that are available are often in stations that are a long distance from the call site. You have been assigned to assess the operation's performance and make recommendations about how to improve the service's responsiveness to calls for service while reducing response times to less than what is contractually required. You are not sure why the service cannot meet these obligations despite the fact that you currently staff seventeen ambulances. Is the problem related to enough ambulances? Is the problem where you are placing the ambulances? Is the problem related to how you are managing the time it takes to get ambulances available and ready for another call? Is the problem a combination of these concerns?

▓ INTRODUCTION ————————

The proper matching of supply and demand is a fundamental component of any EMS service's ability to respond reliably to calls for service in life-threatening situations. The goal for today's EMS manager should be to provide a community with reliable and cost-effective service within the local requirements to produce positive patient outcomes in an equitable manner. This reliability factor can and should be achieved in accordance with any reasonable response time requirement.

Often, the traditional EMS management response to increases in demand has been to add ambulances and personnel by placing them in an equidistant manner relative to each other and without considering variations in geospatial patterns. However, simply increasing the number of available ambulances without proper management of both their placement and daily utilization can lead to marked increases in expenses, little or no operational performance improvement, and potentially reduced clinical outcomes for patients should an ambulance service become overpopulated with paramedics, thereby resulting in reduced assessment and intervention opportunities.

■ COMPONENTS OF MODERN DEPLOYMENT

Modern deployment considers workload and factors that utilize available resources to achieve a balance between geographic coverage, response times, and crew satisfaction. Many factors must be considered when developing a deployment plan:

- Required response performance
- Level-of-care requirements
- Population density
- Geographic density
- Call-demand patterns
- Call acuity
- Road networks and traffic patterns
- Locations of health care facilities

To further the concept of deployment and an organization's ability to provide reliable service, managers must understand the factors that can impact the organization's ability to provide optimal service. Included in this is the organization's ability to accurately measure all the time interval subcomponents that make up a task time, productivity factors (**unit hour utilization [UHU]**), human factors, and control of ambulance resources (control of dispatch center processes).

Decisions pertaining to dispatching and vehicle location are critical to success. If the EMS service cannot do both of these well, there will be inefficiencies in the system. These decisions must be made in a dynamic environment. Measures of timeliness and cost effectiveness are used to assess the effectiveness of any ambulance deployment and staffing plan. When designing ambulance deployment and staffing plans, the following assumptions are made:

- There is a standard time, T, such that if the first vehicle arrives on scene within T minutes, then the call service is deemed a success. The specific value of T may vary with the type of call as more serious calls have lower T values.
- A service area is partitioned into zones of any shape, but all calls from a zone originate in the population center. All travel to and from the zone is measured from the zone center point. Data are collected and aggregated at the zone level.

Timeliness is measured in many ways, including the following:

- *Minimum response time:* Minimize the total average time to serve calls.
- *Minimum travel time:* Minimize the maximum travel time to any single call (ensures that no demand point is too far from an ambulance).
- *Maximum area coverage:* Cover as many zones in the area as possible within T minutes of travel.
- *Maximize call coverage:* Cover as many calls in the area as possible within T minutes of travel.

Note that the third and fourth metrics are not equivalent since some zones in the area may have markedly different call loads.

Besides timeliness, there are other objectives for EMS deployment systems:

- *Minimize cost:* Cost is primarily a function of the amount of labor (person-hours) needed to staff the unit-hours per year, the number of stations that must be opened and maintained, and the number of vehicles that must be purchased, supported, and serviced. Labor is typically the largest cost incurred by any ambulance service.
- *Maximize coverage equity:* The manager must balance area performance against performance in a smaller group of zones.
- *Maximize labor equity:* The manager must balance the workload for all employees in the organization. This helps to reduce employee dissatisfaction. *Source: Reprinted by permission from Health Analytics.*

ANALYZING DEMAND DATA

Demand is considered in two distinct ways: temporally (by time of day and day of week) and geospatially (by location). Ambulance service managers must appropriately analyze demand in both circumstances in order to successfully deploy reliable ambulance services.

COMMON DEMAND PATTERNS

Ambulance capacity planning decisions involve both long-term and short-term considerations. Long-term decisions relate to overall level of ambulance capacity planning over a defined period of time (such as 1, 3, or 5 years), response performance requirements, and any other contractual considerations (e.g., mandated ambulance locations related to political considerations, or mandated ambulance additions keyed by population changes). Short-term considerations relate to probable variations in capacity requirements created by, for example, seasonal changes in population and random, irregular fluctuations induced by temporary events such as a road closure. Short term in the EMS industry can be defined as an hour, day, week, month, or any other amount of time less than a year.

In ambulance capacity planning, short-term seasonal variations can occur in two ways. First, daily demand patterns are predictable, from low volume overnight to high volume in the afternoon and evening, with the pattern repeated daily (Figure 7.1). The demand pattern usually fluctuates from weekday to weekday, but it will typically follow the same pattern for each day of the week, with some variation in overall daily volume. For example, in many organizations, demand may be lower on Monday through Wednesday than on Thursday through Saturday, and this pattern might be predictable on a weekly basis.

The second form of short-term seasonal demand can also occur within a cycle due to

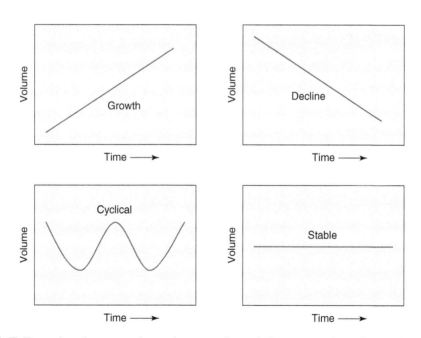

FIGURE 7.1 ■ Examples of common demand patterns for ambulance operations. *Source: Reprinted by permission from Sedgwick County EMS.*

local fluctuations in population volume and type of populations. This can occur in areas that see a large number of seasonal visitors, such as beach vacation communities. For planning purposes, it is very important to understand this type of seasonal variation, especially when using historical demand data. Failure to recognize these seasonal changes can lead to understaffing during periods of high seasonal demand and overstaffing during slower periods based on previous demand that is not representative of the next planning horizon.

These basic demand patterns can be complicated by irregular variations that are sometimes difficult or impossible to predict. This irregularity is created by undefined call clustering, mass casualty incidents, weather emergencies, and so on. This type of irregularity is very difficult to plan for and can have significant impact on an organization's ability to maintain reliable response performance.

The issue of call clustering and the resulting performance degradations was studied in the Santa Barbara, California, EMS system in 2006. Chang and Schoenberg (2006) examined the ability of the ambulance service to reliably perform under load, especially at times when many calls for services were clustered in their arrival to the ambulance service. The researchers found that when significant clusters of calls occurred both temporally and spatially, this random variation in demand load had significant negative impact on the service's ability to maintain effective levels of service. Specifically, "for calls which were preceded by at least one other call within the previous hour and within 20km, the proportion that are violations is 4.56 percent compared with 2.96 percent for calls without such predecessors" (p. 9). Chang and Schoenberg also note that this effect is very pronounced at times when the system is already under high demand loads. This example indicates that ambulance managers must account for the potential of random demand patterns within normal demand, although this issue can

be very difficult to quantify and account for in capacity planning scenarios (Figure 7.2).

Today, technologies are available that can assist EMS managers in monitoring this type of demand variation. The variation depicted in Figure 7.2 is from an EMS service that operates a hybrid deployment system while covering a 1,080-square-mile service area that ranges from dense urban area to sparsely populated farmland. The blue-shaded background denotes the historical incidences of late response. Notice the propensity of late responses after spikes in hourly demand, particularly around 10:00 a.m. This graph also provides a visual representation of the possible mismatch of ambulance peak staffing, as denoted by the red staffing line in this particular example. This matter will be more fully discussed later in this chapter.

■ TEMPORAL DEMAND

Temporal demand analysis focuses on demand based on occurrence counts arrayed and aggregated into weekly demand, daily demand, and hourly demand. Correct interpretation of a temporal, or time-of-day, demand analysis will allow for a determination of the number of ambulance unit hours needed for each hour of the day and each day of the week. When completed, this analysis will supply the manager with staffing needs for a total of 168 hours or the total number of hour for each week. From this analysis, an ambulance staffing model can be built that will appropriately match the demand for ambulance service in a jurisdiction.

FUNDAMENTAL ASSUMPTIONS

Several fundamental assumptions must be understood and managed appropriately when using the temporal demand analysis model:

* Assume each call takes 1 hour to complete.
* Adjust each ambulance service accordingly.

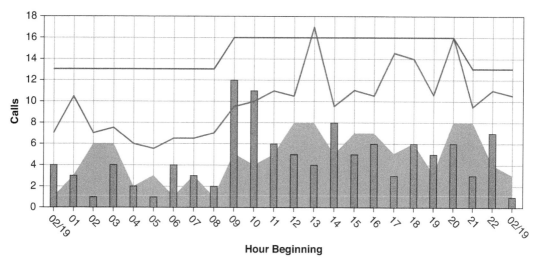

Legend:
Red Line: Hourly staffed ambulances
Blue Line: Historical Average Peak Hourly Demand
Grey Bars: Current Hourly Demand
Blue Background: Historical incidence of calls outside of performance standards each hour

FIGURE 7.2 ▓ Daily demand pattern analysis: Sedgwick County, Kansas. *Source: Reprinted by permission from Sedgwick County EMS.*

* Make adjustments to the number of ambulance resources based on task time if the average is more or less than 60 minutes.
* Ambulance services with lower task times require fewer ambulance resources.
* Ambulance services with higher task times require more ambulance resources.
* Adjustments can be made through demand multipliers or through the performance of a task time analysis.

It is important to note that the proper management of a service's task time can have a significant impact on staffing costs. For example, if an ambulance service has a variable unit hour cost of $80 per staffed ambulance unit hour, transports 50,000 patients per year, and has an average per call task time of 1 hour, the service must expend $4 million per year in direct unit hour costs to accomplish its mission. However, if the task time were to increase to 90 minutes

per transport, the same service would have to spend an additional $2 million per year to accomplish the same mission of 50,000 transports per year with the same reliability.

Task time, as defined previously, is the time the ambulance resource is committed to a call for service until the current call is completed and the ambulance resource is available for another call for service. Within a **total task time** are numerous individual time segments that must be understood and that can be effectively controlled in a balanced manner. Included within these time segments are recommended benchmarks. It is important to understand that the outlined time segments pertain only to the actual capacity planning functions associated with determining the number of ambulances needed at any particular time of day and on any particular day. There are additional time segments to consider, including the dispatching functions prior to the notification of an ambulance resource. These prenotification functions are important when considering the performance of the EMS system overall, but they are not usually considered when planning for ambulance capacity to meet demand for service (Figure 7.3).

PERFORMING A TEMPORAL DEMAND ANALYSIS 4

Temporal demand analysis starts with a query on historical demand. The demand period used in the analysis is typically the 20 most recent weeks of data. However, the exact historical data to be analyzed can and should

vary if the organization routinely experiences significant seasonal variations in overall demand. For instance, in areas with a large influx during summer months of tourists who generate significantly more calls for service than during winter months, it would be more prudent to review data from previous summer months than from slower winter months.

To pull the correct data, the EMS manager must understand several matters pertaining to a computer-aided dispatch (CAD) database schema, including the following:

+ What format the data will be provided in, and whether or not it will need to be converted
+ How the data are stored

Description of Time Interval of Measure	Recommended Fractile Benchmark to Measure
The elapsed time between the crew ~Chute Time~ receiving the call and being en route to the call (wheels turning)	< 60 seconds (90th percentile reliability)
The elapsed time between the crew being en route and arriving at the incident scene (stopped in front of requested location or staging point)	Actual travel time (in an 8:59/90th percentile total response time, this component would be 434 seconds). This will vary slightly both by location and by system design choice.
The elapsed time between the crew's arrival at the location and arrival at the patient	Benchmark for QI purposes—critical, high-rise, and inaccessible patients
The elapsed time between the crew's arrival at the scene and departure for the destination	< 15 minutes, 90th percentile reliability (protocol dependent)
The elapsed time between crew departure from the scene and arrival at the destination	Actual travel time
The elapsed time between the crew's arrival at the destination and its availability for further work	15–30 minutes typically (90th percentile reliability). Call acuity (severity) may require additional benchmarks.
The elapsed time between crew availability and crew departure from destination	Measure to establish internal benchmark
The elapsed time between crew departure and arrival at designated post/location	Measure to establish internal benchmark

 Post Drop (handwritten margin note)

FIGURE 7.3 ■ Typical EMS timing segment benchmarks. *Source: Reprinted by permission from Sedgwick County EMS.*

- How the CAD table relationships and keys work
- What fields must be used to get the correct information
- What table(s) the data are in

In addition, an understanding of the agency's reporting hierarchy and code files within the CAD system must be obtained, including these:

- Agency response areas
- Call types and/or call priorities
- When the clock starts and stops for each call
- Call-cancelled types
- How any call considered for inclusion is captured within the CAD system

Typically **Structured Query Language (SQL)** or Open Database Connectivity (ODBC) connections to the database are used to extract the needed data. The raw CAD data can be extracted to Excel, Access, Crystal, and other such software programs to manipulate them into a usable format for the analysis.

Side Bar

Connecting to Different Data Bases

Open Database Connectivity (ODBC) is a standard database access method developed by the SQL Access group in 1992. The goal of ODBC is to make it possible to access any data from any application, regardless of which database management system (DBMS) is handling the data. ODBC manages this by inserting a middle layer, called a database *driver*, between an application and the DBMS. The purpose of this layer is to translate the application's data queries into commands that the DBMS understands. For this to work, both the application and the DBMS must be *ODBC compliant*—that is, the application must be capable of issuing ODBC commands and the DBMS must be capable of responding to them (Webopedia.com, n.d.).

To correctly array the data for use, manipulation of the data should be by day of week and hour of day. This can be accomplished by using pivot tables in Excel, Access, and so on. Figure 7.4 is an example of the end product that will be used as the template for further temporal demand analysis.

Figure 7.4 is interpreted as follows:

- *Date Column:* Each row in the first column on the left contains a date (in military format), and each represents a day of the week for each of the 20 consecutive weeks analyzed. Figure 7.4 depicts 20 consecutive Mondays.
- *Hourly Data Columns:* Each column beginning 1, 2, 3, etc., represents an hour of each day. Note that this is the hour ending such that column (1) represents the hour from midnight to 1:00 a.m. At the bottom of each column is a total of the number of calls for hour of the day for 20 weeks.
- *Rows:* Each cell with a row of data that corresponds with a date in the first column represents the amount of hourly demand for each day represented. For example, for (20091012) at "1" or hour ending 1:00 a.m., there were five units of demand.
- *Total Column:* The far-right column depicts the total amount of defined demand for each 24-hour period, or day, being analyzed. For example, the total demand for the 24-hour period 20091012 was 134.

It is important to note when selecting data that the EMS manager must determine and know what type of data are being selected. The demand counts represented in Figure 7.4 can either be transports from a scene or total responses to a scene, irrespective of transport determination. This is typically a local decision, but it must be understood. Rationale for inclusion of only transports includes the determination that transports generate revenue. Rationale to capture all responses to a scene includes the fact that the response required a unit of ambulance supply and must be accounted for in the demand analysis.

Hr Ending	1	2	3	4	5	6	7	8	9	10	11	12	13	14	15	16	17	18	19	20	21	22	23	24	Totals
20091012	5	4	6	0	2	2	3	8	6	4	7	7	10	10	6	6	5	8	5	6	9	7	1	7	134
20091019	3	5	3	2	1	4	4	2	6	7	6	10	16	7	5	4	11	6	11	6	8	8	7	6	148
20091026	7	5	3	3	1	1	2	2	4	6	5	1	0	7	3	9	9	8	3	2	5	6	2	3	97
20091102	4	4	3	2	1	1	4	3	4	5	4	8	8	6	9	3	5	5	6	3	3	5	3	3	102
20091109	4	4	3	1	0	2	4	1	7	7	6	5	9	2	0	7	8	6	10	5	5	5	6	3	110
20091116	1	2	4	1	3	2	3	8	6	1	4	5	3	4	7	8	3	5	7	5	9	3	4	5	103
20091123	5	3	5	3	0	2	0	4	4	3	5	9	6	4	3	12	9	7	7	8	5	2	7	6	119
20091130	1	7	5	3	3	8	1	5	4	1	5	8	13	6	6	5	3	6	3	3	4	5	1	3	113
20091207	5	6	0	5	2	2	2	3	5	4	5	5	6	8	10	4	4	8	7	4	4	4	5	6	114
20091214	4	4	3	2	1	0	3	6	7	2	7	6	7	2	4	7	8	4	11	5	2	2	3	7	107
20091221	6	3	0	1	3	1	4	2	3	8	8	2	0	8	6	8	7	14	5	7	9	5	5	6	120
20091228	0	3	7	4	2	4	2	2	4	2	7	9	5	4	6	14	8	5	5	9	4	5	3	5	118
20100104	1	6	0	2	1	3	7	4	2	6	6	7	4	13	3	6	8	5	8	6	8	2	7	4	119
20100111	3	4	3	0	2	0	4	4	5	8	5	7	2	8	7	7	8	6	5	5	5	5	7	13	120
20100118	6	4	2	3	3	0	0	2	7	4	5	5	6	5	7	1	6	2	3	11	3	6	4	6	99
20100125	5	0	4	2	4	3	2	6	3	16	9	6	0	15	7	3	6	4	11	8	7	2	4	7	132
20100201	3	4	3	3	3	4	3	4	7	6	5	4	8	4	4	2	4	6	5	5	3	8	5	6	109
20100208	8	8	5	6	2	6	6	3	6	8	6	11	5	4	6	5	5	4	9	8	3	6	8	4	139
20100215	8	1	1	3	6	1	3	5	3	6	5	6	6	3	3	4	3	3	4	4	6	2	3	8	95
20100222	3	7	3	2	4	2	1	4	11	7	3	4	9	3	8	6	6	6	4	7	3	5	6	1	115
Total	82	84	63	44	44	43	58	78	108	111	112	125	123	123	107	121	126	118	131	117	102	93	91	109	2313

FIGURE 7.4 ■ 20-week temporal demand count for Mondays: Sedgwick County, Kansas. *Source: Reprinted by permission from Sedgwick County EMS.*

A complete temporal demand analysis will include data aggregation as depicted in Figure 7.4 for each day of the week such that seven identical tables are produced.

DATA ANALYTICS FOR TEMPORAL DEMAND

Figure 7.5 corresponds to the data array previously reviewed in Figure 7.4 in that each column represents the hour of the day aggregately for the 20 weeks being analyzed. These calculations are used to determine the number of ambulance units required for each hour of the day and each day of the week (in this case for Mondays). The following subsections present an overview of the specific formulas and calculations needed to generate the "Staff To" line at the bottom of the formula sheet.

Excel Functions

The first six formula rows to include Min, Max, Mean, Median, Mode, and Stdev are standard Excel functions. These formulas are as follows:

* *Min* is the minimum number of call for all hours.
  * Excel Formula: Min(CR:CR) where CR indicates cell reference in the excel worksheet. For example the CR is defined as "cell reference" and could reference cell E42 in an Excel spreadsheet.
* *Max* is the maximum number of calls for all hours.
  * Excel Formula: Max(CR:CR)
* *Average* is the average number of calls for all hours.
  * Excel Formula: average(CR:CR)
* *Stdev* is the standard deviation of calls for all hours.
  * Excel Formula: stdev(CR:CR)
* *90th percentile* is a statistical ranking method used to determine the demand at X percent.
  * Excel Formula: percentile(CR:CR,.9) where .9 = 90 percent

Specific Temporal Demand Analysis Formulas

The remaining formulas were originally developed by Jack Stout and have been proven to be statistically reliable. Experience shows that the Average Peak formula process will generally result in an accurate prediction of 90th percentile (90th%) of demand.

Side Bar

Predicting Call Volume

Predicting the number of crews needed for deployment in any community and when those crews will be scheduled, based on anticipated call volumes, is not a completely accurate process. However, because of the vital nature of EMS services, managers are charged with ensuring consistent levels of service within budgeted constraints. Researchers at UCLA examined the accuracy of call volume predictions calculated utilizing demand pattern analysis, including those techniques described in this chapter. Brown, Lerner, Larmon, GeGassick, and Taigman (2007) examined seven EMS systems utilizing 73 consecutive weeks of hourly call volume data. The first 20 weeks were used to calculate three common demand pattern analysis constructs for call volume prediction: average peak, smoothed average peak, and 90th percentile rank.

The researchers compared actual call volume in the last 52 weeks of the study to the predicted call volumes by using descriptive statistics. The group concluded that generally demand pattern analysis estimated or overestimated call volume, making their use a reasonable predictor for ambulance staffing patterns. When call volumes were overestimated, predictions exceeded actual call volume by a median (interquartile range) of 4 (2–6) calls for average peak, 4 (2–6) calls for smoothed average peak, and 3 (2–5) calls for 90th percentile rank. Call volumes were underestimated 4 percent of the time using average peak, 4 percent using smoothed average peak, and

Total	141	146	108	80	83	76	99	140	189	193	196	219	203	214	191	213	214	203	227	212	174	155	163	196	4035
Min	0	0	0	0	0	0	0	2	2	1	3	2	0	2	3	1	2	2	3	3	2	2	1	1	33
Max	82	84	63	44	44	43	58	78	108	111	112	125	123	123	107	121	126	118	131	117	102	93	91	109	2313
Mean	9	9	7	5	5	5	6	9	12	12	12	14	13	13	12	13	13	13	14	13	11	10	10	12	252
Median	5	4	3	3	3	2	3	4	6	6	5	6	6	5	6	6	6	6	7	7	4	5	5	6	117
Mode	1	4	3	3	3	2	3	4	7	8	5	5	6	4	7	8	8	6	5	5	3	2	4	6	119
StDev	20	20	15	11	10	10	14	19	26	27	27	30	30	29	25	29	30	28	31	28	24	22	22	26	550
Avg High	20	20	16	11	11	12	14	20	26	28	27	30	30	32	26	31	30	29	32	29	25	22	22	27	537
90th Percentile Rank	8	8	6	5	5	6	7	7	10	12	8	10	11	14	9	13	9	11	10	9	9	7	8	11	136
TMT Multiplier	1	1	1	1	1	1	1	1	1	1	1	1	1	1	1	1	1	1	1	1	1	1	1	1	1
Avg Peak	51	52	40	28	27	29	37	49	67	68	68	77	78	78	67	78	78	76	82	74	64	57	56	70	1217
2x StDev + Mean	48	49	37	26	26	26	34	46	63	65	66	73	72	72	63	71	74	69	77	69	60	54	53	64	1352
Smoothed Average Peak	12	50	40	30	28	30	38	50	64	68	70	76	78	76	72	76	76	77	79	73	64	58	59	64	208
Blended Demand	23	35	28	20	20	21	26	34	45	48	48	53	54	54	48	53	53	53	56	51	44	40	40	29	565
UH Adj/Eff Buffer	4	4	4	4	4	4	4	4	4	4	4	4	4	4	4	4	4	4	4	4	4	4	4	4	96
Staff To	16	54	44	34	32	34	42	54	68	72	74	80	82	80	76	80	81	81	83	77	68	62	63	18	1456

FIGURE 7.5 ■ Application of demand analysis formulas. *Source: Reprinted by permission from Sedgwick County EMS.*

7 percent using 90th percentile rank predictions. When call volumes were underestimated, call volumes exceeded predictions by a median (interquartile range; maximum under estimation) of 1 (1–2; 18) call for average peak, 1 (1–2; 18) call for smoothed average peak, and 2 (1–3; 20) calls for 90th percentile rank. Results did not vary among organizations.

It is important to note also that the models did underestimate call volume between 4 percent and 7 percent of the time. When using these methods, EMS managers need to determine if these rates of over- and underestimation are acceptable given local resources and local priorities.

* *Total Mission Time* (TMT Multiplier) is the average task time for an EMS organization to complete a call for service. This is typically calculated as the average of the difference between the time the call is received by the organization until the ambulance assigned to this call is ready for either the next call or assignment into the organization's geospatial deployment plan.
    * Example: 60 minutes average task time/60 minutes in an hour = 1
    * 90 minutes average task time/60 minutes in an hour 5 1.5
    * 45 minutes average task time/60 minutes in an hour = .75

In our example, the TMT is 1, or 1 hour, for simplicity.
* *Average High* represents approximately 75 percent of demand and is calculated by taking the maximum number of demand counts in each consecutive group of five 4-week periods of a 20-week analysis, then dividing the sum of these numbers by 5. This number is then multiplied by the TMT Multiplier.
    * Excel Formula:

$$((max (CR:CR) + max (CR:CR) + max (CR:CR) + max (CR:CR))/5)* \text{ TMT multiplier}$$

* *Average Peak* represents approximately the 90th percentile of demand. It is calculated by taking the maximum number of calls in each

of the two consecutive 10-week periods of a 20-week analysis, then dividing the sum of these by 2 (or average of the two periods).
    * Excel Formula:

$$((Max (CR:CR) + Max (CR:CR))/2)* \text{ TMT Multiplier}$$

This number is then multiplied by the TMT or Total Task time multiplier to adjust for the average time on task.
* *Smoothed Average Peak* is a statistical smoothing of the Average Peak and is used to "blend" the severity of hour-to-hour demand fluctuations for easier peak-load scheduling. It is calculated by taking 20 percent of the previous hour + 60 percent of the current hour + 20 percent of the next hour.
    * Excel Formula:

$$(CR*.2) + (CR*.6) + (CR*.2)$$

* *2x StdDev + Mean* is a statistical process control methodology used as an upper control chart limit. It represents approximately the 95th percentile of demand. It is calculated by taking the standard deviation calculated previously for the hour, multiplying it by 2, then adding it to the previously calculated average for the hour. This result is then multiplied by the TMT multiplier to adjust for task time.
    * Excel Formula:

$$((std dev*2) + (avg))* \text{TMT Multiplier}$$

* *UH Adj/Eff Buffer* allows the manager to adjust the staffing line to accommodate unique service concerns and/or inefficiency factors. Included within this are items such as contractual minimum staffing levels. For example, in the table above the Staff To line shows a staffing level of 10 ambulances during the overnight hours. Should this service be under a contractual obligation to maintain a minimum staffing of 12 ambulances, this constraint can be factored into this buffer.
In addition, this buffer calculation allows EMS managers to account for inefficiencies, or **lost unit hours** and other variables. Specifically, lost

unit hours are units of time that an ambulance is unavailable for calls within the deployment plan for any reason when it otherwise would be expected to be available. This can include off-load delays at hospitals beyond expected time frames, vehicle failures, administrative needs, employee injuries, supply chain/logistics problems, and so on. Often it is very difficult for managers to capture the time allocated to these issues because of CAD system deficiencies or lack of awareness. However, these types of system design inefficiencies are often a large component of both response time exceptions and deficits in organizational performance and capacity planning.

• *Staff To* is the number of unit hours or staffed ambulances required for that hour of that day. It typically defines the minimum number of expected demand at Xth percentile based on the particular demand formula chosen. In this example, we are using the Average Peak + UH Adj/Eff Buffer to calculate the required staffing levels. This is equivalent to the 90th percentile of demand in the period analyzed.

The output of these calculations is depicted graphically in Figure 7.6.

Of note here is the fact that the Staff To line (green line) does not match exactly the Current Staffing line. This mismatch occurs both as overstaffing and understaffing comparative to the model. This is not unusual since it is very difficult to create a schedule that exactly matches the demand model. Schedule to demand line variation can range from as little as 3 percent in a well-managed service to as much as 20 percent in services with fixed schedules that may or may not include peak-load staffing models. The goal with this or any capacity modeling technique is to approximate as closely as possible the supply and demand within defined cost constraints, crew work load requirements, and response time requirements placed on the service.

UNIT HOUR UTILIZATION

Too often, managers work diligently to match supply and demand without understanding the

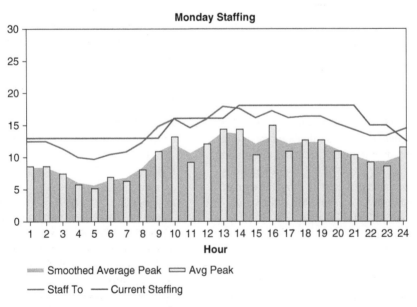

FIGURE 7.6 ■ Temporal demand graphical output. *Source: Reprinted by permission from Sedgwick County EMS.*

workload effects on the service's staff, both aggregately and on an individual unit basis. To assist in the balance of employee needs and service needs, managers must understand and calculate unit hour utilizations (UHUs). The typical ratio is number of transports/number of staffed hours for a period of measurement, or:

> UHU = number of transports per period/total number of hours staffed per period

> *Example:* An ambulance crew is on duty and in service for 12 hours and transports 6 patients during this 12-hour period, or:

> UHU = 6 transports/12 ambulance staffed hours = .5 UHU

The underlying assumption in this calculation is that each call and transport again takes 1 hour to complete. Should the manager find that the time to complete the call is actually 1 hour and 30 minutes on average, this must be factored into the UHU calculation since the ambulance crew will actually be engaged on each call for an additional 30 minutes. This translates to a calculated UHU of .75, or a relation of 9 of the 12 hours being utilized to transport 6 patients. Conversely, if a crew can transport each patient in 45 minutes, this translates to a UHU of .375, or a relation of 4.5 of the 12 hours being utilized to transport 6 patients.

This measure, although simplistic in appearance, is very misunderstood and difficult to explain, especially to policy makers, the public, and EMS providers. In manufacturing processes, utilization rates can and should approach 100 percent within the effective capacity of a well-designed process. This can occur in this instance because the process is designed to experience very little variability and because, in the manufacturing environment, machines and technology, rather than human beings, are often the primary components of the process.

Conversely, in service environments such as EMS and health care, humans must carry out the service and clinical processes and are by their nature subject to more variability in their service product output and the time that it takes to produce this output while at the patient's side. In addition, service environments suffer from increased variability to include (Cachon and Terwiesch, 2006):

* *The inflow of units or patients requesting service.* The biggest source of variability comes from the market itself. Although the general pattern of service requests are predictable, uncertainty always remains about when exactly the next patient will require service.
* *Variability in activity times.* Whenever we are dealing with human operators as a resource, some variability in their behavior is likely. Another source of variability is activity time specific to the EMS service environment in that in most EMS operations the customer is involved in many of the tasks constituting activity time. This is especially true in the EMS environment, considering that each patient will require varying levels of on-scene care that can extend scene times. EMS customers in general have a choice of health care institutions. This may create some variability in service times due to longer or shorter than expected transport times.
* *Random availability of resources.* Ambulances are subject to random breakdowns even with the best maintenance programs employed. In addition, ambulances might not be available to a service for a myriad of other reasons that must be understood and managed.
* *Random routing in the case of multiple flow units in the process.* If an organization does not have the ability to adequately determine which is the closest ambulance to a call for service, variability is created by virtue of a less-than-optimal candidate selection process. In addition, variability may result from the flow of a patient to a more distant tertiary facility that is not in the locale of the ambulance service in question for specialized care of the patient, such as a trauma patient. (p. 105)

An understanding of the foundations of service sector utilization limitations is important for the EMS manager to understand. Generally, the UHU for an organization can range anywhere from .1 or lower in static, low-performing organizations up to .5, or higher, in systems that tightly control the number of available units based on demand. It is important to remember that in a service sector—and particularly in the EMS setting when utilization rates and system failure rates increase in the form of delayed ambulance responses, crew burnout, accidents, and/or patient care errors—customer satisfaction with the quality of services rendered may decrease rapidly as well. Although this failure will depend on the effectiveness of the analysis and system design employed, this increased risk can occur well below utilization rates normally seen in the manufacturing environment. Thus,

the EMS manager must carefully monitor and manage workload while communicating to both employees and policy makers the impacts of increased workload and the corresponding utilization rates.

■ GEOSPATIAL DEMAND ANALYSIS

Geospatial demand, like temporal demand, occurs in a variable manner within a predictive pattern. Generally, demand for EMS services is correlated with population density (Figure 7.7).

Because people and their activities generate demand for EMS services, it is important to understand that geospatial demand will change based on these activities, population demographic types, and the movement of population centers during specific time periods. In Figure 7.8,

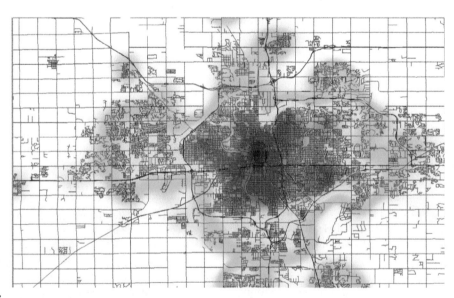

Legend:
Green: Low historical call volume
Yellow: Medium historical call volume
Red: High historical call volume
Purple: Highest historical call volume

FIGURE 7.7 ■ Cumulative demand density analysis: Sedgwick County, Kansas. *Source: Reprinted by permission from Sedgwick County EMS.*

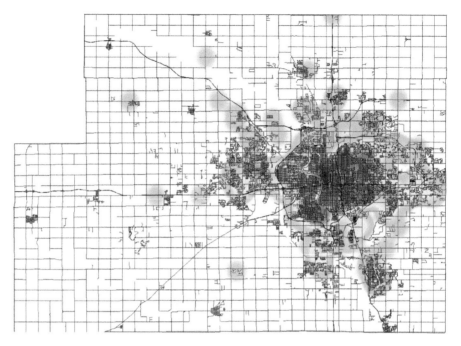

Legend:
Green: Low historical call volume
Yellow: Medium historical call volume
Red: High historical call volume
Purple: Highest historical call volume

FIGURE 7.8 ▨ Demand density for Tuesdays, 1400–1500 hours: Sedgwick County, Kansas. *Source: Reprinted by permission from Sedgwick County EMS.*

this demand is measured over a 2-year period in a cumulative manner and is consistent with the population centers within this community. The darker areas toward the center of the metropolitan area depict the highest levels of demand, whereas the lighter (green) areas depict the areas of lowest historical demand.

Analysis of different time frames reveals distinct changes in the overall demand pattern, location, and intensity. The data in Figure 7.9 were collected over the same time frame as the overall 2-year demand assessment interval and reveal distinct changes in the geospatial distribution of demand for EMS services over differing days and hours.

When analyzing these changes, it is important to understand potential factors driving demand pattern changes. These factors can include general movement of population centers, such as daily movement or people from suburban residential areas to core business areas of a community. Does the community in question have other unique qualities, such as special populations—for example, skilled nursing facilities; major traffic arteries; mass gathering facilities; concentrations of bars or other nightlife activities; hospitals (if they are transfer generators); areas of high poverty or low normative health care access; and so on. Analysis may reveal a general correlation of demand to the factors driving it. This is important because EMS managers generally fail to appreciate unique underlying demand drivers in a community. As a result, ambulance deployment patterns and plans

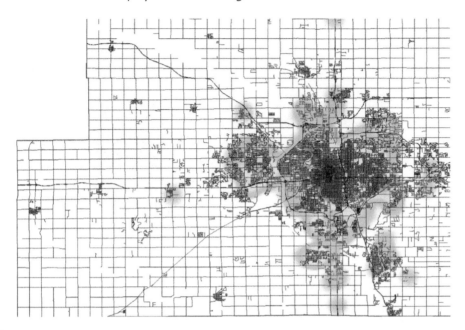

Legend:
Green: Low historical call volume
Yellow: Medium historical call volume
Red: High historical call volume
Purple: Highest historical call volume

FIGURE 7.9 ■ Cumulative demand density for Mondays, 0400–0559 hours: Sedgwick County, Kansas Hours. *Source: Reprinted by permission from Sedgwick County EMS.*

will often be mismatched to specific geospatial demand pattern changes (Figure 7.10).

TRADITIONAL GEOSPATIAL MODELING TECHNIQUES

As EMS has evolved, so has our ability to use modeling techniques to understand and respond to demands for service. Ambulance deployment modeling techniques range from simplistic deterministic models that account for limited variables, such as aggregate demand only, to advanced mathematical models that include heuristic probability factors or hypercube modeling techniques that can account for multiple variables in varied combinations, such as variability of demand, the potential for

an ambulance to be busy and unavailable on a random basis, and the need for dynamic redeployment of ambulances. The math that the more sophisticated models utilize is beyond the scope of this text: It is very complicated, requires intensive computer-based technologies to utilize correctly in a dynamic environment, can be very expensive, and is often beyond the ability of most EMS organizations to acquire. Because of these factors, and due to the need for ease of use, the set covering and maximal covering are the most utilized models. These latter two models also have the potential to be the least accurate in environments that are more dynamic. Thus, it is important for EMS managers to understand the basic premises of these two models and the limitations in their practical use.

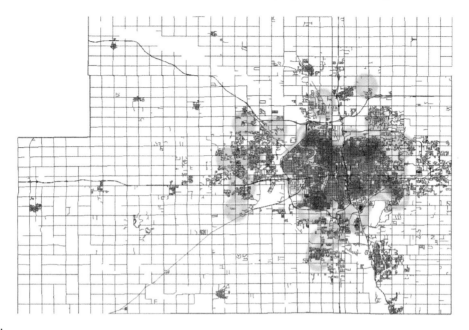

Legend:
Green: Low historical call volume
Yellow: Medium historical call volume
Red: High historical call volume
Purple: Highest historical call volume

FIGURE 7.10 ▪ Cumulative demand density for Thursdays, 1400–1500 hours: Sedgwick County, Kansas. *Source: Reprinted by permission from Sedgwick County EMS.*

The **set covering model** seeks to minimize the number of vehicles that is needed to cover all specified zones. A zone can be any geospatial area designated by the planner. The premise of this model is to minimize cost and provide equitable coverage. Analysis allows each vehicle to have a unique of demand data that it covers and all demand points are considered equal in importance irrespective of the any associated acuity level for each individual demand point. This model generally overestimates an organization's ability to cover demand because it fails to account for times when the unit being analyzed is busy.

The **maximal covering model** takes a slightly different approach in that it holds the number of vehicles fixed, then locates the vehicles to cover as many calls as possible within a required response time. This objective can result in some zones or areas of a response district being uncovered. Again, there is no allowance for the vehicle(s) being analyzed already being busy.

The key deficiencies in the set covering and maximal covering models are (Goldberg, 2004):

♦ The use of a single objective, when in fact both cost and performance are key.
♦ The inability to consider sometimes busy vehicles and therefore uncovered demand even though the model claims full coverage. This also leads to the assumption that the closest vehicle to each zone is the only vehicle that ever answers calls for that zone.
♦ All demand, travel time, and service time data are assumed to be deterministic. In reality,

demand timing and location are both random but predictable and modelable based on past data. Service times and travel times are also random and sometimes highly variable.

♦ Using single sets of data leads to a single set of locations and hence these models have no ability to analyze dynamic real-time decisions such as repositioning. (pp. 26–27) *Reprinted by permission from Health Analytics*

Coverage models have been used frequently by researchers and service managers for the following reasons:

♦ The concept is simple to communicate to decision makers and the public (a call is either covered or not).
♦ Many EMS services use the percentage of calls covered as a performance measure. Perhaps the most common EMS standard is to respond to 90 percent of all urgent calls within 8 minutes, although there is no clinical evidence to support this standard.
♦ Deterministic coverage models typically result in integer programs that are easy to solve using standard optimization software.

AMBULANCE DEPLOYMENT PLANNING

Ambulance deployment plan methodologies can range widely but generally fall within three categories: fixed (static geographic-based) deployment, dynamic-demand-based deployment, and hybrid-demand/geographic-based deployment.

Fixed (Static Geographic-Based) Deployment

Plans of this nature involve the placement of ambulances within equally distributed geographic zones or call areas typically within a station-based plan. These placements may or may not coincide with the geospatial demand load on a whole system or during specific times of the day. This mismatch, compounded with the fact that ambulances are generally busy in a random pattern, can lead to coverage and response-time problems, especially in areas of increasing demand for service. Generally organizations

that utilize this type of deployment plan depend on the dispatch of the first due ambulance within the zone that a call for service occurs in and will always assign the first-due ambulance to the call despite the location of other ambulances within that zone at the time of the request for service. If another call occurs within this same zone, then another ambulance from outside of the original zone, or the next due ambulance, is assigned to the call. This process can continue with gradual degradation of coverage and response-time effectiveness for both the area immediate to the call location and for a service area in general if calls continue to occur within the same general area until the original unit assigned to this zone returns to service or until there are no ambulances left to respond. This process can also repeat itself sporadically as calls for EMS service occur within the larger service area. If demand continues to rob geographic coverage, eventually large geospatial holes will occur, leaving large geographic areas with high historical demand uncovered. For instance, if an organization's only available ambulance within an area of high historical demand is assigned to a static plan, the organization will not be able to respond to that demand; in addition, response times will probably increase due to the likelihood that this last ambulance resource will be consumed followed by additional calls for which there will be no ambulance available to respond (Figure 7.11).

This type of deployment plan has its basis in the origins of ambulance deployment and system design before the advent of the modern high-performance or dynamic ambulance deployment methodologies and the technologies to support these plans. This type of planning is still used in many places for many reasons—some valid, others not. Static-based plans can be useful in very low-volume organizations where demand for EMS services is limited and where geospatial demand patterns are fairly static, meaning that the demands for service tend to occur from the same locations. Generally, this type of plan overemphasizes geographic

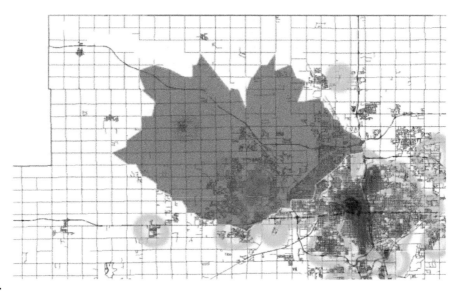

Legend:
Green: Low historical call volume
Yellow: Medium historical call volume
Red: High historical call volume
Purple: Highest historical call volume
Red Polygon: Expected drive time coverage of positioned ambulance

FIGURE 7.11   Static ambulance placement example: Sedgwick County, Kansas. *Source: Reprinted by permission from Sedgwick County EMS.*

coverage of a service area, underemphasizes response-time equity, and fails to recognize that the geospatial demand for EMS services is fluid rather than static, as depicted in the demand analysis graphs in Figures 7.8, 7.9, and 7.10.

In areas where geospatial demand fluctuates or where temporal demand is increasing each year, a static plan will either become very inefficient due to lack of coverage and response-time equity or it will become very expensive because of the need to add more ambulances than are needed based on a temporal demand analysis. This cost is compounded if these ambulances are placed within stations that must be built or leased and maintained.

Dynamic Demand-Based Deployment

Dynamic-demand based deployment processes are the extreme opposite of static-based

deployment plans. These plans focus solely on demand and tend to deemphasize the need to provide overall geospatial coverage and, hence, equity of service. This approach can lead to ambulance crews spending time changing post locations without a call assignment, increased costs of fleet maintenance due to excess mileage from the deployment plan, increased fuel costs, unneeded stress on ambulance crews, and the potential for frequent, unacceptable, and even life-threatening response times to peripheral areas of a service district.

Hybrid-Demand/Geographic-Based Deployment

This deployment practice starts with the allocation of geographic-based units in order to maximize both the demand and geography of a service area that is covered (Figure 7.12).

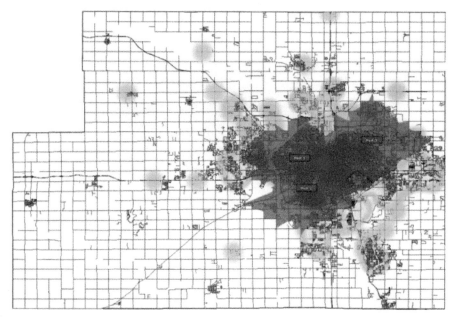

Legend:
Green: Low historical call volume
Yellow: Medium historical call volume
Red: High historical call volume
Purple: Highest historical call volume
Blue Polygon: Expected drive time coverage of positioned ambulances

FIGURE 7.12 ■ Ambulance placement relative to demand. *Source: Reprinted by permission from Sedgwick County EMS.*

Typically, a planner will place one ambulance such that it covers as much demand and geography as possible. Then this process will be repeated until both a maximal amount of demand and geography is covered with the number of ambulances that are available to the organization. The amount of "service area" overlap can and will vary, as is depicted in Figure 7.12. Once the geographic base is in place, the planner can begin to examine demand-based post points that are typically in the areas of highest demand and that are interspersed within the geographic posts that were assigned earlier in the process. The location and number of demand-based units/posts will depend on variables that include the intensity of the historical demand in the area

being analyzed, the probability of ambulances in an area of high historic demand being unavailable for call, or to the amount of anticipated variation in drive time to a call based on changing road conditions and traffic patterns.

The goal in this approach is to balance an organization's ability to maintain equitable response times with equitable and reasonable individual crew workloads while deploying an appropriate number of ambulances into an area in a cost-effective manner. Properly utilized, this approach will allow the crews to have some downtime at a physical post while still allowing a changing demand pattern and a deployment plan that allows flexibility through the utilization of demand-based street-level deployment points.

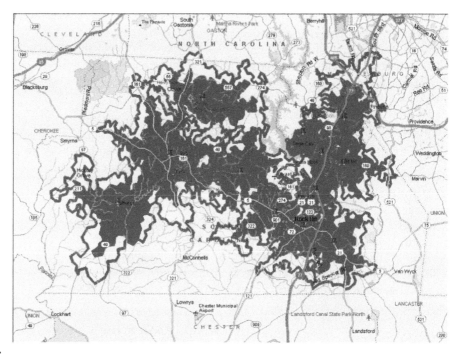

Legend:
Blue: 7-minute drive time from assigned post
Yellow: 9-minute drive time from assigned post

FIGURE 7.13 ▦ Seven-minute versus ten-minute drive time coverage. *Source: Reprinted by permission from Sedgwick County EMS.*

When attempting to maintain geographic coverage equity, it is important to understand that the amount of coverage based on the distance that an ambulance can travel will vary based on road network changes. Thus, it becomes very important to be able to incorporate modeling into the plan based on GIS mapping and knowledge about actual travel-time variation. This information can be obtained by utilizing actual GPS data from ambulances, if available, as they carry out daily activities. Incorporating this information with demand data will allow for a much more precise estimate of coverage and the organization's ability to provide reliable response time based on changing conditions. Figure 7.13 shows a defined difference in this organization's ability to respond in a 7-minute versus a 10-minute time frame. The blue areas

indicate a 7-minute drive-time coverage capability while the yellow areas indicate a 10-minute drive-time capability.

Modeling techniques such as this, supported by good geographic information system data, will allow for a much more realistic understanding of the demand for service in a jurisdiction and an organization's ability to respond in an effective manner. For example, if the organization depicted in Figure 7.13 incorporates a 10-minute drive-time expectation and can only achieve 7 minutes reliably, then a change in the deployment plan might be warranted.

Redeployment of ambulances in a dynamic fashion presents a very difficult problem for EMS mangers. Plans that are too aggressive as calls for service are received tend to cause needless domino-style move-ups of available ambulances. In a properly utilized hybrid plan, all geographic posts should be covered first as units become available. Subsequent units can then be assigned as required to demand-based posts within the plan. Thus, if a geographic coverage unit is activated for a call, coverage can either be reestablished with a proximate demand-based unit or with a unit that becomes available from a hospital or other site. Conversely, if a demand-based unit is activated with properly placed geographic-based units also in place, rarely is there a need to redeploy other local units.

It is important to understand that this type of plan is dynamic and should be designed to flex and contract in a logical manner over specific periods of time and unit availability. These changes should correlate with the known geospatial demand patterns within the organization's service area responsibility.

GEOGRAPHIC INFORMATION SYSTEMS

Geographic information system (GIS) technology integrates tabular data with geographic features to assess and better understand real-world problems. This real-world problem for EMS providers is the proper allocation of a specified number of ambulances in both space and time in order to provide a reliable level of service as measured by response-time performance in a cost-effective manner. Unlike a paper map, a GIS-generated map can incorporate many layers of varied information that provide unique views of a geographic space. GIS layers for EMS providers can include population characteristics, such as age demographics and overall population locations and trends, as well as locations of the following:

- Streets
- Land parcels
- Topography
- Lakes, rivers, other bodies of water
- Hospitals
- Ambulance stations

- Other emergency services, such as fire and law enforcement
- Specialty-care and long-term-care facilities
- Schools
- Public venues, such as shopping malls and theaters

GIS can also assist in analysis of incidents within a jurisdiction in order to display trends, illustrate patterns, and identify areas of high call volume. Incident data utilized can include the following:

- Incident type
- Incident cause
- Date of the incident
- Time of the incident
- Unit that was dispatched
- Unit that arrived on scene

AMBULANCE SCHEDULING

Once the EMS manager has measured the temporal demand for ambulance services, a schedule must be built that manages this demand factor within the expected and accepted risk level. This risk is usually measured as a response-time requirement, such as 90 percent of all responses within 9 minutes, and within some form of an EMS provider workload requirement, such as a system unit hour utilization, or UHU, such as .4. These requirements will vary from system to system, and there is no set or recommended threshold for either measure outside of the 5-minute threshold for responses to cardiac arrest patients. UHU workload requirements can vary from less than .1 to as high as .5. Managers must consider schedule patterns, the required time on task for each assignment, the total time deployed per shift, and other factors to achieve efficiency and avoid crew exhaustion (Fitch, 1991). Generally, schedules should be designed and managed in consideration of clinical effectiveness, the support of healthy and well-rested crews, the ability of the organization to support the schedule requirements logistically, and the constraints of a budget.

Consequences of Shift Work

The body's internal clock is controlled by circadian rhythms that regulate various functions, including wakefulness, over each 24-hour period. Working nights and on rotating shifts can disrupt one's normal circadian rhythm and result in sleep debt, which can have serious consequences for personnel health and can affect a service's level of risk and liability. Cognitive function and body temperature are at their lowest between the hours of 2:00 a.m. and 6:00 a.m. Thus, for staff working the night shift, the greatest risk of error or injury can be during these early morning hours when lower body temperature increases the risk of drowsiness and fatigue.

EMS managers must be aware of the impacts and effects of circadian rhythms and work to design schedules that help to limit any adverse impact on personnel. These rhythms affect the following as well as other human functions:

- Body temperature
- Digestion
- Hormone levels
- Mental alertness
- Sleeping patterns

The following body functions show more activity during daytime hours and decrease in function during nighttime hours:

- Body temperature
- Heart rate and blood pressure
- Respiration rate
- Adrenaline production

Effects of Fatigue In 2007 the Australian Council of Ambulance Authorities indicated that shift workers need at least 8 continuous hours of sleep to maintain optimal levels of cognitive and functional performance. A routine lack of sufficient sleep cycles will build what is called sleep debt and result in both short-term and chronic fatigue. The more sleep debt a person accrues, the more likely he is to suffer the effects of fatigue. Fatigue affects a person's judgment skills, clear thinking, and ability to gauge one's own ability to monitor self-fatigue. This lack of effective cognitive ability may lead to a decline in job performance characterized by increased risk of error and unsafe work practices. The most notable effects of fatigue include the following:

- Desire to sleep
- Lack of concentration
- Irritability
- Poor judgment
- Reduced hand–eye coordination
- Impaired memory in relation to timing and events
- Reduced visual perception
- Reduced alertness
- Slowed reaction times
- Increased risk-taking behavior

Research related to shift work and fatigue generally indicates that errors are linearly related to levels of fatigue. A decrease in cognition is associated with increases in error rate and has been related to the effects of alcohol. Fletcher, Lamond, van den Heuvel, and Dawson (2003) found that after about 17 hours of being awake, fatigue-related impairment is equal to .05 percent blood alcohol concentrate, with 24 hours without sleep being equivalent to .1 percent blood alcohol concentration. This relationship is important for EMS managers to consider when designing work schedules because fatigue and alcohol impairment exhibit similar impacts on performance, including delayed reaction time and impaired reasoning. Impacts to employees engaging in shift work can occur both on duty and off duty as personnel attempt to return home or to other off-duty activities.

Recommendations for Designing Shift Work
EMS managers must plan very carefully both the timing and duration of shifts. It is no longer acceptable to plan only for supply and demand to minimize cost irrespective of the needs of the workforce or the desire for quality outcomes for

patients. Shift design must be a balanced process of supply and demand matching personnel needs while ensuring workforce health, patient safety, and safety of the public with whom EMS providers interact daily. In the 24/7 environment, there is no perfect schedule. All hours of the day must be covered in order to ensure adequate levels of service, response time compliance, and clinical patient outcomes. However, EMS managers can have significant negative impacts on a service's operations through poor shift design and work practices. The following is a set of general recommendations concerning shift design:

+ Night shifts should be limited to two shifts per week of no more than 12 hours per shift. If this is not possible, then the maximum shift length should be limited to 8 hours.

+ Shifts of 12 hours should be limited to no more than two consecutively.
+ Maximum hours worked in one day should be no more than 12, including any overtime.
+ Total hours scheduled in a week should not exceed 48.
+ Overtime should be limited to 12 hours per week.
+ Extended shifts should be accompanied by longer rest breaks.
+ Days off between shifts should be evenly distributed.
+ Shift changes should be moved forward, rather than backward, on a 24-hour clock.
+ Shift patterns should be consistent and predictable.
+ Mechanisms should be in place to allow for appropriate shift-change activities.

Best Practice

Responding to Growing Demand in Sedgwick County"

Sedgwick County EMS is located in Wichita, Kansas. The organization is the exclusive EMS provider for both the County of Sedgwick, including all municipalities and the City of Wichita, with a diverse geographic response area of 1,080 square miles and responsibility for the prehospital health care and emergency services for 525,000 citizens.

The response time requirements are divided into urban, suburban, and rural zones, each with a different response time target (Figure 7.14). The urban zone target is 8 minutes and 59 seconds, in the 90th percentile. The organization in 2009, as depicted by Figure 7.14, was experiencing a growing demand for service that its geospatially based deployment plans were not keeping up with, resulting in increased response times. An identified opportunity for improvement to service levels provided and the need for improved response time reliability under the contract prompted the management team

to begin the process of evaluation and redesign of deployment and ambulance staffing plans.

The organization began by educating all members of the management staff and members of the field provider staff in the concepts of ambulance demand analysis and modern geospatial deployment plans. So that both the operations managers overseeing the plan and the field staff executing the plan could understand the logic and the intended outcomes once implemented, it was important that every employee involved in the process have a foundational understanding of modern concepts of ambulance deployment and staffing prior to making any substantive changes to the current plan.

During the investigative phases of the project, it is was quickly determined that the current static deployment plans, with intermittent ambulance moves to cover open geographic territory after busier ambulances were assigned to calls, was resulting in high demand areas being uncovered for extended periods of time and causing longer-than-expected responses to calls for service (Figure 7.15).

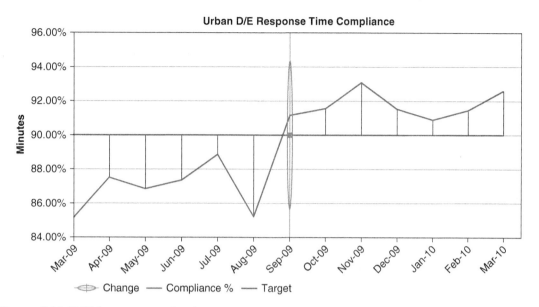

Figure 7.14 ▪ Urban response-time improvements, life-threatening calls: Sedgwick County, Kansas. *Source: Reprinted by permission from Sedgwick County EMS.*

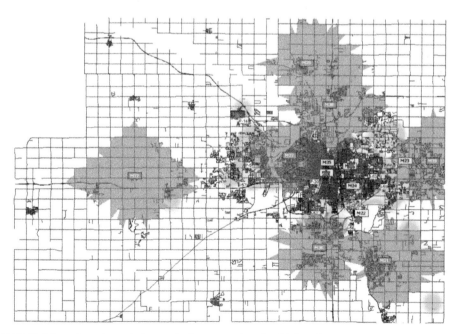

Figure 7.15 ▪ Map of static ambulance deployment showing high-volume areas uncovered by an available ambulance. *Source: Reprinted by permission from Sedgwick County EMS.*

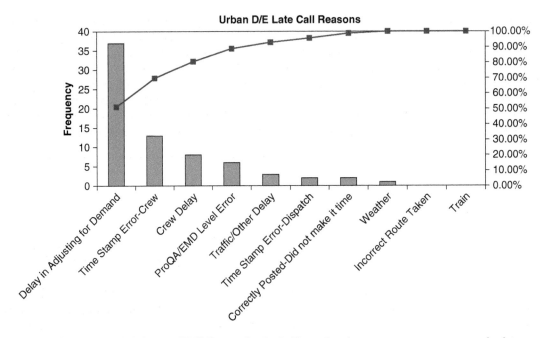

FIGURE 7.16 ■ Sedgwick County EMS Pareto Analysis Chart showing common cause reasons for late responses. *Source: Reprinted by permission from Sedgwick County EMS.*

This methodology is equivalent to the deterministic and static deployment plans described in this chapter. Based on the information gathered, the management team designed a new hybrid deployment plan that took advantage of the locations of the current physical EMS facilities in the urban areas and added strategically located street corner posts to supplement high-demand areas. The intent of the plan was to ensure that high-demand urban areas were serviced with ambulance responses within the required time frame while maintaining appropriate levels of available ambulances both to the urban high-volume centers and to the peripheral suburban and rural areas of the county. The service utilized advanced geospatial analysis software to assist in designing the deployment plan.

In late August 2009, the new deployment plan was invoked and monitored. As indicated in Figure 7.16, the service began to see improvements in its response-time compliance, along with noticeable improvements in high-demand areas maintaining adequate available ambulance coverage. During the

subsequent weeks and months, the service continued to monitor the performance improvements through the use of real-time data-monitoring services designed to alert the management team to outlier response times and trends and changes in performance.

To ensure that the improvements in performance continued, a full-time ambulance deployment manager was added to the management team and was dedicated to analysis of the service's operational response-time performance. Utilizing quality-management techniques, the organization began intensive reviews of performance with daily, weekly, and monthly summaries of both current period performance and, more important, information was presented to all members of the organization about causes of long response times. Figure 7.16 depicts a process known as Pareto analysis. This methodology is designed to give decision makers information about common-cause errors that are most likely to negatively impact response-time performance. The most common reasons for delays in responses, as shown in Figure 7.16, were delays in adjusting the deployment plans. Armed with this information, the management team continued to analyze specific late calls for service with the intent of understanding why the plans were not adjusted to the design and intent of the plan. Over time, the service noted reductions in out-of-compliance responses, a decrease in actual response times, and increases in contractual compliance not only in the urban areas of its district but in all response zones. Since the change in deployment methodologies combined with the implementation of technologies and modern quality-improvement techniques, the service has improved its response-time performance from 86 percent to 93 percent to 94 percent compliance consistently, based on its requirement of 8 minutes 59 seconds for life-threatening calls in its urban-response zone.

CHAPTER REVIEW

Summary

No single factor or consideration will produce an effective ambulance deployment plan and crew staffing model. EMS managers must account for many factors when planning for the effective delivery of EMS services. At the core of this service delivery is the ability of the EMS organization to respond to requests for service in a reliable and predictable manner, whatever that defined parameter might be. To allow for a high level of reliability, the EMS organization must understand the demand loads placed on it both temporally and geospatially; it must then deploy ambulances in an effective and logical manner that best matches a limited supply to a known demand level. In addition, the organization must provide patients with paramedics and EMTs who are capable of providing a high level of care that is oriented to defined patient outcomes and done in a safe and appropriate manner. All of this must be done a dynamic environment that is subject to variability. Thus, the EMS manager must be adept at managing risk and uncertainty in a logical manner so as to produce a consistently high-quality product operationally.

WHAT WOULD YOU DO? Reflection

A review of the ambulance deployment plan and the demand loads on the system revealed a mismatch of ambulance supply in relation to the demand for service at certain times of the day and days of each week and in how the available ambulances were deployed into the system. This problem was compounded by the fact that your managers did not have timely information available to them to adequately monitor the service's ability to meet its response time and ambulance coverage. Thus, your management team was not able to correct for deficiencies in either the number of ambulances deployed over the course of a day or their placement relative to changing geospatial demand patterns. You spent considerable time studying the demand loads on the system such that you were able to redeploy existing resources, both in terms of timing and physical placement of the ambulance supply. This resulted in your organization being able to cover calls for service within the required time frames, resulting in a reduction of the service's response time to within the contractual requirements.

Review Questions

1. Define temporal demand analysis and relate how it impacts an EMS organization's ability to determine proper ambulance levels during the course of a day.

2. Define deterministic ambulance deployment modeling and its limitations regarding the correct deployment of ambulances to maintain effective coverage levels and response times.

3. Compare and contrast a static deployment plan versus a hybrid ambulance deployment plan.

4. Describe seasonality in demand analysis and its potential impact when performing a temporal demand analysis.

5. An ambulance in your organization has an average task time of 1 hour and 30 minutes. During the preceding 12 hours, this ambulance was in service the entire time and transported four patients. What is the UHU for this unit?

6. Define UHU buffer and its impact on an EMS organization to adequately meet demand for service based on the number of units deployed into the system.

7. Identify reasons for lost unit hours in your organization and their potential negative impact on your system performance, then suggest what could be done to mitigate the situation.

8. Define GIS and its impacts on ambulance deployment planning and demand analysis.

9. Based on your understanding of the body's circadian rhythm, define the negative impacts to the health of EMS professionals when shifts are improperly designed.

References

Anantharaman, V., D. Andersen, S. Lim, F. Ng, M. Ong, et al. (2009, March). "Geographic-Time Distribution of Ambulance Calls in Singapore: Utility of Geographic Information System in Ambulance Deployment (CARE 3)." *Annals of the Academy of Medicine Singapore*(3), 184–191.

Aufderheide, T. P., K. M. Vrotsos, R. G. Pirrall, and C. E. Guse. (2008, July/September). "Does the Number of System Paramedics Affect Clinical Benchmark Thresholds?" *Prehospital Emergency Care* 12(3), 302–306.

Bayley, R., M. Weinger, S. Meador, and C. Slovis. (2008, January/March). "Impact of Ambulance Crew Configuration on Simulated Cardiac Arrest Resuscitation." *Prehospital Emergency Care* 12(1): 62–68.

Brachet, T., and G. David. (2009, June). "Retention, Learning by Doing, and Performance in Emergency Medical Services." *Health Services Research* 44(3), 902–925

Brown, L., E. Lerner, B. Larmon, T. LeGassick, and M. Taigman. (2007). "Are EMS Call Volume Predictions Based on Demand Pattern Analysis Accurate?" *Prehospital Emergency Care* 11(2), 199–203.

Budge, S., E. Erkut, and A. Ingolfsson. (2008). "Maximum Availability/Reliability Models for Selecting Ambulance Station and Vehicle Locations." University of Alberta, School of Business.

Cachon, G., and C. Terwiesch. (2006). *Matching Supply with Demand: An Introduction to Operations Management.* New York: McGraw Hill.

Chang, J., and F. Schoenberg. (2009, February). "A Statistical Analysis of Santa Barbara Ambulance Response in 2006: Performance Under Load." *Western Journal of Emergency Medicine* 10(1), 42–47.

Coontz, D., A. Garza, M. Gratton, J. Ma, and E. Noble. "Effect of Paramedic Experience on Orotracheal Intubations." *Journal of Emergency Medicine* 25(3), 251–256.

Dean, S. (2008, March/April). "Why the Closest Ambulance Cannot be Dispatched in an Urban Emergency Medical Services System." *Prehospital and Disaster Medicine* 23(2), 161–165.

Erdogan, G., E. Erkut, A. Ingolfsson, and G. Laporte. (2008). "Scheduling Ambulance Crews for Maximum Coverage." The University of Alberta, School of Business.

ESRI.com. (2007, January). "GIS for Fire Station Location and Response Protocol." See the organization website.

Fitch, J. (1991, August–September). "Schedules and Deployment: A Stress Factor for EMS." *Ambulance Industry Journal.*

Fitch, J., R. Keller, D. Raynor, and C. Zalar. (1993). *EMS Management: Beyond the Street,* 2nd ed. Carlsbad, CA: JEMS Communications.

Fitch, J. (2002, February). "Strategic Deployment: Two Decades of Experience Provide Important Lessons on How to Deploy Emergency Resources." *Journal of Emergency Medical Services 27*(2), 36–45.

Fletcher, A., N. Lamond, C. J. van den Heuvel, and D. Dawson, D. (2003). "Prediction of Performance During Sleep Deprivation and Alcohol Intoxication Using a Quantitative Model of Work Related Fatigue." *Sleep Research Online 5*(2), 67–75.

Goldberg, J. (2004). "Operations Research Models for the Deployment of Emergency Services Vehicles." *EMS Management Journal 1*(1), 20–39.

International Association of Fire Chiefs. (2007, June). "The Effects of Sleep Deprivation on Fire Fighters and EMS Responders." See the organization website.

Motohashi, Y., and T. Takano. (1993, December). "Effects of 24-Hour Shift Work with Nighttime Napping on Circadian Rhythm Characteristics in Ambulance Personnel." *Chronobiology International 10*(6), 461–470.

Stevenson, W. (2007). *Operations Management.* New York: McGraw Hill.

Stout, J. "System Status Management: The Strategy of Ambulance Placement. *Journal of Emergency Medical Services 8*(5), 22–32. See the organization website.

Teow, K. (2009, June). "Practical Operations Research Applications for Healthcare Managers." *Annals of the Academy of Medicine Singapore 38*(6), 564–453.

The Council of Ambulance Authorities. (2007, May). "Shift Hours in the Australian Ambulance Industry: An Issues Paper on Workforce Health and Safety, Patient, and Public Safety." See the organization website.

Webopedia.com. (n.d.). "ODBC." See the organization website.

Key Terms

geospatial demand Occurs in a particular location in a service district such as a city or county.

lost unit hours The number hours in a period of time that an ambulance is unavailable to respond to calls for service for some reason, such as mechanical problems, crew issues, administrative issues, or patient off-load delays at a hospital that are longer than expected.

maximal coverage model Holds the number of vehicles fixed, then locates the vehicles to cover as many calls as possible within a given response-time requirement.

set covering model Seeks to minimize the number of vehicles needed to cover all specified ambulance response zones.

Structured Query Language (SQL) A database computer language designed for managing data in relational database management systems (RDBMS), and originally based on relational algebra and calculus. Its scope includes data insert, query, update and delete, schema creation and modification, and data access control.

temporal demand Volumetric demand or demand that occurs in a specific hour of the day or day of the week irrespective of the geographic location of the demand.

total task time The amount of time the ambulance resource is committed to a call for service until the ambulance resource is completed with the current call and available for another call for service.

unit hour utilization (UHU) The ratio of the number of transports per period divided by the total number of hours staffed per period.

Human Resources Administration

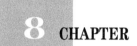

8 CHAPTER

CHRIS COLANGELO, M.S.H.R., NREMT-P; FORREST WOOD, EMT-P;
ERNESTO RODRIGUEZ, EMT-P

Objectives

After reading this chapter, the student should be able to:

8.1 Provide a brief history of human resources as a profession.

8.2 Identify the functional (subspecialty) areas of human resources as a profession.

8.3 Identify legal mandates that provide the foundation for employee management.

8.4 Describe the importance of job descriptions and how they are used for employee management.

8.5 Identify and describe the selection and hiring process to include job posting, application/applicant review, interviews, background check, and job offer.

8.6 Identify and describe the functional life cycle of an employee to include new employee orientation, performance improvement, progressive discipline, promotion, and employee departure (voluntary and involuntary).

8.7 Describe discipline and the process of progressive discipline.

8.8 Describe the process of employee mentoring and succession planning.

Overview

Ambulance services in the United States range in size from one ambulance operated by volunteers and managed by a community board of directors to large governmental agencies and even larger, private, for-profit corporations. This text presents information that the manager of an ambulance service, large or small, needs in order to keep the business solvent and provide clinically excellent service to the community.

Key Terms

Americans with Disabilities Act (ADA)	**Fair Labor Standards Act (FLSA)**	**KSAs**	**preferred qualifications**
Civil Rights Act of 1964	**Family Medical Leave Act (FMLA)**	**mentoring**	**progressive discipline**
	job descriptions	**minimum qualifications**	**succession planning**
		performance improvement	

WHAT WOULD YOU DO?

You are the manager of an urban ambulance operation. One of your supervisors comes to you obviously irritated and upset. He starts the conversation by saying, "You remember I talked to you about George and you asked me document his tardiness and performance issues? I haven't documented it, yet, but he did it again. When I was talking to him, he kept making excuses, and I lost my temper. He made me so mad I gave him two days off without pay!"

■ INTRODUCTION

For ambulance services, as for many service organizations, the single largest investment and largest continuous budget item is personnel. Working with people can also be the biggest challenge. Organizational structure, recruitment and retention, crew supervision, professional development, compensation and benefit management, and staffing all push supervisors and administrators to their limits. Common personal beliefs about what people expect and how employees gauge job satisfaction can be challenged, and supervisors are often forced to adjust their practices and beliefs about the management of human assets at the most fundamental levels. Many supervisors begin this phase of their career without any special training. Yet as new supervisors, they are confronted almost immediately with personnel management challenges that have the potential to be problematic and even explosive. Supervisors can quickly find themselves dealing with such issues as pay incentives and increases (compensation), recruitment and retention, and interpersonal conflicts. **Performance improvement** (disciplinary) issues can also surface early in the career of a new supervisor. Whatever the issue, the untrained or undertrained supervisor will be in unfamiliar territory. Most new supervisors make the best of a bad situation by tapping into readily available resources or by just following their gut instincts. Unfortunately, those resources and instincts may not provide the most appropriate answers, and the situation can quickly become very uncomfortable for the new supervisor.

With knowledge and planning, the supervisor can avoid many uncomfortable situations. Understanding the role that human resources management plays, and knowing what areas a supervisor should handle on his own or with the assistance of outside resources, are key to the long-term success of the new supervisor.

HUMAN RESOURCES MANAGEMENT

Like many professional disciplines, human resources management (HRM) has evolved to keep pace with the ever-changing business environment. HRM, in its most basic but recognizable form, can be traced back to the early part of the twentieth century. As labor issues began to peak in major manufacturing industries, union development and government regulation began to appear.

Early human resources professionals were responsible for documentation and compliance with respect to personnel management. Most of today's workforce has had to complete required employment paperwork when accepting a job offer. Much of this paperwork is required for the organization to be in compliance with government regulations. Over time, HRM has changed as regulations and workforce expectations have changed. HRM practices have become more complex as laws governing compensation and equal opportunity (discrimination) were introduced. The development of labor unions and collective bargaining agreements have also affected HRM. Globalization of the marketplace, increased workforce competition, and increased workforce demands have also added

to the value of a strategic and well-developed HRM program/department for most organizations. The broader the scope of the supervisor's HRM knowledge, the more success he will have in navigating the modern workplace.

HUMAN RESOURCES BASICS

One of the first lessons supervisors should learn with regard to human resources is the legal foundation for employee management. Legal mandates do not exist for all facets of employment practices; for instance, they do not provide supervisors with guidelines for developing **job descriptions**.

LEGAL MANDATES

Over time, numerous federal and state laws have been enacted that impact the employer-employee relationship. Supervisors must have a basic understanding of these legal mandates and how they affect the daily work environment.

Fair Labor Standards Act (FLSA)
Established in 1938, the **Fair Labor Standards Act (FLSA)** created the concept of minimum wage and the first standards for overtime compensation.[1] It also addressed the issues of child labor. Like the Civil Rights Act and its many variants, a basic understanding of its guarantees is also essential to HRM. This includes the definitions of *exempt* and *nonexempt* as well as rules pertaining to overtime. Generally, unless specifically exempted by law or regulation, the FLSA requires all employers to pay time and one-half of the employee's hourly salary for every hour worked over 40 in a 7-day pay period. Extensive regulations detail and implement specific FLSA provisions.[2]

---

[1] 29 U.S.C. Chapter 8.
[2] 29 C.F.R. Chapter 5.

Employment Discrimination

The civil rights events of the 1960s and 1970s brought about some of the greatest fundamental changes in how individuals are viewed and treated since the Civil War. The **Civil Rights Act of 1964**, Section 703(a) (and updated in 1991), made it unlawful for an employer to "fail or refuse to hire or to discharge any individual, or otherwise to discriminate against any individual with respect to his compensation, terms, conditions or privileges of employment, because of such individual's race, color, religion, sex or national origin."[3] The Equal Employment Opportunity Commission (EEOC) was created as a result. When combined with other federal laws and regulations that have been enacted over time, the Civil Rights Act's impact has been profound and continues to impact employees and employers almost daily. Organizations have structured policies and maintain records in order to comply with the mandates of the act. Hiring processes, promotional processes, and workplace culture have all been affected by this regulatory framework. In 1967 Congress passed the Age Discrimination in Employment Act, which added age as a protected class. Protections are provided for worker over the age of 40.[4]

Discrimination cases are usually grouped into two main classifications: disparate treatment and disparate impact. In disparate treatment cases, the discrimination action is directed at an individual because of his protected class (i.e., race, religion, sex, etc.). For example, an employer may decide not to promote a woman to a supervisory position because of a belief that women cannot effectively supervise men. In other words, the decision is made based on the person's membership in a protected class.

---

[3]Civil Rights Act of 1964 § 7, 42 U.S.C. § 2000e et seq (1964).
[4]29 U.S.C. Chapter 14.

In disparate impact cases, employers have implemented some type of employment practice that is neutral on its face but, nonetheless, discriminates against a protected class and is not sufficiently job related to withstand challenge. For example, an ambulance service that implemented a physical ability test that required the performance of six pull-ups to pass might be challenged because women as a class have less upper body strength than men or because pull-ups or similar activities are not closely related to the job duties of an EMT or paramedic.

Regardless of the organization's intent, if a business practice, such as a hiring standard, creates a disparate impact on a protected class, the organization may be liable. Legal precedents change periodically, including measures to determine disparate impact. Supervisors should regularly consult with human resources experts or legal counsel with regard to current precedents.

Sexual (Gender) Discrimination

Although addressed in the Civil Rights Act of 1964, workplace discrimination based on sex often is discussed as a separate topic. Sex discrimination cases, like other discrimination cases, are usually classified as either disparate treatment or disparate impact cases. In addition, sex discrimination encompasses the concept of sexual harassment. The two primary classifications of sexual harassment are *quid pro quo* harassment and hostile work environment harassment.

- The concept of *quid pro quo* (Latin for "this for that") sexual harassment implies that an action, either positive or negative in outcome, will result for granting or refusing to grant sexual favors. Quid pro quo sexual harassment typically involves a supervisor and a subordinate, with the supervisor using, or being perceived to use, a position of authority to coerce compliance with demands (Figure 8.1).

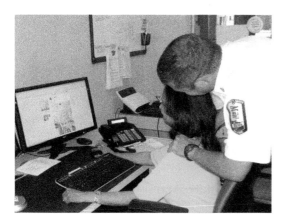

FIGURE 8.1 ■ Inappropriate physical contact between supervisor and subordinate greatly increases the risk of a sexual harassment claim at a later time. *Source: Official Wake County EMS photo by Mike Legeros. Used with permission.*

* Hostile work environment sexual harassment is a concept in which a person feels threatened or ill at ease because of actions or activities of others in the workplace. For example, an employee might allege harassment of the hostile workplace variety based on other workers' hanging sexually explicit pictures in the workplace, or by other employees' repeated use of racial slurs or epithets. The person alleging harassment need not be one of the parties involved in the activity and can simply be someone who witnesses the activity or action. Hostile work environment sexual harassment can involve workers at any level and across any levels of an organization.

Supervisors should pay particular attention to claims of sexual harassment. Inaction on the part of a supervisor who has received a sexual harassment complaint can lead to personal liability for that supervisor. If you are the supervisor to whom this type of activity is reported, you have a duty to act immediately. Organizations should have a well-developed sexual harassment policy, including reporting pathways and investigatory

plans. It is recommended that sexual harassment investigations be conducted outside of the department in which the complaint was generated. Ideally, a team comprised of external senior leadership and human resources professionals would be utilized to investigate sexual harassment complaints.

Family Medical Leave Act
The **Family Medical Leave Act (FMLA)** outlines requirements for when an employee is entitled to time off and is protected from discharge up to a total of 12 workweeks of unpaid leave during a rolling 12-month period.[5] Qualifying requirements must be met in order to be eligible. In 2009, the FMLA protections were expanded to provide 26 weeks of unpaid leave for qualifying active-duty military personnel and their family members.

Americans with Disabilities Act
Since its passage in 1990, the **Americans with Disabilities Act (ACT)** extended and provided protections to citizens for discrimination based on disabilities.[6] The ADA requires accessibility to facilities for both employees and the general public. Even though the ADA has been in place for two decades, it still is an area of the law that changes fairly frequently. Supervisors should seek assistance from human resources experts and legal counsel any time an employee requests an ADA accommodation or a claim is made against the organization for failure to comply.

Uniformed Service Employment and Reemployment Rights Act
The Uniformed Service Employment and Reemployment Rights Act (USERRA) provides that military service veterans have certain

---

[5]P.L. 103-3; 29 U.S.C. Section 2601; 29 CFR 825.
[6]P.L. 101-336, § 12101(a)(8), 104 Stat. 327, 329 (1990) (amended 2008).

rights to reemployment on return from service.[7] Specific conditions apply. This is another area where supervisors would benefit from seeking counsel from their human resources professional. Of particular interest to EMS employers is the fact that, since 2003, USERRA rights also apply to members of disaster medical assistance teams (DMATs) and similar organizations when called to federal service (National Association of Disaster Response Teams, n.d.).[8]

National Labor Relations Act

In 1935, Congress enacted the National Labor Relations Act (NLRA).[9] The purpose of this act is to protect the rights of employees and employers, to encourage collective bargaining, and to curtail certain private sector labor and management practices, which can harm the general welfare of workers, businesses, and the U.S. economy.

Under the NLRA, the rights of employees to form, join, decertify, or assist a labor organization, and to bargain collectively, are protected. Employees may also act together to improve their working conditions without a union. Together, these activities are called "protected concerted activity." Federal, state, and local governments, including wholly owned government corporations, are excluded from the NLRA. However, some states, using their plenary police powers, have applied the NLRA to themselves and their political subdivisions.

Many ambulance service managers will find themselves called on to work in a collective bargaining environment. In those situations, the collective bargaining agreement (CBA) will be well established, and the manager will need to learn to work within the rules that the agency and the union have agreed on.

It is important to note that, from the managers' perspective, the union and the CBA are not necessarily "the enemy." Although the CBA may require the employer to follow procedures that at times seem onerous, it is important to remember the following points:

+ Those provisions were previously and *voluntarily* agreed to by the organization's management.
+ Many of those provisions became bargaining unit demands because of perceived unfair treatment of employees by management.
+ Those provisions are subject to negotiation the next time the contract is re-negotiated.

Managers charged with implementing the CBA must be diligent in following its provisions, or risk "unfair labor practice" litigation. Those same managers must also step up at contract negotiation time to ensure that the important interests of the organization are not overlooked.

It is also important to keep in mind that not all labor-management interactions are negative, and that a cooperative relationship can benefit all parties. The International Association of Fire Chiefs (IAFC)/International Association of Fire Fighters (IAFF) *Labor-Management Initiative* is a well-known fire service program that trains chief fire officers and union officials to improve trust and work together better (IAFC and IFFC, 1999–2013). Participants focus on shared goals, relationships, and developing action plans on issues of mutual concern.

It is beyond the scope of this book to provide a complete course in collective bargaining and labor-management relations under the NLRA. A course in labor-management relations is recommended for ambulance service managers who will be called on to administer collective bargaining agreements, and all supervisors and managers should be trained, preferably by the organization's legal

---

[7]Public Law 103-353, codified as amended at 38 U.S.C. §§ 4301–4335.
[8]See 42 U.S.C. § 300hh-11(e)(3).
[9]29 U.S.C. §§ 151-169.

counsel, in the specifics of an agency's collective bargaining agreement.

JOB DESCRIPTIONS

At their most basic level, job descriptions establish the responsibilities, **minimum qualifications**, **preferred qualifications**, and reporting relationships for each position. With these fundamental components of each position established, job descriptions provide the basic building blocks for the organization. Job postings, selection criteria, and performance expectations are derived from the job descriptions. In addition, job descriptions can be used to compare positions in order to determine organizational structure and compensation differences.

The development of job descriptions often begins with a needs assessment, possibly as part of a strategic planning process. Utilizing human resources professionals in the needs assessment process is recommended. As each job is defined, a description for that position must be reviewed (an already existing position) or developed (a newly identified position). The job description will spell out the knowledge and skills required to successfully perform the task and/or objectives that must be met in order to perform successfully. There may also be specific physical characteristics that must be met. These are often described as minimum qualifications. They are usually listed in the job requirements or job description and include knowledge, skills, and abilities (physical requirements), also known as **KSAs**.

Frequently, additional knowledge, skills, attributes, and/or abilities that enhance the ability of an individual to perform the job are also included in job descriptions and job postings. These are listed as preferred or recommended qualifications.

As mentioned, another use for job descriptions is the evaluation of existing jobs.

One example would be using job descriptions to compare similar jobs within the same organization in order to evaluate salary/wage levels. For an existing job, the job description may be evaluated through an observation process. A human resources professional or supervisor may observe several employees performing in the position being evaluated. Once the observation is complete, an assessment is conducted and the identified job KSAs are documented and quantified. It is important to note that it is often not the frequency of a particular KSA that dictates the relative value assigned to a position but, instead, the diversity of KSAs. For example, one supervisor may have 50 employees who do the same job using low-level knowledge and skills. Although the number of employees assigned is high, the knowledge and skills to supervise are limited because there is little variety in the position types. Someone who supervises a small number of employees who have a wide range of skills may have a higher level of compensation because of the demands required to supervise these diverse positions.

Together, the legal mandates and the position job descriptions form the fundamental building blocks for the management of employees. However, supervisors need to clearly understand that neither of these foundation pieces remains static. Laws are constantly being challenged in the courts and changed in the legislature. Supervisors should attend regular employment law updates. Likewise, job descriptions should not be created and forgotten. Job descriptions should be living documents that change as the organization grows and position needs change. Forgotten and static job descriptions often come back to haunt supervisors at the most inopportune moments, such as when a candidate challenges the validity of a hiring or promotional process. If the process is based on an outdated job description, the organization may face legal liability. At the least, the organization's public image could suffer. At the worst, the organization could face a civil penalty. Supervisors need to regularly revisit both of these fundamental components of employee management.

■ EMPLOYEE SELECTION AND HIRING————————————

Once a position has been approved and the job description completed, it is time to hire. Once the applications have been received, the next step is to process the applications. Most organizations use some type of interview during the selection process of applicants. On completion of the assessment testing and interviews, candidates should undergo an extensive background investigation. Once a selection has been made, an offer of employment is extended.

JOB POSTING

Job posting usually involves several steps. The first step is to advertise or post the position. Most organizations have standard policies governing the posting of positions. The following are some of the questions that may come up and should be addressed by such policies:

* Will this position be posted internally, externally, or both?
* For what time period will the job be available (posted)?
* How will the job be posted?
* What media will be used for advertising?

In addition, supervisors should be aware of any requirements dictated by a collective bargaining agreement or organizational personnel policies.

Though it should have been determined prior to the job being posted, supervisors often fail to address how the applications and applicants will be processed until after the job is posted. Supervisors must use a consistent process to evaluate applications and applicants. This includes using defined criteria to evaluate and select candidates. Also, prior to receiving the first application, supervisors should determine what assessment process they want to use.

APPLICATION AND APPLICANT PROCESSING

One of the primary concerns in reviewing applications is to ensure that each applicant meets all of the minimum qualifications (MQs). One of the common errors that may subject organizations to possible litigation in the hiring process is failing to evaluate applicants to ensure they meet minimum qualifications. When reviewing applications, supervisors should confirm that they have properly identified the MQs as they were stated in the job posting and that each applicant meets the MQs.

In the event a supervisor finds a candidate who meets the majority, but not all of, the minimum criteria for a position and he wants to consider that candidate, the supervisor should tread very carefully. Ideally, the supervisor would cancel the recruitment and then repost the position with the reduced set of minimum qualifications. If this is not an option, the supervisor should consult with his human resources specialist to determine the best course of action. In the worst case, the supervisor may be able to screen all candidates based on a reduced set of minimum criteria; however, this still may not hold up if challenged legally by a candidate who did have the full set of posted minimum qualifications. Ultimately, the supervisor will have to justify why the candidate who did not meet the minimum qualifications was so uniquely qualified as to warrant a deviation from the established standard.

Often, on completion of the application review for minimum qualifications, more than one qualified candidate is identified. To sort the remaining candidates and determine who participates in the rest of the assessment process, a scoring system is often developed. In an attempt to quantify the process, points are assigned to various elements of each candidate's application. Points are awarded for education, job experience, and perhaps certifications or course completion certificates (ACLS, PHTLS, and so forth) beyond the minimum qualifications. Point systems provide an objective way to value (quantify) the qualifications determined to be the most important to the organization. The key is consistency in applying the point system to all applicants in the process.

In addition to the application review, other assessment tools may be used. It is not uncommon in EMS for candidates to have to complete a written examination of medical knowledge, a practical EMS skills exam, a physical agility exam of some type, and an interview process.

Side Bar

A Word about Physical Agility Tests

Over the years, physical agility testing allegedly has been used as a barrier to entry into the profession, especially against women. Various physical performance evaluation instruments have been successfully challenged by women, alleging that the physical abilities required by the test were not legitimately connected to the physical requirements of the job. The key guidance which has emerged from these challenges is that physical capability test evolutions must be related to job requirements. Called job-related job duties (JRJDs), these requirements must be commonly occurring skills. If only infrequently required, they cannot be used as a barrier to job entry.

On the other hand, if required as part of regular job performance, the skill not only can

be, but should be, included in a physical abilities test (Figure 8.2). The best example for EMS is the requirement to be able to lift a certain amount of weight. The requirement that an individual, regardless of gender, be able to lift 150 pounds is commonly accepted as realistic. Recent changes in response practices and equipment are changing that, however. Multiple–unit response (first responders as well as transport crews), stretcher innovations, and loading devices may not only reduce employee on-the-job injuries but may modify lifting requirements on JRJDs as well.

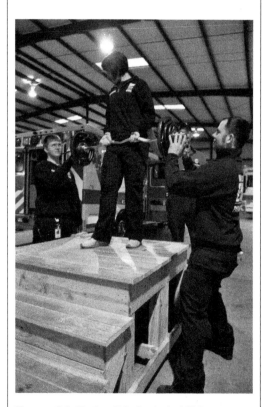

FIGURE 8.2 ■ A valid physical abilities test will ensure that new employees can meet job-relevant physical standards prior to being offered employment. *Source: Official Wake County EMS photo by Lee Wilson. Used with permission.*

Similar to the application points system developed to rank candidates prior to the testing process, candidates are also ranked based on their test scores. Those who advance in the process are chosen based on the ranking process. Many organizations, especially civil service or governmental agencies, require that at least three qualified candidates be interviewed prior to final selection.

INTERVIEW PROCESS

Interviews can range from peer interviews to supervisor interviews or general interviews to technical interviews. Organizations should take great care in developing their interview process. Most supervisors have little background in the development of valid and reliable employment selection tools, so formal interviewer training by a qualified trainer should be conducted if at all possible. Although most supervisors put great trust in a general job interview, it has been shown to be one of the most unreliable predictors of employee performance and success. Structured interviews (where a standard set of questions is asked of all candidates) provide a little more validity in predicting employee success; however, most supervisors do not like the format of the structured interview. When developing an interview component to hiring, supervisors should reach out to human resources professionals who specialize in selection methods.

BACKGROUND AND REFERENCE CHECKS

Laws governing background investigations are varied from state to state, so a little research by supervisors prior to developing background investigation policies is advisable. As a general rule, background investigations should be completed prior to job offers being extended. The most common (and recommended) components of the background investigation include these:

- Driver's license verification
- Criminal history check

- Driving record check (usually required by the insurance company).
- Certification verification with the appropriate state and national agencies
- Drug screening
- Previous employment verification
- For employers who bill the Medicare program for services, each employer must be checked against the National Practitioner Data Bank and Healthcare Integrity and Protection Data Bank (n.d.).[10]

Additional checks can be performed, including listed character references and verification of education.

Reference checks can be time consuming, and in the past they have often provided little value. This is mostly due to a risk-adverse trend resulting in the establishment of policies that only permitted supervisors to provide information such as position held, dates of employment, and salary at time of separation. In recent years, state legislatures have been reviewing and modifying laws to encourage the disclosure of employment information to potential employers, which may result in more value coming from reference checks. North Carolina's job reference law is a relevant example:

§ 1-539.12. Immunity from civil liability for employers disclosing information.

a. An employer who discloses information about a current or former employee's job history or job performance to a prospective employer of the current or former employee

---

[10]The National Practitioner Data Bank (NPDB) and the Healthcare Integrity and Protection Data Bank (HIPDB) have been created by the federal government to serve as repositories of information about health care providers in the United States. Federal law requires that adverse actions taken against a health care professional's license, including disbarment from the Medicare and Medicaid programs, be reported to these data banks. See 45 C.F.R. Parts 60 and 61 for details.

upon request of the prospective employer or upon request of the current or former employee is immune from civil liability and is not liable in civil damages for the disclosure or any consequences of the disclosure. This immunity shall not apply when a claimant shows by a preponderance of the evidence both of the following:

1. The information disclosed by the current or former employer was false.
2. The employer providing the information knew or reasonably should have known that the information was false.

b. For purposes of this section, "job performance" includes:

1. The suitability of the employee for re-employment;
2. The employee's skills, abilities, and traits as they may relate to suitability for future employment; and
3. In the case of a former employee, the reason for the employee's separation.[11]

Properly conducted, background checks can provide an employer with a wealth of information about prospective employees, with little attendant risk. A good deal of skill and devotion of time are required to conduct an effective background check. Given that ambulance service employees are provided virtually unlimited access to the persons and property of some of society's most vulnerable members, investment of staff training time or the use of an outside contractor to conduct a professional background investigation is highly recommended. If your ambulance service believes that a candidate for an EMT or paramedic position should meet the same standards of character as a candidate for a law enforcement position, then an investment of 20 to 80 hours of staff time in a background investigation will not seem an unreasonable investment.

---

[11]North Carolina General Statutes § 1-539.12.

EMPLOYMENT OFFER

The offer of employment is usually in writing, but it may be initially extended verbally. The complexity of the offer is tailored to the position and the circumstances of the offer. At the entry level, the offer typically takes the form of a letter that outlines pay, benefits, and other conditions of employment pertinent to the position. More complex offers may include an actual employment contract. Supervisors must make sure the offer letter is detailed and accurate prior to presenting it to the candidate.

The offer letter may also include additional conditions or requirements that must be completed prior to final hire. Many organizations include drug screening, medical screening, and physical requirement testing after the offer is made but prior to the first day of employment. These types of conditions should be included in the offer letter with very clear deadlines for the candidate.

EMPLOYEE LIFE CYCLE

The orientation process is the organization's first opportunity to formally introduce the newly hired employee to performance expectations. Employee performance is dependent on many factors. Some of them are controlled by the employee, such as attitude, effort, and knowledge; some of them are controlled by the employer, such as setting expectations, environment, and culture. Among the most exciting events that can happen in anyone's career is getting promoted to the next step up the ladder of success. There are generally two ways employees leave an organization: voluntarily or involuntarily. Among the highest priorities of ambulance service leaders should be the planning for the long-term sustainability of the organization.

NEW EMPLOYEE ORIENTATION

The complexity of the orientation process depends largely on the complexity of the job the employee will be required to perform. At the very least, employees should be familiarized with the organization's history; its mission, vision and values; policies, procedures, and performance expectations; employment requirements such as certifications and licenses; and any necessary operations-based training that may be specific to the work area in which the employee will be assigned.

When developing an orientation program, it is most beneficial to begin by defining the performance expectations that a new employee must be able to meet when he enters the work area. Expectations are commonly defined as the quality and quantity of work the employee needs to produce based on the skills associated with the employee's position. For example, "Newly oriented paramedics shall be able to complete a medical record within 15 minutes after patient contact without missing more than one essential item at least 95 percent of the time." By compiling a list of statements such as these, an orientation program that prepares personnel to meet performance goals can be designed with greater confidence.

A well-planned and executed orientation program can be completed efficiently and reduce the cost of preparing newly hired paramedics to enter the work area quickly (Figure 8.3). An orientation program that prepares employees thoroughly will reduce the potential that new employees will experience performance problems in their new role. It also reduces the risk of workplace misunderstandings, job-related accidents, and the organization's liability related to poor customer service.

PERFORMANCE IMPROVEMENT

The likelihood that an employee will meet minimum performance expectations increases

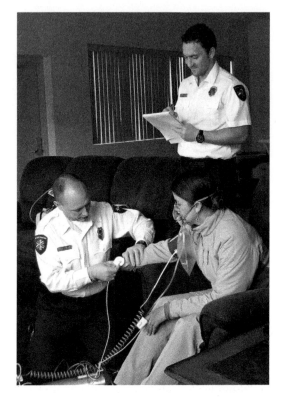

FIGURE 8.3 ■ A formal field training and evaluation program ensures effective employee integration into the new organization, documenting compliance with standards and progress toward achieving performance benchmarks. *Source: Courtesy of Zach Brown/Ada County Paramedics.*

with the organization's ability to define expectations, measure employee performance, and communicate both clearly and effectively. Organization leaders also need to set reasonable performance expectations and provide a work environment conducive to success. For example, requiring billers to find certain missing information on medical records but not providing adequate research tools for that purpose reduces the employee's chances of being successful.

Establishing minimum performance expectations is a responsibility of the organization. The best approach is for supervisors to evaluate what activities must be done well as a whole in order to satisfy customer needs. Once those areas are identified, they should be used to develop organization-level key performance indicators, which can then be used to determine what employees need to do well on individually. For example, if customers expect an ambulance to arrive promptly to scheduled appointments, then the organization can establish a key performance indicator such as "On-time arrival to scheduled appointments equal to or greater than 95 percent of the time." This measure can be easily monitored each day. In order for the organization to meet this customer expectation, each employee must pay close attention to dispatch information to avoid arrival at a wrong address and must know how to read maps effectively. Counting and reviewing the number of times an employee arrived on time at the address where he was dispatched to can be used to measure how well the employee performs in these areas. Performance goals should be set so that employees clearly understand what is expected of them.

Feedback to employees about their performance is vital to improving and sustaining top performance. Companies that find ways to provide rapid and effective feedback about performance are most likely to attain higher levels of employee performance. Employees in those companies also tend to achieve higher levels of job satisfaction since they are able to successfully achieve measured performance indicators.

Feedback can be provided in an assortment of ways. How an organization chooses to provide feedback depends on a variety of factors. Some of these factors include the following:

+ Number of employees in the organization
+ Ratio of employees to supervisors
+ Available resources for communication (e-mail, message boards, databases, intranets, etc.)

Organization leaders need to make feedback an important part of their success strategy and to explore methods to provide frequent and timely feedback. Surveys conducted by Gallup, Inc., indicate that a supervisor recognizing good performance is among the most effective measurement methods (Buckingham and Coffman, 1999).

Still, what if an employee doesn't meet performance expectations? How does a supervisor improve employee performance? Is it time for discipline?

Side Bar

Progressive Discipline

What is discipline? Unfortunately, for most people discipline describes a negative outcome for personal actions. But what is the origin of the word *discipline*? It is a derivative of the word *disciple*. What is a disciple? One definition is a teacher. How is it that a word derived from *teacher* has come to be associated with a negative outcome? Shouldn't discipline be a philosophy, not an outcome? Shouldn't it address both positive and negative behavior?

It has been demonstrated repeatedly that performance improves and desired behavior is achieved faster when the focus is on positive rather than negative feedback. Rewards and incentives are examples of positive discipline programs. Supervisors should also be acutely aware of the negative connotation of the word *discipline* and work to establish a more positive attitude within the workplace with regard to discipline and its many forms.

Most organizations subscribe to a process of **progressive discipline**. Progressive discipline is comprised of escalating steps of penalty for unacceptable performance or behavior. In line with the progressive discipline philosophy is the idea that the "punishment should fit the crime."

Before a supervisor can answer the question "Is it time for discipline?" the supervisor must determine whether the issue is one of conduct (behavior) or performance. Conduct issues involve breaches of integrity, tardiness, absenteeism, insubordination, gross disrespect of the community or colleagues, and other issues with a "right or wrong" component. Conduct issues are issues less tolerated by employers, and they often allow shortcutting the typical progressive discipline ladder. Immoral, unethical, or other behavior that is offensive to the agency and the community often enjoys less due process protection than do performance-based issues. Most people understand that egregious conduct simply does not have to be tolerated in most places, and that the ability of employers to correct these issues is limited.

Issues of unacceptable job performance (or performance issues) require a different approach. Before undertaking progressive discipline, supervisors and managers must determine if the performance expectations are reasonable, have been clearly communicated (or taught), and are being measured effectively. Supervisors should also question whether organization policies, procedures, tools, or equipment could be a contributing cause of employees not achieving top performance. Discipline must be considered only after work situations are carefully examined, documented, evaluated, and corrected if necessary. Sometimes, organization leaders write policies that conflict with each other or that cause confusion about priorities. For example, if employees are required to clean their station, check their vehicles, and complete their station log before their first assignment, what happens if customer needs take priority over these things? Should the employees be disciplined if they couldn't get those things done because of a competing priority? What kind of training would help employees "understand" why they need to get those things done

faster when they conflict with other priorities? Is getting those things done physically possible? Supervisors must remain diligent to identify systems that generate or promote poor performance based on their design. It is dangerous to assume that an employee who does not meet work expectations simply has a behavioral problem, because that could result in overturned disciplinary actions and failure to improve employee performance.

After evaluating these criteria, if the supervisor believes the root cause of the poor performance is the employee in question, then discipline is probably warranted. At the first level of discipline (often called coaching or verbal warning), the supervisor must focus on ensuring that the employee truly understands what is expected and that there are no external barriers to performance. This is typically achieved through a face-to-face meeting between the employee and his supervisor. During this meeting, supervisors should work with the employee to develop a plan for improvement, which may include additional training or education.

If employee performance fails to improve after verbal coaching, the next step may be a written warning. This step involves a formal document, usually in the form of a letter or memorandum to the employee. At a minimum, this document should specifically include the performance expectation, the examples of the employee not meeting the expectation, the corrective actions that must be taken, and the timeline for improved performance. The document should also clearly articulate that if the employee's performance does not improve, further discipline up to and including termination may result.

If the employee's performance continues to fail to meet expectations, discipline continues based on the organization's additional progressive discipline steps. In some organizations, this includes additional written warnings. In others, it includes suspensions and/or demotions. All progressive discipline eventually leads to improved employee performance or termination.

In some situations, employees simply make poor choices. Job and other personal frustrations can lead to behavioral issues, which must be faced directly and without delay. Supervisors need a background in conducting crucial conversations in order to achieve absolutely clear understanding about the organization's behavioral expectations (Patterson, Grenny, McMillan, and Switzler, 2011). Undesired behavior can rapidly affect an organization's standing in the community and its reputation with customers. Failing to address behavioral issues sends a strong message to all employees within an organization, and they must be handled quickly, fairly, and consistently.

A well-written discipline policy establishes clear guidelines about when discipline will be used and how it will be conducted. Supervisors must be well informed about the organization's disciplinary policy and each step in the process. First-line supervisors need training on how to write disciplinary documents and who in the organization must review them before delivering them to employees. Legal advice from a firm with human resources expertise, in-house counsel, or human resources specialists regarding the content of disciplinary communications can help reduce liability and protect the organization should legal action result in response to disciplinary measures.

Replacing employees is an expensive venture. It can be avoided by making sure that the right people are selected during the hiring process, setting clear performance expectations, providing timely feedback about performance, and coaching to improve performance. If all of this is handled in an explicit and genuine fashion, organization leaders will be faced with a more important problem: who to promote into leadership positions.

PROMOTIONS

Often promotions mean higher pay, recognition of a job well done, and broader responsibilities (Figure 8.4). A promotion can be a gateway to even more exciting opportunities for an employee and for the organization. With new leadership come new ideas, new energy, and opportunities to change the status quo of an organization. Just as it is important to select the right people to bring into the organization, it is also important to select the right employee for promotion.

Similar to external selection and hiring processes, promotional processes should be conducted in a consistent and objective manner. Qualifications should be clearly established and communicated in a written job description for the position. Relevant experience to be considered should be specific enough to discern what is really needed and yet not so specific that employees are disqualified unfairly. Evaluations of previous job performance should be included in the selection process with consideration for both positive (commendations) and negative (disciplinary actions) aspects. Previous job performance

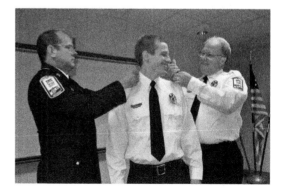

FIGURE 8.4 ■ The significance of an employee's promotion to a position of new responsibility should not be overlooked. Persons being promoted, families, and co-workers should be included in promotional events. *Source: Official Wake County EMS photo by Mike Legeros. Used by permission.*

should be specifically evaluated for evidence that an employee is growing, maturing, and learning, even from mistakes.

As previously noted, the validity of general interviews is less than optimum. However, few organizations would select a candidate for promotion without an interview process. Therefore, interview boards should be carefully selected and trained in the interview process. Subject matter experts should be identified and used to evaluate candidate responses to scenario-based questions. Some companies have had great success by requiring candidates to submit written solutions to problem statements. This gives the assessment team an opportunity to consider the candidate's use of innovation, writing skills, organizational ability, and persuasive talent. Another assessment tool that is often used is to require candidates to deliver a presentation about particular subject matter to gauge their ability to deliver a message in an interesting and credible fashion. Another option is an inbox exercise, during which a candidate must respond to a variety of problems in a short period of time, often using written, e-mail, or phone communication. Complex scenarios such as dealing with media questions or employee conflict management can test capabilities that the organization considers extremely important.

All this said, if an organization's leadership team has done its job correctly, much will be known about internal candidates for promotions. That is, if they have taken **mentoring** and **succession planning** seriously.

MENTORING AND SUCCESSION PLANNING

Succession planning is achieved through the mentoring of leaders who will manage the service in the future and planning for the succession of existing leaders with new individuals who are prepared for the rigors the service will face as it grows and prospers.

Mentoring takes many forms, ranging from formal mentoring programs to occasional contact between employees and current leaders. Experienced leaders should take opportunities to share information about what skills employees must master to become successful leaders. Formal programs often define these areas as competencies.

Defining competencies is the process of determining what knowledge, skills, abilities, and characteristics a leader needs to have in order to achieve the organization's mission and vision based on its value system. These competencies can then be used to develop training programs, internships, and other experiences for employee career development programs. Experienced leaders can use competencies to guide them through assessing employees whom they are mentoring.

> ### Side Bar
>
> **A Word about Mentoring Programs**
>
> An effective mentoring program should be managed like any other program or project. The two parties should conduct an initial meeting and outline exactly what the expectations of the process should include. This should involve learning objectives, benchmarks, measures, and time lines, to include the end point of the mentor-protégé relationship.
>
> Although the relationship developed in a mentorship can often extend over a lifetime, the actual formal mentoring program should have a clear end, generally a year or less. Remember, this is a program designed to develop the future needs of the organization.

Succession planning involves evaluation of existing leadership to determine if there will be a need to change organizational structure to meet future needs as well as preparation for the departure of existing leaders due to changes in interests, lateral movements within the organization, promotions, and retirements. This aids in developing future leaders with greater specificity and setting priorities on career development and talent searches within the organization. A needs assessment of both organizational and individual needs should be performed. Identified needs should be prioritized. After a personnel inventory, potential candidates are then identified and their strengths and weaknesses are assessed. Finally, a development and training plan is formulated that should include both formal education and organizational training. This may also include assigning a mentor to assist with the individual development process.

One thing to note is that professional development, such as medical continuing education and compliance with operational educational mandates (many from the Occupational Safety and Health Administration [OSHA]), is not the same as succession planning and career development. Often organizations focus too much on immediate needs and just-in-time education. Very often, long-term planning and professional development are cut due to tight budgets; however, losing leaders and not having readily available internal replacement candidates constitute a failure on the part of the management team to prepare for the future.

As employees progress through their life cycle with the organization, expectations for performance naturally become progressively higher as they attain knowledge and skills commensurate with their experience. Graduated pay scales should be developed to accommodate increased performance expectations—not just a pay scale based on time in grade but an increased expectation for competencies as well. Supervisors should also be prepared for increased expectations resulting from employees looking for new growth and professional opportunities. Failure to provide increased opportunities often leads to the loss of valuable talent and organizational knowledge.

EMPLOYEE DEPARTURE (SEPARATION/ TERMINATION)

A good supervisor should know the costs associated with employee turnover. Like the costs associated with on-the-job injuries, the costs for replacing employees can often justify many things, including, to name just a few, pay increases, increased benefits, additional time off, recruitment bonuses, and relocation allowances.

Separation (Voluntary Departure)

Employees leave employment for many reasons. In all cases, valuable information about the organization can be gained from an exit interview.

Exit interviews should occur as soon as possible after the employee resigns and should address topics such as working conditions, schedules and working hours, supervision and leadership, physical conditions, vehicle maintenance, and personal and organizational safety—in other words, everything that impacts the daily working life of an employee. Exit interviews are most productive when they are conducted by someone the employee considers to be neutral (i.e., not in the direct chain of supervision). Remember, studies show that the primary reason people leave an organization is their supervisor.

Termination (Involuntary Departure)

Typically, termination should be the last option after all other remedies have been attempted. As a general rule, disciplinary meetings leading up to a termination should involve at least two supervisors. Having two supervisors in the disciplinary meetings eliminates the possibility of a "he said/she said" situation if the terminated employee claims supervisory misconduct occurred during the meetings. Having an organizational policy that dictates the termination process and is approved by the organization's legal counsel is preferable. Regardless, termination actions should be discussed with the organization's human resources department/agency and legal counsel.

Once the decision to terminate has been made, the action should be swift, complete, and without debate. A full disclosure of entitlements, appeal rights, and actions (including benefits and pay) should be available and communicated in writing to the employee. Remember to include procedures for the return of equipment, such as uniforms, keys, or other materials; termination of any access to buildings and computers (especially HIPAA-related databases); and any other organization resources that should be addressed.

Don't forget COBRA benefits. Most benefits-earning employees are entitled to the continuation of medical benefits at the time of separation from an employer. Typically, supervisors do not have to deal directly with this process; however, supervisors should be aware that COBRA benefits exist and how to refer the employee to the organization's human resources professional responsible for benefits administration.

The person being terminated should be escorted until he has departed the building. If the person must return to a duty post to retrieve personal materials, an escort should be provided. Although we like to assume that the majority of people are reasonable, high stress and emotional turmoil can cause people to do strange things. Be safe, not sorry . If the individual is being terminated for cause, decide before the action whether the person will be eligible for unemployment benefits, or whether the organization will dispute an unemployment insurance request. Again, this is a discussion for your organization's legal counsel and human resources department/agency before the termination action takes place.

■ ORGANIZATIONAL DEVELOPMENT AND STRATEGIC HUMAN RESOURCES MANAGEMENT

The human resources function and its staff specialists are frequently called on to assist in organizational development. This includes anything from organizational structure (reporting protocols, such as who answers to whom, compensation structures, position development, etc.) to addressing individual employee needs (professional development, performance improvement, etc.). To fulfill these requests, human resources professionals have become experts at analyzing and comparing organizations against benchmarks. In recent years, the push has been for human resources professionals to become an integral part of the management team and provide a strategic focus on the management of personnel. Supervisors who embrace the expertise of the human resources professional will find a very capable ally in the management of an organization's most valuable resource: its employees.

■ HUMAN RESOURCE PROFESSIONALS

Just as other professions have grown and developed specialties, so has HRM. Within the umbrella of HRM, there are subspecialties. These subspecialties include benefits, classification and recruitment, compensation, employee relations, employee training and development, payroll, and labor relations. In smaller organizations, a human resources generalist may fill several or all of these roles; however, larger organizations may have several human resources professionals assigned to each of the separate subspecialties. Another alternative for smaller organizations is to outsource some or all of these human resources functions. In recent years, a new industry of independent human resources companies has developed to provide human resources services to smaller organizations. Each organization must evaluate the advantages and disadvantages with regard to how human resources functions are structured and provided.

BENEFITS SPECIALISTS

Benefits specialists are typically experts in the ever-changing world of employee benefits. This includes everything from insurance (health, dental, life, disability, etc.) to retirement benefits/programs. It is difficult for supervisors to maintain an accurate knowledge base considering the complexity of today's benefits market. A good benefits specialist can provide a significant return on investment for an organization.

CLASSIFICATION AND RECRUITMENT SPECIALISTS

Classification and recruitment (C/R) specialists are typically known as recruiters. These human resources professionals are experts in creating and evaluating job descriptions, crafting job postings, and conducting application/applicant evaluations. Supervisors should seek out their recruiters and establish a good relationship prior to needing the C/R specialist's expertise. C/R specialists should also be knowledge experts regarding the organization's human resources policies and standards for recruitment and selection. C/R specialists can also be valuable assets when evaluating or creating a new organizational structure.

COMPENSATION SPECIALISTS

Compensation specialists are experts in evaluating and managing compensation systems. This includes salary structure development and maintenance, raise programs (merit/pay for performance, cost of living, etc.), and legal standards with regard to compensation. Compensation specialists are typically adept at benchmarking salary systems and compensation for like positions (internally and externally). One caution should be made for supervisors of organizations who are using "specialty" compensation mechanisms such as "fluctuating workweek" or the 207(k) exemption (for firefighters and law enforcement). These types of compensation systems are not in the mainstream for the majority of the nation's workforce. Therefore, many compensation specialists are not familiar with the specifics of these compensation programs and may require acclimation time. Moreover, the 207(k) exemption, in particular, has proven problematic for the fire service and non-fire providers alike, and attempts by employers to reduce costs through creative payment schemes have cost governmental subdivisions, particularly cities, millions of dollars in back wages and penalties for violation of the overtime provisions of FLSA.[12]

EMPLOYEE RELATIONS SPECIALISTS

Employee relations (ER) specialists provide support to both the supervisor and the individual employee. ER specialists typically work to limit the organization's exposure in situations such as sexual harassment, wrongful discipline/termination cases, and unemployment claims. They do this through policy development, organization-wide education programs, and record keeping. ER specialists work closely with legal counsel and supervisors to make sure discipline practices are conducted in a fair and consistent way per organization policy.

---

[12]See, for example, *Lawrence v. City of Philadelphia*, 527 F.3d 299 (3rd Cir. 2008), where a group of fire-paramedics did not meet the responsibility clause of 207(k) because firefighting was not one of their job duties, as laid out in their job descriptions and in organization operating practices.

EMPLOYEE TRAINING AND DEVELOPMENT SPECIALISTS

Employee training and development specialists are regularly considered trainers within the organization and typically have adult education credentials. Although they are not certified to set up an organization's continuing medical education program, they can assist with the creation of a professional development program for the organization's next generation of leaders. They may also use stock programs for employee compliance issues, such as sexual harassment and diversity training.

PAYROLL SPECIALISTS

Payroll specialists may or may not be located within the human resources department in a large organization; in smaller organizations, this function is routinely outsourced. With that being said, payroll specialists are experts in running the periodic payroll run, maintaining

Best Practice

Field Training and Evaluation Program

Even graduates of the best EMT or paramedic educational program are not fully prepared to go to work in your ambulance service. Similarly, experienced EMTs or medics who have never worked in your organization may not be ready to staff your ambulances. A program is necessary to ensure that the essential competencies required by your service are possessed by every new employee.

For years many ambulance services have utilized some form, often informal, of a field training program. However, informal field training programs are subject to a variety of problems, inconsistencies, and biases that may subject the employer to liability for negligent hiring, negligent retention, or wrongful termination.

Based on a well-established and legally sound program developed in the law enforcement community, the EMS Field Training and Evaluation Program (EMS-FTEP) evolved in a number of respected EMS agencies in the late 1990s and the early 2000s. The program has been adopted by the National EMS Management Association (NEMSMA) as a best practice program.

EMS-FTEP is structured to provide valid, reliable, and consistent training and evaluation to each new employee, in a manner that meets the content validity requirements for the use of tests as a basis for employment decisions. It is built upon a three-pronged program of core elements: the standardized evaluation guidelines, which establish the organization's standards for evaluation of new personnel; the daily observation report (DOR), which is the instrument for documenting daily performance in each guideline area; and the recruit training manual or phase guide, which specifies the competencies required of all new employees and the timeline on which they are to be developed. EMS-FTEP is a sound, legally defensible approach to the training of new employees, aimed at ensuring operational as well as clinical competence before the employee is fully ready to serve his or her community.

NEMSMA offers two courses to assist ambulance services and other EMS agencies interested in implementing EMS-FTEP. "Developing and Managing the EMS Field Training and Evaluation Program" is a 2.5-day course for senior managers, training officers, and supervisors who are responsible for field operations and will be involved with FTEP. The Basic FTO Course is a 3-day course for experienced field personnel who will be responsible for instructing and evaluating newly hired staff members.

Best Practice

Credentialed Human Resources Professionals

One way an ambulance service can ensure the competence of candidates for HR positions is to look for certification from the Human Resources Certification Institute (HRCI; www.hrci.org). HRCI offers two certifications that cover all HR disciplines.

* Senior Professional in Human Resources (SPHR)
* Global Professional in Human Resources (GPHR)

The possession of an HR credential may help an ambulance service to identify the most credible candidates from a stack of many applicants' résumés. Certified HR professionals can be expected to know the most current principles and core practices of HR management. An employer that insists on certification for its professional HR staff helps to ensure updated HR programs and policies in the organization.

Source: Adapted from content provided by the Human Resources Certification Institute, www.hrci.org.

---

compliance with federal and state withholding requirements, and producing annual employee tax documents.

LABOR RELATIONS SPECIALISTS

Labor relations (LR) specialists are typically experts in collective bargaining practices. For supervisors working in a collective bargaining environment, the LR specialist will be an invaluable resource for working within the bounds of the collective bargaining agreement. Just as the ER specialist was closely aligned with the organization's legal counsel, so is the LR specialist.

CHAPTER REVIEW

Summary

For most ambulance services, personnel represent the single largest budgetary item. Employees also constitute the single most valuable resource for all service industries. Therefore, supervisors and managers must make effective HRM a top priority. Unfortunately, most supervisors in the EMS and ambulance industry begin their supervisory career prior to receiving any supervisory training. The structure of human resources support for supervisors depends on the size and structure of the organization, but all supervisors should know how to access this support and should understand their limitations with regard to human resources issues.

Supervisors should have a basic understanding of the legal foundations for personnel management to include the Civil Rights Act, Family Medical Leave Act, Fair Labor Standards Act, sexual discrimination, and veterans' rights. Supervisors should also be familiar with the creation and development of job descriptions and how job descriptions then drive the creation of job postings, application and applicant review, and even organizational structure. Selection and hiring processes should be conducted consistently and per organization policy.

Supervisors should also be familiar with the employee life cycle and how human resources can play a role at each step in the process. Supervisors should be comfortable with performance improvement and progressive discipline of employees. Ideally, supervisors will establish an organizational culture that embraces mentoring and succession planning.

The human resources profession has been moving toward the role of strategic partner for many organizations. With the creation of subspecialties within the human resources profession, experts are available in all specialty areas to support supervisors. Each organization must determine how the human resources function is provided (i.e., internally within the department, as a separate department within the organization, or outsourced). However, regardless of the method, successful supervisors will be familiar with their human resources support and how to access that support.

WHAT WOULD YOU DO? Reflection

Background:
This supervisor has spoken with you in the past about "George." George has been his regular "problem child." He is continually late to work, his written reports are sloppy and incomplete, and he and his partner have a reputation for keeping a sloppy unit. You know the supervisor has spoken to him before; however, the supervisor has been remiss in following through with his counseling session reports (there is nothing in the personnel file), even after you have discussed this need with him. Your supervisors, by following standard operating procedures, have the authority to send someone home with pay, pending outcome of an investigation, but they cannot take away pay without review and confirmation. In training, you have stressed to your supervisors not to make decisions while emotionally stressed, in particular when they are angry.

Conclusions:
This action cannot stand. It is against organizational policy and represents bad personnel practice.

You must counsel your supervisor, stressing the following points (at a minimum):

1. There is no documentation to support such a severe progressive disciplinary action.
2. He cannot give time off without pay until the action is reviewed by higher authority.
3. He was wrong to take such a strong action while in such an emotional condition. He was not under control emotionally.

You can also discuss the process of progressive discipline as well as the difference between formal and informal actions.

Review Questions

1. What two components form the fundamental buildings blocks for managing employees?
2. What new concept and standards did the Fair Labor Standards Act create in 1938?
3. What legislation outlawed discrimination on the basis of race, color, religion, sex, or national origin?
4. How much protected time off is guaranteed as a result of the Family Medical Leave Act for employees with a qualifying condition that does not relate to military service?
5. Compare and contrast the differences between quid pro quo and hostile work environment as it relates to sexual harassment in the workplace.

6. Explain the purpose of job descriptions.
7. An applicant has all of the preferred qualifications, but lacks one of the minimum qualifications. What options does the hiring manager have to offer this candidate the position? Justify your response.

References

Brittle, L. R., and J. W. Newstrom. (1990). *What Every Supervisor Should Know: The Complete Guide to Supervisory Management*, 6th ed. New York: McGraw-Hill.

Buckingham, M., and C. Coffman. (1999). *First, Break All the Rules: What the World's Greatest Managers Do Differently.* New York: Simon & Schuster.

Buhler, P. (2002). *Human Resources Management: All the Information You Need to Manage Your Staff and Meet Your Business Objectives.* Avon, MA: Adams Media.

Desimone, R. L., J. M. Werner, and D. M. Harris. (2002). *Human Resources Development.* Fort Worth, TX: Harcourt College Publishers.

Goldsmith, M., and L. Carter (Eds.). (2010). *Best Practice in Talent Management: How the World's Leading Corporations Manage, Develop, and Retain Top Talent.* San Francisco: Pfeiffer, an Imprint of Wiley.

IAFC and IFFC. (1999–2013). "Labor-Management Initiative: LMI." See the organization website.

Jackson, S. E., R. S. Schuler, and S. Werner. (2009). *Managing Human Resources*, 10th ed. Mason, OH: South-Western Cengage Learning.

Moran, J. J. (2008). *Employment Law: New Challenges in the Business Environment*, 4th ed. Upper Saddle River, NJ. Pearson Education.

National Association of Disaster Response Teams. (n.d.). "Mission Statement." See the MedicCom website.

National Practitioner Data Bank and Healthcare Integrity and Protection Data Bank (n.d.). See the organization website.

Noe, R. A. (2010). *Employee Training and Development*, 5th ed. New York: McGraw-Hill/Irwin.

Patterson, K., J. Grenny, R. McMillan, and A. Switzler. (2011). *Crucial Conversations: Tools for Talking When Stakes Are High*, 2nd ed. New York: McGraw-Hill.

Wrighton, S. (Ed.) (2005). *Effective Supervisory Practices: Better Results Through Teamwork*, 4th ed. Washington, DC: International City/County Management Association.

Key Terms

Americans with Disabilities Act (ADA) Federal legislation that expanded the scope of discrimination protection initially provided by the Civil Rights Act to include individuals with disabilities. Disability is defined as any physical or mental impairment that substantially limits a major life activity.

Civil Rights Act Federal legislation that outlawed discrimination in schools, the workplace, and public facilities on the basis of race, color, religion, sex, or national origin.

Fair Labor Standards Act (FLSA) Federal legislation that established employer responsibilities and national standards with regard to employee compensation and child labor.

Family Medical Leave Act (FMLA) Federal legislation that provided for unpaid leave for employees experiencing certain qualifying medical or family related issues.

job descriptions Written documents that establish roles and responsibilities, minimum and preferred qualifications, and reporting structure with regard to other positions.

KSAs Knowledge, skills, and abilities, usually used with regard to a job description or job posting.

mentoring The process of an experienced or senior member of an organization working with a less experienced or new employee to develop knowledge, skills, and abilities.

minimum qualifications The lowest knowledge, skills, or abilities necessary to perform a job.

performance improvement A method of bettering productivity (human or business) by establishing metrics and then providing feedback based on those metrics.

preferred qualifications Knowledge, skills, or abilities a supervisor/manager would like a candidate to have for a position.

progressive discipline A method of modifying employee performance though escalating steps of penalty for unacceptable performance or behavior.

succession planning The process of developing programs designed to identify and prepare employees to step into key positions within an organization.

Ambulance Specification and Procurement

Jonathan A. Olson, M.B.A., M.H.A., NREMT-P, EFO

Objectives

After reading this chapter, the student should be able to:

9.1 Describe a methodology to define the desire and need for a new ambulance for an EMS agency.

9.2 Identify the applicable regulations for an ambulance to be credentialed and placed into service in the state and local EMS systems.

9.3 Discuss the limitations in the physical vehicle based on where it will be utilized and stored.

9.4 Identify key features that will be required inside the ambulance module to meet the operational and clinical needs of the ambulance service.

9.5 Identify different ambulance construction materials, and discuss techniques for identifying the specifications that best suit the needs of the ambulance service

9.6 Discuss the reasons for properly specifying the electrical requirements of an ambulance.

9.7 Identify the regulations that stipulate what emergency equipment, such as lights and sirens, are required or prohibited for use on ambulances.

9.8 Evaluate different designs and equipment to enhance the safety of paramedics working in the ambulance, and include them within the specification document.

9.9 Estimate the required payload for the ambulance based on the operational and clinical needs of the ambulance service, and use this information in selecting the appropriate chassis

9.10 Develop a thorough plan for inspecting an ambulance prior to delivery, based on the specification and vendor build plans.

Overview

Ambulance services in the United States range in size from one ambulance operated by volunteers and managed by a community board of directors to large governmental agencies and even larger, private, for-profit corporations. This text presents information that the manager of an ambulance service, large or small, needs in order to keep the business solvent and provide clinically excellent service to the community.

Key Terms

applicable requirements and regulations	angle of departure final inspection	gross vehicle weight rating (GVWR)	prebuild conference

WHAT WOULD YOU DO?

The general manager of your ambulance service has come to you with a task that you have been hinting at for quite some time. It has been several years since the service purchased a new ambulance, and the current fleet is showing its age. Maintenance costs are on the rise. The service is looking for a vehicle that will provide many years of service, meet the current and future needs of the service, and remain within budget. You have thought about what a new ambulance should look like and contain, but you have no experience in actually buying one. The whole department will be depending on you to get this right.

1. Who are the stakeholders in this process?
2. What are possible sources for regulations that may help you determine the capabilities required in an ambulance in your jurisdiction?
3. What limitations may need to be included in designing the ambulance?

■ INTRODUCTION

The process of procuring an ambulance requires planning, research, and strict attention to detail. These steps are all necessary to ensure that the delivered vehicle meets all the needs of the agency, is practical to operate, and will provide reliable service. It presents an opportunity to look at current technology and advancements in the ambulance market, and to review any issues that the service's paramedics have found with the existing ambulance design or configuration. It also presents an opportunity for an ambulance service to review anticipated changes that will provide or require additional capabilities for the vehicle or its support systems.

■ NEEDS AND WANTS

When starting the procurement process, one must first identify what the necessary features and capabilities of the vehicle (the needs) are and what features and capabilities the paramedics using the vehicle feel are desired (the wants). Identifying the needs should start with a review of the **applicable requirements and regulations** that govern transport vehicles in the jurisdiction where it will be used. If the agency is bound to use a vehicle that meets the current federal ambulance specification, this must be noted in the agency specification document. The federal ambulance specification, known as the KKK standard, are published by the General Services Administration.[1] (The current version of the document, KKK-A-1822, can be located on the Internet at www.gsa.gov/automotive.) Although an agency may be bound to operate a vehicle that carries the KKK certification, this standard only represents the basic requirements for an ambulance being procured by a federal agency and that most likely will not serve as the end product of the procurement process. The regulatory agency that licenses ambulances in a jurisdiction (usually the state EMS office) is another source for the capability requirements for the ambulance. Most states have defined detailed regulations that govern basic requirements and capabilities. These regulations should be very closely studied prior to preparing a vehicle's specification, as it would be quite detrimental for a delivered vehicle to be found ineligible for state licensure. Some jurisdictions stipulate, through regulation, the total weight of a vehicle or the required payload of a completed vehicle. This factor must be clearly stipulated in a specification document.

The specification for a new ambulance will also be driven by the role the vehicle will play within the local EMS system. There will likely be significant differences between a vehicle that is intended to provide basic life support or nonemergent interfacility transport and an ambulance that is intended to provide paramedic-level emergency response in a 9-1-1 system. The intended staffing and crew configurations (size and functions) on the vehicle will have ramifications on the end product. Clearly defining the role of the vehicle is the first step in directing the procurement process.

The paramedics who will be using the vehicle are an excellent source for identifying the wants list. A good approach involves asking field paramedics to look at the existing fleet and identify items that could be changed for practicality and safety. Websites from the various ambulance manufacturers are a good source for seeing what new features are being offered throughout the ambulance manufacturing industry. Many vendors will bring demonstrator vehicles to an ambulance service's location so that staff can examine features, or they will arrange for newly delivered vehicles in the area to be available for viewing. EMS and fire expositions or conferences are a good opportunity to see multiple vendors at one time. Once the paramedics have developed their list of wants, priorities should be defined for consideration later in the process, when vehicle cost issues are considered. The culmination of determining the needs and wants will prepare you to start the process of designing the ambulance.

■ LIMITATIONS

Once the needs and wants are identified, the next step is to evaluate the limitations—for example, the space in which the vehicle would be stored. On more than one occasion an emergency vehicle has been delivered, after a thorough research and procurement process, only to find that it will not fit within the

---

[1]At the time of this writing, the federal government has decided to allow the current GSA specification to expire. The National Fire Protection Association (NFPA) has undertaken to develop a consensus statement that is a work in progress. NFPA standard 1917, Ambulance Design and Construction, should be available by the time this book is published. Whether or not the individual state regulatory agencies will adopt NFPA 1917 in their jurisdictions remains to be seen.

confines of the station or post for which it is intended, or that it is unable to fit under the portico at local health care facilities. This assessment should include not only defining the maximum height, width, and length of the vehicle but should also take into account the angle of the apron leading from the street into the apparatus bay or other garaging structure. Constructing a vehicle that has any length behind the rear axle can precipitate issues of clearing the entrance to the bay, either rubbing on the top or dragging on the bottom. This is not usually an issue with aprons that are at the same grade as the apparatus floor; however, any changes in the grade should be taken into account when designing the vehicle. The **angle of departure**, defined as the maximum angle (from the ground) that a hill or obstacle can have (Figure 9.1) and that the front of your vehicle can still clear, must be calculated to determine if the rear step bumper will drag along aprons that angle up from the entrance to the apparatus bay.

Failure to account for this will result in the bumper dragging on every exit and entrance. Likewise, for aprons that angle downward, rather than the bumper dragging, the top of the ambulance might impact the overhead door or the threshold over the entrance. Both of these situations must be considered when determining a safe overall length for the vehicle.

In determining the overall maximum length of the vehicle, not only does the available space pose a limitation, but what remaining space is available to the front and rear also should be considered. Do paramedics routinely remove the stretcher inside the building for decontamination or cleaning? Will there be room behind this vehicle to accomplish this without having to pull the vehicle partly outside? The discussion of overall vehicle length must include both a review of local practice to ensure that current procedures can be continued and a careful evaluation of options should alteration be necessary.

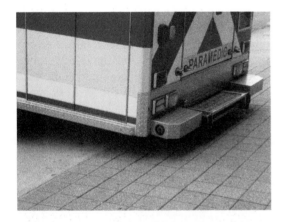

FIGURE 9.1 ■ Along with the height, length, and width considerations for parking a truck inside an apparatus bay, one must also consider limitations once the truck leaves the station. In this example, the length required behind the axle to accommodate a bariatric lift poses potential problems when crossing different surface grades. *Courtesy of the Author.*

■ DESIGNING THE MODULE———

The first step in developing the specification must focus on the work end of the ambulance. The needs list will help to craft this process. A priority throughout this phase is ensuring the safety for those working in the ambulance module. This will include looking at how equipment and supplies are stored and ensuring that everyone will have a seat with appropriate restraint devices.

STORAGE

To begin, review the standard equipment that must be stored in the module. This should include all equipment and stock that are kept on shelves interior to the ambulance as well as ensuring safe storage for portable equipment. A good rule of thumb to start this process is to establish up front that everything will have a designated home and that on the floor is unacceptable. It is essential that space be designated for keeping portable equipment secure should the vehicle be involved in a collision (Figure 9.2). Anything that is not secured in the vehicle is apt to become a projectile capable of rendering mortal injury. The standard approach to the portable equipment compartment is having doors, either single- or double-hung panels or a roll-up tambour style, inside the patient compartment. Regardless of the style, it is essential that doors include a device to secure them in the closed position and that they be constructed from a material that will

withstand impact from anything stored inside the compartment.

Another approach would be the use of cargo-style netting to cover the compartment opening (Figure 9.3). The netting offers the advantages of paramedics being able to quickly and clearly see all the contents of this compartment and improved air circulation for items affected by climate. The netting is infinitely configurable to the user's needs using buckles or latches, allowing access to the entire area at once or individual portions. The netting also will not suffer over the years from damage from impact or loosening of hinges, as can occur with doors.

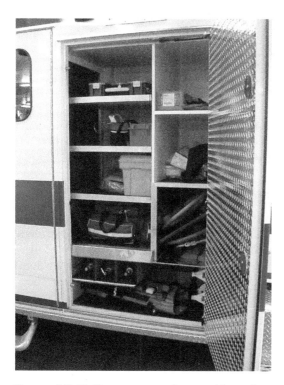

FIGURE 9.2 ■ Compartments for portable equipment must be designed around the particular needs of the agency. This design contains a single transverse compartment for the low-height storage of backboards. *Courtesy of the Author.*

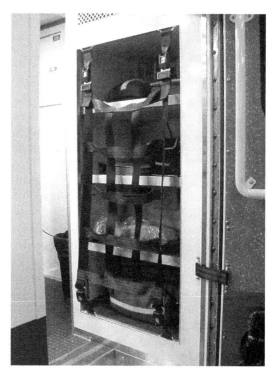

FIGURE 9.3 ■ The use of web netting allows for clear view of an equipment cabinet content. This design allows the net to be released from either the top or the bottom. *Courtesy of the Author.*

SEATING

The next step in designing the interior should focus on the location from which the primary attendant intends to work. The intent here is to define a location where the primary attendant will be seated, in order to then build out from that location the necessary cabinetry, controls, and fixtures in the module to minimize, as much as is possible, that person having to stand or move about the vehicle when it is in motion.

Traditionally, ambulances have been outfitted with a bench-style seat that served many purposes, including the primary attendant location. Not only did it provide a seating point for providers and workspace for equipment, but many were outfitted to affix a second supine patient on a litter. Many bench designs also accommodated storage space underneath. If an ambulance service intends to include storage space underneath the bench seat, include hydraulic cylinders with a lift rating greater than the weight of the seat and one at each end. The bench seat specification should also include a positive latching device that will keep the lid securely shut in time of collision.

Although the bench provides a multipurpose surface, it also presents the challenge of safely restraining those seated there. New seating options are available for ambulances that can provide the ability to face forward while providing patient care while also retaining the ability to transport a second litter or backboard-restrained patient (Figure 9.4). These seats can be installed in place of the traditional bench seat. They offer the advantage of rotating into a forward-facing position when facing the patient is not necessary. The current research on ambulance crashes indicates that the safest way to be seated in the module of an ambulance is in either a forward- or rear-facing position (Levick, 2008). Seats should be outfitted with a secure lap

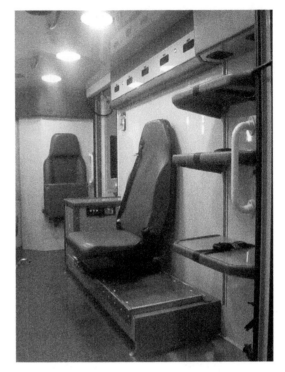

FIGURE 9.4 ■ Seating can be specified to meet the particular needs of an agency. In this example, the seat slides horizontally to better align with different patients. *Courtesy of the Author.*

belt and a single over-the-shoulder seat belt. In her article Dr. Levick cites an Australian study that determined the use of four- or five-point harnesses as being "highly hazardous when seated sideways." Should your specification maintain the standard bench seat configuration, it should include secure lap belt restraint devices for three occupants.

Another option for seating the primary attendant is on the street side of the vehicle in what has traditionally been referred to as the CPR seat. (It is an industry convention to use *street side* and *curb side* for driver and passenger, respectively.) The advantage to this location is that most of the traditional controls that require utilization during transport are located on this wall, usually within reach of this seat, including climate control, lighting, communications equipment, suction devices, and onboard oxygen systems. Although each of these have traditionally been located on the forward street-side bulkhead, they can all be relocated, or replicated, on the curb side of the module, allowing their use without paramedics having to move around while the vehicle is in motion. The integration of solid-state electrical systems in ambulances in the last decade has opened up new opportunities for redundant switch locations in vehicles. Placing light switches not only where paramedics will be seated, but also inside the doors, may help to reduce injury while enhancing convenience. Many mobile radios can be configured with two or more control heads, to allow the radio to be utilized from different locations, again eliminating the need to move somewhere to conduct a primary business function while the vehicle is in motion.

For all seating within the module of the vehicle, some standards must be met regarding upholstery. Federal Motor Vehicle Safety Standard (FMVSS) 302 governs the flammability of materials used in the interior of vehicles. Upholstery used in the module of an ambulance should meet this standard. To be compliant with occupational safety and health standards (42 CFR 1910.1030), upholstery should be made of a material that can be thoroughly decontaminated and applied without exposed stitching or welting where fluids can accumulate and absorb. Most ambulance manufacturers utilize a nylon-reinforced vinyl material that is compliant with both of these standards. These materials are available in a variety of colors and are resistant to wear and tearing.

WITHIN ARM'S REACH

Regardless of where the primary attendant will be seated, the interior of the module

should be designed outward from that point. The next step would be to determine what equipment and supplies the primary attendant would need to have within arm's reach, and then to design storage cabinets to meet those needs. Although most ambulance manufacturers have standard shelving and cabinet configurations, custom placement and changes are possible. The use of drawers is becoming more popular, in that they can be located adjacent to the primary seating location (Figure 9.5). Depending on the size of the drawer, a large share of the equipment and supplies used during transport can be kept within arm's reach, eliminating the need to move around or have portable equipment bags sitting on the floor or adjacent seating space. Drawers can be configured with tabs to hold them open once pulled out, should always include a positive mechanism for securing them shut, and should be operable with one hand.

Outlets for the onboard oxygen and suction system should likewise be placed both

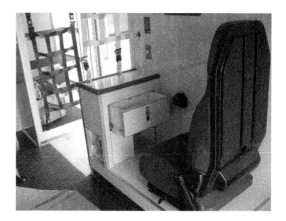

FIGURE 9.5 ■ The attendant seating in this unit can be adjusted to face forward, sideways toward the cot, or toward the rear for a seated patient. Note the easy access to a drawer for often-used supplies and equipment. *Courtesy of the Author.*

within arm's reach of the attendant seating location and close to the patient cot. Thought should be given to placement of oxygen outlets, such that they are placed for quick access from each potential patient location as well as to facilitate the operation of devices such as continuous positive airway pressure (CPAP) equipment. Access to the main oxygen cylinder (particularly its control valve) should be easy from within the module. Although placing this cylinder within arm's reach of the attendant may be difficult, some of today's systems can be controlled remotely through an electric valve switch. Many of these electric valve systems also provide a remote indicator of the remaining content within the oxygen tank.

One challenge to this process is finding suitable locations where the cardiac monitor/defibrillator can be placed and secured, while remaining fully functioning for patient care. To address this issue, several manufacturers now market specially designed mounts to secure these devices in the mobile environment (Figure 9.6). If a mount is chosen, it would be necessary to designate where that mount is to be placed, with the necessary plating underneath to withstand the stress and torque should the vehicle be in a collision while the cardiac monitor is secured. If the cardiac monitor used by the agency provides for recharging from an 110V AC-power source, locating an outlet in close proximity to this mount also should be a requirement.

ADDITIONAL CABINETRY

Although it is desirable to place as much of the equipment and supplies within arm's reach of the attendant, it is unlikely that all of the equipment and supplies either required or desired in the module can meet this test. Any additional cabinetry should be designed around the needs of the agency and the specific equipment and supplies that are to be stored (Figure 9.7). In building a specification document, detail should be provided for each cabinet to include the approximate dimensions as well as intended utilization. This can be accomplished best through a detailed chart and sketches of the layout. The

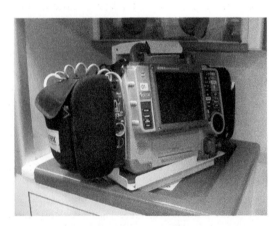

FIGURE 9.6 ■ Locking mounts are available for every EMS cardiac monitor defibrillator. These devices safety secure the unit while maintaining access for use while in the rear of the ambulance. *Courtesy of the Author.*

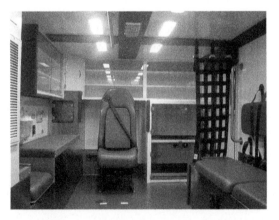

FIGURE 9.7 ■ This interior design utilizes the seat at the head of the cot as the primary location for the attendant; therefore, the cabinetry is concentrated behind and beside this location. *Courtesy of the Author.*

sketches do not have to be of computer-aided-design (CAD) quality; however, the more clearly an agency can portray its needs and desires, the better are its chances of receiving an ambulance that meets its needs and wants requirements.

It is also recommended that during the assessment phase of reviewing bids or offers, the ambulance service should require the vendor to provide CAD renderings of your descriptions. Although seeing something in one dimension on paper does not equate to seeing it after it has been built, this will give those involved with procurement a good opportunity to evaluate what the service has asked for against what the vendor is offering so that and necessary changes can be discussed prior to the beginning of construction.

One important safety consideration when reviewing cabinetry designs is cabinet placement in relation to the heads of seated paramedics and patients. Cabinets should be spaced far enough from seated individuals to minimize the possibility of them striking their heads during an impact. All exposed corners should be rounded and padded to prevent injury.

Certain cabinetry needs require additional research when developing the overall vehicle specification. For example, if space for the storage of controlled substances is designated inside the vehicle, special requirements may apply to the security of that cabinet. This cabinet will likely require key access or other limited access measures. Should local regulations require key access, each vehicle should be keyed differently to ensure security and to limit access only to those issued the key for their assigned vehicle. Some of today's systems integrate a variety of security technology into this process (Figure 9.8). From card-reader-based systems to keypad locks with individually coded combinations to systems that remotely open the compartment by way

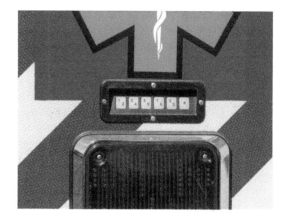

FIGURE 9.8 ■ A variety of technology solutions exists for ensuring ambulance security. This unit has external keypads installed at the rear of the unit to allow quick unlocking of the module for patient loading. *Courtesy of the Author.*

of radio or data connectivity, each agency should look at its individual requirements and needs to ensure that the appropriate standard is adopted and installed.

Many of the pharmaceuticals carried on advanced life support (ALS) vehicles now require refrigeration until time of administration. A variety of manufacturers builds refrigeration units of all sizes that will operate on either 12V DC or 110V AC power systems. Should the clinical objectives of the agency involve the induction of hypothermia via chilled IV fluids, the ambulance service should be aware that most *refrigeration* units will not cool to a temperature low enough to maintain fluids in the therapeutic range. To maintain the fluids between 34°F and 37°F at all times (current recommendations for hypothermia), a *freezer* unit is required (Figure 9.9). The ambulance service should carefully specify the required capabilities of the refrigerator or freezer unit, and test those capabilities, before accepting the unit for delivery. Freezer and refrigeration units are

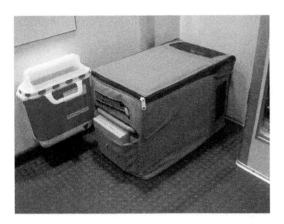

FIGURE 9.9 ■ Refrigerators or freezers are often required to properly store certain medications or clinical treatments. This freezer from Engel can be securely affixed to the floor for safety while allowing ease of access and, should the unit fail, quick exchange. *Courtesy of the Author.*

available that either can be built into the factory cabinetry of the unit or mounted within available compartments or floor space in a manner that will withstand a collision. Built-in devices have an advantage in that they can be designed into the vehicle around other cabinetry needs, and they do not utilize space that is otherwise needed for other equipment or supplies. The disadvantage to these units over portable or removable units is that a malfunction of a built-in unit renders the entire ambulance out of service until it can be repaired. With removable freezer and refrigerators, one would simply need to remove the defective unit and replace it securely with a functional one. If you choose the removable device, ensure that the location for the mount has the necessary plating underneath to withstand the stress and torque should the vehicle be in a collision and that the appropriate power source is available in close proximity.

Side Bar

Specialized Equipment: Permanent versus Fixed

If you have a clinical need for specialized equipment in an ambulance, give some thought to whether it is necessary to have it built in or mounted in the vehicle. A good example would be temperature regulation and monitoring equipment that is needed to properly maintain medications and fluids. By having refrigerators or freezers built into the cabinetry of the vehicle, you run the risk of having a unit out of service should that equipment malfunction or fail. By mounting a portable unit, you provide the same capability, but you have the option of swapping out a failed device with a spare and not losing the entire ambulance from your fleet.

Look for devices that can be safely affixed in a vehicle, either in available floor space or on a large shelf, which will meet the clinical needs of the service but can be quickly replaced in a time of failure. Many of these devices offer options for power supply and can provide external temperature regulation and monitoring.

Ambulance cabinetry has traditionally been constructed of wood; however, several manufacturers now offer cabinets made of aluminum. The aluminum cabinetry is lighter and less apt to damage from exposure to moisture. Aluminum cabinetry can also be welded to the modular frame of the ambulance, providing additional structural integrity within the body. The disadvantage to the aluminum is the increase in cost compared to wood cabinets. Cabinetry of either wood or aluminum can be custom designed to the needs of the agency. Should your design for cabinetry include any larger cabinets with internal shelving, it is essential that the shelves be securely held in place while also adjustable for future needs. One type of suitable construction would require the use of aluminum tracks, two per side, to which the shelves can be affixed with adjustable screws. Shelves that are attached with clips may work well in the home or office, but they often lack the integrity to withstand the mobile environment. As many supplies on shelves are stored within boxes or bins, the inclusion of a 1-inch lip on the side of the shelf facing the interior of the ambulance body will help to keep items from sliding up against and potentially damaging the ambulance body or hindering opening the cabinet.

Cabinets can be specified with a restocking feature that will allow the entire frame to fold upward to provide more of an opening for restocking supplies. If you desire to have this feature, ensure that the manufacturer installs a positive locking mechanism on both sides of the cabinet to securely hold the cabinet shut should the vehicle be involved in a collision.

The interior surfaces of the cabinets and shelves should be coated with a material that is impervious to liquids. Wooden cabinets and shelves often are coated with a laminate material, and aluminum can be powder-coated. Both of these options provide a surface that can be cleaned and can be color-coordinated with the interior of the ambulance. The installation of lighting within cabinets has become popular in recent years with the advancement in LED lighting. This feature provides a low amperage solution that makes it easier to locate equipment and supplies within deep cabinets that may not be sufficiently illuminated by the ceiling lights inside the ambulance module.

Some ambulance services may wish to have additional cabinets and portable equipment that can be accessed from both the outside and the inside of the ambulance. Special attention should be paid to these spaces to ensure that the seal on the exterior door is sufficient to prevent moisture or fumes from reaching the patient compartment. As these spaces are likely to be larger than the other cabinets, the use of cargo netting may be beneficial over doors opening into the patient compartment.

HEADLINER AND CEILING

The headliner and equipment installed on the ceiling of the module are important for a number of reasons. Properly installed grab rails are essential to ensuring the safety of those who have to move around in the ambulance while it is in motion. Grab rail material should be strong enough to support the weight of paramedics and properly anchored into plating welded to the modular structure at multiple points. Aluminum tubing is commonly used for this purpose due to its high strength and lightweight properties. The aluminum also provides a surface that is easily decontaminated of residue. Grab rails should be placed where they are easily reached by paramedics in all seating positions, but as close to the ceiling as possible to minimize their being an overhead strike hazard.

In addition to the overhead grab rails, handles should be placed at each door to facilitate safe entry to and exit from the ambulance. Ensure that in each location that a grab rail or handle is placed, sufficient plating is welded underneath to properly support the stress under use. Any other hardware that is attached through the walls or headliner should be properly supported from behind. All support materials should be thoroughly welded to the modular structure. Although this can often be difficult to determine on a one-dimensional drawing, those responsible should ensure that there are sufficient handles for staff and civilians to safely enter and exit the vehicle and that they are placed so that people of all heights can safely use them.

The headliner of the vehicle should be made of a nonporous material that is easily cleaned and decontaminated. Since fluids and other contaminants can be sprayed or projected

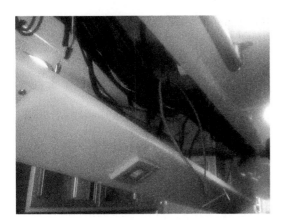

FIGURE 9.10 ■ Having a designated corridor within the ceiling for cables, coaxial antenna lines, and other wiring is necessary for post-delivery installation and repair. In this example, the corridor is installed centerline in the ceiling for ease in installing antennas through the modular roof. *Courtesy of the Author.*

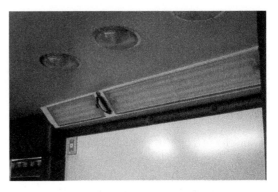

FIGURE 9.11 ■ Lights can be specified and installed based on the particular needs of an agency. In this example, a bank of fluorescent lights is mounted in the upper corner of the module wall in addition to standard lights in the headliner. *Courtesy of the Author*

onto the headliner, the design should minimize seams that will hinder thorough decontamination. Many ambulance manufacturers utilize solid sheets of **ABS** plastic or other solid material that may be coated with an antimicrobial compound to improve the ability to keep them clean and sanitary. The headliner should provide necessary points of access for installing antennas to the module roof (Figure 9.10).

LIGHTING

Interior lighting in an ambulance is a very important feature that should not be minimized for the sake of budget. For many years, modular lighting was accomplished with dual-intensity incandescent or halogen lighting. Both incandescent and halogen lighting, although meeting the need, were often plagued with the ongoing need to replace bulbs (Figure 9.11). With the advent of LED lighting, the lights are virtually maintenance

free and require much less power to operate (Figure 9.12). Regardless of the type of light used, sufficient lighting over the patient cot, seating area, and side entrance doorstep well is essential. The side entrance steps should also be sufficiently illuminated for safe entry and exit whenever that door is opened. For

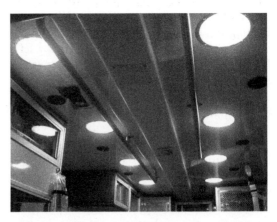

FIGURE 9.12 ■ The installation of LED lighting in the headliner can create a bright, shadow-free workspace and uses minimal electricity. *Courtesy of the Author.*

patient comfort, it should be possible to turn off unneeded lights, as well as have two levels of illumination. Lighting should also be configured to automatically illuminate at the brightest setting whenever any exterior door is opened.

Another beneficial feature is the installation of a check-off light circuit controlled by a timer switch. This circuit, with the switch installed adjacent to either the side or rear doors, allows a group of lights to be illuminated directly from the battery so that paramedics can inventory equipment and supplies without having to engage the master switch in the cab. A timer is utilized so that the lights are not inadvertently left on, potentially draining the batteries to the point that the vehicle will not start.

FLOORING

The floor of the ambulance body is one of the more important features of the vehicle, second only to safe seating. Regardless of what equipment is used in the vehicle, the flooring is subject to constant use and should be designed to provide many years of trouble-free operation. Regulation will often dictate the actual height of the vehicle floor in relation to the ground height outside the rear of the ambulance. (This topic, as well as the means to address such regulations, will be presented later.) The floor should be constructed of aluminum, marine-grade plywood, or a combination of both. In addition to the primary materials, the use of a moisture barrier should be specified as well as an appropriate insulation material. The insulation will serve not only to enhance the climate control systems but also will provide a degree of soundproofing. The flooring substructure should be integrated into the overall modular construction to ensure the proper support and integrity. All cot-fastening hardware should be installed into support plates welded between the frame members of the vehicle to ensure the strength and integrity of the mount for patient and attendant safety.

It is essential that the floor of the vehicle prevent moisture and fumes that originate underneath the vehicle from getting inside the module and that the exterior surface of the flooring is made from a material that will prevent the absorption of any liquid materials inside the vehicle. This is accomplished, first, by ensuring that the entire underbody is thoroughly coated with a material that will resist moisture and salt as well as provide a measure of soundproofing. Second, the floor covering should be a seamless material that will endure constant exposure to the elements inside the ambulance. A number of different materials in use will meet this requirement, of which the most commonly used is a heavy-duty no-wax vinyl. Such flooring is available in different colors and slip-resistant texture patterns. The flooring should be installed so that it extends up at least 3 inches along the sides (in a baseboard-like configuration) to prevent liquid material or contaminants from seeping underneath the cabinetry and seating. The flooring should be supported by a solid material where it rolls up the sides in order to prevent it from creating a crease and subsequently cracking.

INTERIOR WALLS

The interior walls of the module should be covered in a material that is highly resistant to damage and will not absorb contaminants. This is commonly accomplished using Formica, aluminum, stainless steel, or a combination of these materials. Each provides a surface that is resistant to damage and can be easily decontaminated. Regardless of the material chosen, it is essential that all seams be thoroughly sealed. To provide a well-lit working environment, bright colors with a polished, light-reflective finish should be chosen for the inside surfaces. By choosing the right combinations of color and material (or combination of materials), a much brighter working environment can be created, without adding to the lighting requirements of the vehicle.

As with the floor of the ambulance, sufficient insulation within the walls and ceiling is necessary to maintain climate control and reduce outside noise. Insulation materials should be complaint with the FMVSS 302 standard. You will want to pay particularly close attention to the insulation when doing a midproduction inspection. All void spaces within the walls and ceiling should be thoroughly filled with insulation material, with the only required minimum gaps around installed electrical equipment. A variety of materials are used for insulation in ambulances, and your choice should be made based on the environment where the ambulance will be used. Fiberglass bat insulation is the most common type of insulation and is often constructed with a reflective backing material to aid in deflecting heat from the sun. Other materials used include closed-cell polystyrene (Styrofoam) blocks and sprayed polystyrene foam or fiberglass.

CLIMATE CONTROL

Selection of the climate control system for the module should be researched to best meet the environment in which the ambulance will be utilized, including where the ambulance will be stored. For many years, heating and air conditioning for ambulance modules were merely extensions of the factory-installed chassis equipment of the original equipment manufacturer (OEM). Chassis heater lines would utilize in-line valves to divert the heated fluid through a separate heat exchanger and blower unit installed in the patient care area. The air conditioner would work much the same way, tapping the chassis condenser and circulating Freon through the rear unit. Equipment using this principle is still available and in use today.

Over the last decade, ambulance builders have adopted new technologies, mostly for the recreational vehicle industry, to provide more efficient heating and cooling of the patient module independent of chassis-installed equipment. The first generation of these independent systems utilized self-contained units that were often mounted on the roof of the ambulance, much as you would see a unit mounted on top of a camper trailer. They required little interior space inside the vehicle and had controls easily accessible to the ambulance occupants. The primary disadvantage of these units was that they added to the overall vehicle height. Many units would add 12 inches or more to the roofline of the vehicle.

The second generation of independent systems was comprised of multiple components, allowing better integration into the cabinetry of the interior of the vehicle. These systems are advantageous for a number of reasons. They pose little or no additional workload on the OEM heating and air conditioning systems, reducing the probability of their failures. Second, these systems provide more robust heating and cooling of the patient care area and can be thermostatically controlled, much as a device would work in a home or facility. They are able to raise or lower the ambient temperature in the patient care area to the desired level much more quickly than the legacy systems. These systems also have the option of being dual-voltage, using either a 12V DC or 110V AC power source, to maintain climate control both while a vehicle is in operation as well as when it is parked with a shoreline power (AC line charging) source. This is important for vehicles that are either parked outside or within facilities that do not provide or maintain sufficient climate control in the apparatus bays.

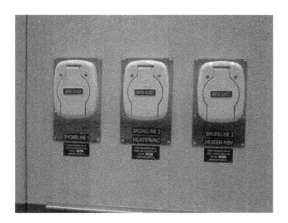

FIGURE 9.13 ▦ The equipment requirements of the vehicle should be matched by the shoreline capacity required to maintain systems. On this particular unit, three 30-amp service lines are required for the specialized equipment that is installed. *Courtesy of the Author.*

These component systems are equipped with an external condenser unit that can either be mounted on the front of the module above the cab or underneath the module body. Many ambulance manufacturers now offer a ducting system for these units that will distribute air flow out adjustable ports from the front to rear of the module in the headliner. This feature provides more balance in the heating and cooling of the module and is especially beneficial in larger vehicles. Should you determine that a dual-voltage system is best suited for your ambulance, the specification must require the installation of the necessary shoreline power to support the amperage requirement of the system chosen. Most of these require independent 20- or 30-amp electrical supplies (Figure 9.13).

EXTERIOR COMPARTMENTS

With the exception of the patient cot, a majority of the larger equipment will be stored and accessible from the exterior of the module. As local research was necessary to properly lay out the interior of the module, a like process is required to properly design the exterior compartments of the ambulance. In building the specification document, detail should be provided for each exterior compartment to include the approximate dimensions, as well as its intended utilization. For certain pieces of equipment—for example a particular make and model of stair chair—it is essential that this information be provided to the builder so that sufficient space can be allocated in the design.

The exterior compartments of the vehicle should be designed with the employee in mind. Equipment required for personal safety, such as turnout gear or other personal protective equipment (PPE), should be stored where is can be easily accessed. Heavy equipment should be stored as low as possible to avoid injury on removal or replacement, and shelves within the compartments should be limited so that all employees can access the necessary supplies without using a step or ladder. If a compartment will have shelves that cannot be easily reached from the ground, they probably need to be redesigned to be accessible from both inside and outside of the module.

If a compartment will have shelves that cannot be easily reached from the ground, they probably should be redesigned so that they are accessible from both inside and outside of the module. One important facet of designing the exterior compartments is determining the location where long spine boards will be stored. Until the mid-1990s, backboards were often stored horizontally from the rear of the ambulance or slid in from the rear underneath the bench seat. Later designs moved them to upright storage on the curb side of the ambulance, which remains very common today. Some newer designs incorporate transverse compartments at the front of the module so backboards can be stored horizontally. The advantage to this approach is that the equipment is easily removed and replaced by people of all heights. Regardless of the storage methodology chosen, it is important that some type of restraint be installed to prevent these devices from falling out when the door is opened. This is commonly accomplished using 1- or 2-inch webbing connected by a seat-belt-style buckle.

Another important detail in designing the exterior compartments is the storage of the onboard oxygen system. The M-size oxygen tank is the most commonly used cylinder for ambulance delivery. When full, these tanks can weigh as much as 100 pounds. This presents an issue of safely replacing empty cylinders. Products are available to assist in this process that either slide out, for horizontally installed tanks, or extend out and drop to ground level by way of a motor-driven device for vertically mounted tanks. Clearly detailing the cylinder that you intend to use in the ambulance is important. Although adjustable retention straps are available, fixed aluminum or stainless steel straps can be installed for their ease of use. When choosing this option, the diameter of the tank must meet the size of the installed strap to ensure it is secured properly in place. Different brands and composites of M-cylinders will have different diameter and height dimensions.

DOORS AND WINDOWS

Exterior doors on ambulances are available in a number of different, and often proprietary, designs. These designs often incorporate different structural approaches to create a smooth external appearance. Keys points for the door specification are a tight-fitting seal to prevent moisture and contaminants from penetrating into the vehicle and compartments and a secure latching mechanism. Door interiors should permit easy access to latching and locking hardware for repair and maintenance. Automotive-style latches are now available

that have improved ergonomic values over paddle-style latches, requiring less force to unlatch the door. For compartments that when opened need to remain open, the use of either hydraulic struts or other hold-open device must be specified. These devices should be firm enough to hold the door in the completely open position, but not so stiff as to restrict easy closure.

For the rear doors of the ambulance, the specification must detail the number and location of hardware to hold the doors open. The placement of this hardware will dictate how widely open the rear doors will be. For example, if there are light heads on the rear of the ambulance, hardware should be located so as to hold the entire door as flush as possible against the rear of the module. Larger doors on taller vehicles may require two sets of hardware per door, especially to ensure that doors stay open when the vehicle is facing downhill.

Windows are a standard feature found on side and rear access doors on ambulances. Most windows can be specified with an integrated sliding section to allow for fresh air ventilation into the vehicle. Depending on the desires of your agency, a variety of window film can be applied from various degrees of tint to colored shading that is transparent from the inside looking out but restricts nearly all visibility from the outside into the vehicle. Most manufacturers offer a wide range of window options and placements, including large windows on the curbside wall of the vehicle.

◼ MODULE ELECTRICAL SPECIFICATION ————————

Over the last 20 years, electrical equipment in ambulances has evolved from mechanical switches, relays, and breakers to solid-state circuitry and computer controls. The key element in establishing an electrical specification for a vehicle is to ensure that the system is capable of generating and maintaining the needed power for all onboard systems and is wired in compliance with all applicable standards.

Tracing an electrical problem in an ambulance does not need to be akin to seeking a needle in a haystack. Specifying wiring that is capable of carrying at least 125 percent of the maximum load for each circuit is a necessity. Overloading circuits on a vehicle is a guarantee of long-term problems. By clearly identifying the need, whether through specifying the exact piece of equipment that will be powered by a circuit or estimating the overall power need for a system, future problems can easily be avoided. Ambulances should be delivered with an as-built set of electrical drawings to aid in any troubleshooting process.

The generation of power for an ambulance commonly initiates with the OEM supplied alternator, or alternators. The electrical generation system should be capable of providing 125 percent of the total power demand of the vehicle. Prior to the introduction of strobe and LED lighting on ambulances, providing 125 percent of the demand was often a significant engineering challenge. Many ambulances required alternators operating in tandem to meet that requirement. With halogen bulbs and mechanical sirens no longer prevalent on most new vehicles, single alternators can often meet the overall electrical needs of the ambulance. For specialized vehicles that require additional power for equipment and devices, independent generators are an option. These generators can be freestanding devices in an exterior compartment or operated by power-take-off systems dependent on the vehicle drivetrain.

KKK standard 3.7 requires a minimum of two batteries on all certified ambulances. These batteries should be installed in a ventilated area, either under the hood or in an external compartment (Figure 9.14). Batteries should be installed so that jump-starting can

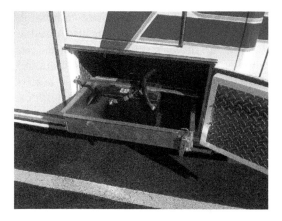

FIGURE 9.14 ■ The location for the vehicle batteries will vary by chassis and ambulance manufacturer. This example shows the auxiliary battery in a pullout tray, with the primary battery under the hood. *Courtesy of the Author.*

be completed without the use of tools or through an installed isolator. To maintain the batteries, vehicles should have an onboard charging system, powered through an external shoreline, that is capable of providing at least 45-amps of output. This system must provide not only power to keep batteries properly charged for the chassis ignition system but also working power to onboard systems such as mobile computers and equipment chargers.

Battery chargers and conditioners can be integrated with an onboard power inverter for energizing the 110V AC outlets in the ambulance module. This is desirable for agencies that perform interfacility transports of patients relying on equipment such as intravenous pumps or those that have cardiac monitors with the ability to function and charge via an AC adapter. These systems can provide 1,000 watts or more of regulated AC power for equipment requiring AC service. Such systems utilize the inverter for AC power when the vehicle is running and automatically transfer to the AC power when the shoreline is established.

The federal standard requires a minimum 15-amp utility power connector, or shoreline plug, on the driver's side of the vehicle. For vehicles with charging needs for installed onboard systems, 15-amp service may not be sufficient. Many ambulances are equipped with 20-amp shorelines for onboard charging and electronics and, as previously mentioned, 20- or 30-amp shoreline connections for 110V AC climate control systems.

SHORELINE CONNECTIONS

Shoreline connections have improved in recent years with the inclusion of ignition-sensing ejectors that mechanically press the plug out of the vehicle receptacle. Traditionally, shoreline connections were located near the front of the module, either on the street side or front face, so that the driver would recognize their presence and disconnect them manually prior to entering the vehicle. With the addition of automatic ejecting outlets, installing them on the front face should be avoided as the plugs ends can become projectiles that break side-view mirrors. Likewise, should the ejection mechanism fail to completely separate the cable from the vehicle, outlets on the side of the vehicle cause the wire to pull at a 90-degree angle from the direction of the vehicle leaving the bay, resulting in damage at the building end of the shoreline. A good option is to install the shoreline connections on the rear face of the vehicle. This approach increases the chance that an incompletely ejected shoreline will pull straight out from the connection as the vehicle moves outward.

Shorelines, regardless of the direction they exit the vehicle, should always be installed with secure anchoring and strain relief to the structure in which they are installed, and they should be equipped with short nontwist-lock pigtails at the end that plug into the vehicle. Pigtails provide a second point of separation to reduce chances of cable or building damage, and they provide an easy solution should the connector on the end be damaged. Shoreline connectors should always have the spring-loaded cover in place and should routinely be wiped down to ensure that a good seal is in place when not in use. Although the connections for the different amperage ratings for shorelines will often differ to the point that they are incompatible, each inlet on the vehicle should be clearly labeled for the intended amperage line that is to be inserted.

ELECTRONIC EQUIPMENT

If the ambulance service intends to have radios and other electronic equipment installed post-delivery, the specification process is a good opportunity to ensure that the installation of this equipment is quick and trouble free. Using local installers as a resource in the specification development phase will make their job easier once the vehicle is delivered. First, determine where in the vehicle you intend to install the electronic equipment. Many radios today have a remote transceiver located in one compartment with two or more control heads elsewhere in the vehicle. Once this location is determined, calculate the total power needs for this equipment. This total power need should be based on the equipment that you intend to install post-delivery as well as any future expansions for equipment such as networking equipment, GPS devices, and so on.

With this information, you can specify the installation of buss bars in close proximity to provide both battery and ignition power. Many radios require constant power to maintain memory (onboard programming) and an ignition source to automatically turn the radio on with the vehicle starting. A grounding point can also be installed at this location. Having the electrical components installed by the manufacturer will keep the installers from having to find power for these systems after delivery—which can be a time-consuming process, involving partial dismantling of the vehicle. This is also an opportunity to have the ambulance manufacturer install conduit within the walls of the vehicle for passing cables to the control heads in the cab and module, and running coaxial cable for antennas to the ceiling area of the module. Each conduit should include semirigid pull wires for each cable that you intend to install within it. Be sure when specifying the diameter of the conduit that you take into account any preinstalled connectors that may be present on the radio cabling, noting that these may have to pass through 90-degree turns within the conduit to reach their final destination.

The ambulance manufacturer can install a removable access panel at the location where the remote radio head is to be installed. For coaxial cable, to ensure proper shielding and to minimize signal loss, specify the correct type of cable that is required for the radio and antenna. This information can often be found in the equipment owner's manual or from your local radio installation staff.

WIRING

Several standards are applicable to the wiring in an ambulance. Section 3.7 of the KKK standard specification details the minimum standard for many of the electrical systems within these vehicles. From general requirements through criteria for installation to battery systems, adherence to Section 3.7 should be stipulated in all specifications. Society of Automotive Engineers (SAE) standard J1292 is the Automobile and Motor Coach wiring standard for primary wiring and distribution systems in vehicles. It should also be a required standard stipulated within an ambulance specification document.

EMERGENCY LIGHTING AND WARNING EQUIPMENT

As ambulances are required to work in all environments, including the dark of night, it is essential that the exterior lighting on the vehicle be sufficient for the intended purpose. The KKK standard requires an ambulance to be equipped with clear floodlights on both sides and the rear of the ambulance, unobstructed by the rear doors. The rear lights are also required to be automatically activated when the back doors of the ambulance are opened.

Side Bar

Warning Equipment

As with nearly everything else in the realm of technology, warning systems for emergency vehicles continue to evolve at a rapid pace. Just a few years ago, the industry introduced the first generation of light-emitting diode (LED) technology to replace strobes and halogen lights. Today's lights are primarily based on the third generation design of LEDs.

When developing the specification for a new ambulance, it is valuable to do some research not only to see what is new with warning equipment but also to find out from those who have installed and utilized this equipment what is truly effective, both operationally and from a cost perspective. One good source for such information is the online discussion boards found at elightbars.org. On the numerous forums available there, people are discussing visual and audible warning equipment, providing readers with information about installation, quality, and general reviews of performance. Participants include manufacturers, dealers, installers, and end users of this equipment.

Halogen bulbs have been the standard for many years for ambulance floodlights. Many vendors utilize specially designed optics within the lens to disperse the light toward the ground to better illuminate the space around the vehicle. With advancements in vehicle headlight systems, technologies such as high-intensity discharge (HID) lighting have emerged for use as scene lighting on ambulances (Figure 9.15). By nature of their function, these lights produce more light per watt of energy required than does a halogen or incandescent bulb. Although these lights produce a brighter light with a wider reach, they result in the production of more glare, which is not always desirable on emergency scenes.

The basic standard for ambulance lighting is set forth in KKK Section 3.8. This should be considered as the minimum requirements for any ambulance. The KKK standard requires an ambulance to have 12 fixed red lights, one fixed clear light, and one fixed amber light, to function in a dual-mode configuration. Eight of the red lights are to be affixed to the upper corners of each side of the module with the clear light on the front in the center and the amber light to the rear in the center. Two red lights are to be affixed to the front grille of the

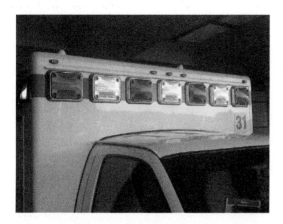

FIGURE 9.15 ■ Using a widely dispersed array of lights on the front of the module in contrasting colors provides long-distance recognition of the ambulance and short-distance attention to drivers. *Courtesy of the Author.*

chassis, at least 30 inches above the ground, and two red lights are to be mounted on each fender, as close as possible to the front edge (U.S. General Services Administration, 2007). The standard does not prohibit additional lighting on the vehicle, such as a lightbar.

Emergency lighting requirements, in particular limitations and colors, are often stipulated by state statute. For example, ambulances in North Carolina are permitted to display red lights (along with fire apparatus), whereas blue lights are reserved exclusively for law enforcement vehicles. In New Jersey, it is permissible for ambulances to display any combination of red, blue, or white lighting. Research should be undertaken to ensure that what is specified for installation on the ambulance meets all local and state requirements. Because of its perceived greater visibility at night, several states (New Jersey, Idaho, Texas, and Oregon) have recently amended their statutes to allow for use of blue lights on all emergency vehicles.

To date, there is no science to clearly support the effectiveness of one color light versus another. In a 1994 study conducted by the Phoenix Fire Department, findings suggested that the amber-colored lighting was less likely to disrupt the vision of approaching motorists or draw their attention to the scene in comparison to red, clear, or blue, therefore reducing the incidence of secondary crashes at highway scenes (U.S. Fire Administration, 2004). Since then, the application of amber lighting to the rear of emergency vehicles has become more prevalent. In the mid-1990s, the amber light was added to the center position on the KKK federal specifications.

Emergency lighting on ambulances has advanced significantly in recent years. Not only have these advancements resulted in better, more recognizable warning lights, but less power from the vehicle is required to operate these newer lights. LEDs offer some significant advantages over halogen, incandescent, and strobe lights. They have a long life span, infrequently requiring replacement or repair, due in part to their construction and its inherent resistance to vibration, which adversely impacts filament bulbs. They require far less current to operate at full brightness. For example, a halogen lamp used as one of the twelve body lights required by the KKK specification will pull as much as 5-amps. The same light in an LED configuration draws less than 2-amps (Whelen, 2010). Using this example, selecting LED over halogen would save 36-amps (or 60 percent) from the overall demand on the vehicle electrical system. The current KKK standard sets a limit of 40-amps for the ambulance warning light system. Performing this calculation for all the lighting needs of the vehicle clearly shows the advantage of using LED lighting over halogen lighting.

One disadvantage to the use of LED lighting is the initial cost. Comparing the body lights used in the previous example, the halogen light is available for around $94, whereas the LED model costs around $285. Although this is a significant difference, the vehicle equipped with the halogen lighting will require a flasher with a cost of around $225 and replacement bulbs that sell for nearly $20. LED lights are available with an integrated flasher device, and these lights commonly do not require an external flasher.

SIRENS

The KKK standard requires that an ambulance be equipped at a minimum with a siren capable of emitting a warning sound of 123 decibels (dB) at a distance of 10 feet. This siren should also include a public address system. The particular brand of electronic siren is left to the preference of the purchaser.

As technology has enhanced the lighting options for ambulances, so has it changed ambulance sirens. The mechanical siren was standard equipment on ambulances through the 1970s before the electronic siren became a popular alternative. Although the mechanical

sirens were loud and clearly recognizable, they also required the electrical system to yield as much as 100-amps when fully engaged. Although introduced in the late 1950s, electronic sirens became common in the late 1970s on ambulances as the functional alternative to the power-hungry mechanical siren.

Today, numerous variations to the standard wail and yelp tones are available, with frequency and duration of each differing among brands. Most brands also provide a third tone option, either a European hi-lo siren or a fast-paced oscillation of the yelp tone. Other sirens available today use digital processors to mimic the sound of the mechanical siren. The latter have become increasingly popular on ambulances as well as fire apparatus due to their recognizable sound with a lower power requirement.

Ambulances are required by the KKK standard to have two speakers mounted on the outside of the vehicle in the vicinity of the front bumper or grille. In the mid 1990s, speakers migrated from the roof of the ambulance chassis to their current location on the front. This was advantageous to the vehicle occupants because it reduced the ambient noise riders were subjected to when the siren was activated, and it minimized the impact of a distracting sound during patient care.

Regardless of the lighting options that are selected for an ambulance, it is important that the control switches, including the siren, be within arm's reach of both front-seat occupants while they are securely seat-belted.

EXTERIOR GRAPHICS AND SAFETY FEATURES

For many years, a majority of the ambulances in the United States were adorned with the standard Omaha orange stripe and blue lettering as specified in the KKK standard. Some would say this offered a distinct benefit for recognizing an ambulance for what it is. Although the specification remain unchanged for federally purchased ambulances, the entire spectrum of colors and designs now exists within the EMS community.

Side Bar

Vehicle Conspicuity

The concept of giving an emergency vehicle a higher degree of visibility continues to generate much debate within the industry. With advancements in vinyl materials, applying reflectivity to a vehicle is virtually limited only by one's desires and imagination. Many agencies attempt to blend additional conspicuity into a branding of such for their vehicles. This branding makes them readily identifiable as "ours" while enhancing the visibility of them to other vehicles.

In developing such a concept on a local scale, agencies must consider what brand they want to attain: something totally new or an upgrade to an existing graphical design. Existing designs can be altered slightly, while maintaining that traditional look of a services fleet. An example of this would be to add white striping to outline the perimeter of the ambulance module. In daylight, the stripe is nearly invisible. In the dark when exposed to the headlights of another vehicle, the entire outline of the ambulance glows noticeably. Another example would be the addition of a single horizontal belt of reflective material, either in the same white mentioned above or in a complimentary but highly contrasting color, to existing striping. Using the contrasting color approach also enhances daytime visibility. Whenever possible, this stripe should extend around the front of the vehicle on the bumper. Another example would be the addition of chevrons to the rear face of the module. This simple addition, when done appropriately using 6-inch-wide stripes applied at a 45-degree angle, will significantly enhance the rear visibility (and safety) of the vehicle at all times.

A U.S. Fire Administration (2009) study examined emergency vehicles and conspicuity to improve responder safety. This report identified some key findings that can be implemented within the ambulance specification. First, the study found that the use of retroreflective materials is key to improving the conspicuity of emergency vehicles and that, by using contrasting colors, emergency vehicles will stand out among the clutter of the roadway. The report cited that reflective materials may best be used to outline vehicles and that these materials should be applied to maximize the reflection from other vehicles' headlights. It also reported that using fluorescent colors offers better visibility to emergency vehicles during daylight hours.

In the 2009 revision of NFPA 1901, the Standard for Automotive Fire Apparatus (National Fire Protection Association, 2009), the fire service took a proactive approach to vehicle conspicuity by requiring 45-degree chevrons on at least 50 percent of the rear-facing vertical surfaces of new fire apparatus. The striping is to be an alternating pattern between red and either fluorescent yellow, yellow green, or reflective yellow using 6-inch stripes (U.S. Fire Administration, 2009). The objective was to begin the establishment of a standard throughout the fire service to improve the visibility of these vehicles at a vulnerable angle, especially when parked in or along roadways. Many departments have expanded this philosophy by installing reflective chevron striping to the front bumpers of apparatus, addressing the other highly vulnerable angle of the vehicle at intersections (Figure 9.16).

Although any agency may have a tried and true graphics design that represents a brand to the agency as opposed to a color scheme, the purchase of a new vehicle is an opportunity to integrate many of the USFA and NFPA recommendations. The rear of an ambulance is better suited for the installation of the chevron pattern than most fire apparatus.

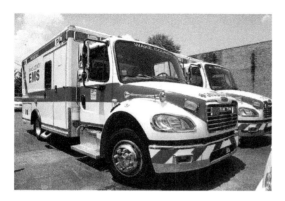

FIGURE 9.16 ■ Properly designed graphics, with contrasting but highly recognizable colors, should be complimentary to any visual warning systems. *Courtesy of the Author.*

With lighting equipment and glass windows being the only obstructions, installing a contrasting pattern of chevrons will greatly enhance the visibility of the rear of the vehicle. This can be taken a step further by installing additional chevrons on the inside of the rear doors for added conspicuity when the doors are open for loading.

The addition of a single retroreflective fluorescent-colored horizontal stripe in the lower third of an ambulance will significantly add to its daytime and nighttime visibility to traffic. The visibility of the vehicle will be significantly enhanced with the installation of 2-inch white reflective tape outlining the perimeter of the ambulance box, although it will remain nearly invisible during the daytime.

An important option that will help to ensure the security of the vehicle while on scene is the ignition bypass device or a transmission interlock. The ignition bypass allows the operator of the vehicle to remove the key once the system has been engaged. This prevents the vehicle from being shifted into gear and will shut down the engine if the brake pedal is applied. The transmission interlock device requires the depression of a button or foot switch to allow the vehicle to be placed into gear. Both systems are effective for ensuring that vehicles do not leave the scene with unauthorized drivers.

Onboard video systems have become a popular tool to assist the safe driving and backing up of emergency vehicles. These systems can include cameras on three sides of the vehicle that activate automatically with the application of the turn signals or on placing the vehicle in reverse. The side cameras, known as blind-spot cameras, are beneficial in larger vehicles that tend to have less visibility just to the rear of the chassis. Cameras can be installed with integrated speakers so that the driver can hear the voice commands of a spotter while backing up the vehicle. Camera systems can be installed with small liquid crystal displays mounted in the cab or with the display integrated into the rear-view mirror. Such systems provide the driver with a 360-degree view of the vehicle from the front seat.

In recent years, more ambulance fleets have been installing onboard computer systems designed to monitor driver performance and ensure compliance with vehicle operation standards. Such systems integrate with the OEM computer on the vehicle to monitor the use of key features such as seat belts and turn signals, while monitoring acceleration, braking, and gravitational forces by way of an integrated accelerometer. These systems log data that can then be downloaded for review of performance and compliance. In addition, such systems can provide the driver with real-time feedback, warning them when they are approaching established parameters and notifying them when those parameters have been exceeded. Users of these systems report a significant cost savings in vehicle maintenance and repair, with the initial investment often being recovered during the first few years of ownership.

The safety of the paramedics and patients in the ambulance should be an overarching tenet in the development of the ambulance specification. From the graphics to improve conspicuity and visibility to the installation of systems designed to enhance driver behavior and performance, the financial investment in these items is nearly always outweighed by the cost of one unfortunate incident.

■ CHASSIS SELECTION

Once the base specifications have been created for the module of the ambulance, consideration can be given to finding the appropriate chassis on which the body can be mounted.

The market for OEM chassis for ambulances is dynamic, often in a manner that is not advantageous to an ambulance service. Ambulances are a very small portion of the light- and medium-duty truck chassis market, so changes occur without much thought to the needs of the ambulance builders and services. In recent years, Ford has stopped producing the diesel-powered, light-duty E-series van chassis, with only a gasoline-powered option remaining. GMC discontinued the C4500 Kodiak/TopKick series, and the Sterling brand has been eliminated. New federal and state emission standards further complicate the issue, with complex emission control systems added to available chassis.

Committees and managers contemplating ambulance procurement must contemplate fuel choice. Will the vehicle be powered by diesel or gasoline? Although it is not possible to specifically describe all the differences, issues such as heat accumulation and dissipation, engine performance (torque, acceleration, and engine operating speed), anticipated fuel economy, repair costs, and anticipated life span also must be considered. A fleet services mechanic or local vehicle service specialist can advise concerning the gas-diesel decision

at the time a selection will be made. Whatever the choice, it must be able to be serviced (both preventive maintenance and regular repairs) somewhere nearby.

The physical size of the module will have a large bearing on the style of chassis that can be utilized in order to meet the KKK minimum payload capacity requirements. The payload capacity is calculated using the **gross vehicle weight rating (GVWR)** and the curb weight. The GVWR is the maximum weight allowed with the vehicle fully loaded for response, including passengers, equipment, and fuel. The GVWR is determined by the manufacturer of the chassis and can usually be found on the vehicle's door frame. The curb weight is how much the vehicle weighs without installed equipment or passengers but with a full tank of fuel. The curb weight is then subtracted from the GVWR to give you the payload capacity. The KKK standard identifies the following minimum payload requirements for ambulances:

Single rear-wheeled van ambulances	1,500 lbs.
Dual rear-wheeled, modular ambulances	1,750 lbs.
Additional/medium-duty modular ambulances.	2,250 lbs

To complete this process, you will need to determine the weight of the equipment that you intend to install or store on the ambulance. You will also need to calculate the average weight of paramedics assigned to the vehicle. The KKK standard assumes an average weight of 150 pounds for each person. You should subtract this additional weight from the payload capacity. If the remaining value is not sufficient to account for the weight of a patient, additional personnel, or other equipment that may be utilized on the vehicle, you should consider a chassis with a higher GVWR rating. At no time should a vehicle be operated where the payload and additional weight exceed the total GVWR of the vehicle as this may result in unsafe operating conditions, impacting the ability to control and safely stop the vehicle.

Once the class of chassis has been determined, there are a number of other specifications to be considered prior to selecting the make and model that the ambulance will be built on. First, the type of fuel to power the engine must be reviewed. If your agency has reliable access to both diesel and gasoline, this will likely not be an issue. In addition, determining who will perform the maintenance and other servicing of the vehicle may steer you toward diesel or gasoline. Diesel mechanics are often not as easy to find as those qualified to work on gasoline-powered internal combustion engines. Consult with whomever currently services your vehicle to ensure that they can meet your future needs should you change from one type of engine to another. Other considerations for chassis selection include items such as the need for four-wheel-drive capability or a limited-slip axle. Once the basic requirements for the chassis have been determined, the choice of manufacturer is up to the preferences of the agency purchasing the vehicle.

Ambulances are often operated by different staff members on different days or shifts. The inclusion of certain electric options, including dual power mirrors, power seats, tilt steering wheel, and adjustable seat belts will facilitate rapid reconfiguration for different-size people. Ambulance services may also wish to include single-button locking systems that allow the locking of all doors and compartments with a single key fob or onboard switch.

▣ DEVELOPING THE SPECIFICATIONS DOCUMENT

A well-developed and detailed specifications document is a key factor in ensuring that what is delivered meets the needs and wants of the purchasing agency. Samples of specifications documents are commonly available for the asking either from other agencies or various ambulance builders. The KKK standard is a good format to use for the development of the document. By maintaining the format and convention of this document, your specifications are easily evaluated by potential vendors and compared with other like documents.

In addition to the outline of the federal document, you will want to include sections specific to your objectives. One such area would be to include specifics for any additional systems, equipment, or supplies you request (in addition to those previously mentioned in this chapter), such as a new stretcher or stair chair. The more information you provide, the more likely it is that the selected vendor will be able to provide helpful suggestions toward meeting your ambulance service's requirements.

In developing the details of each section of the document, be as specific as possible regarding particular items that are desired. For example, if your other vehicles all have a particular brand of suction aspirator installed and you want to maintain consistency to minimize disposables, provide clear details down to the part number regarding what you\ desire. If a particular brand or model of light-head or siren has worked for you, ask specifically for that make and model. If the service has no experience with an item, or the writers are unsure of exactly what the service is seeking (for example a brand of 110V AC/12V AC air conditioning unit), clearly detail the exact functionality and performance that are required from the device and allow the builder to recommend a product to meet these standards. Ambulance builders have a staff of engineers to address customers' needs, modify standard designs for local needs, and maintain the knowledge base regarding the most current and most reliable options available.

Require your builder to provide you with documentation, including CAD renderings of solutions to customization issues, rather than assuming he knows what your team envisions because he says so. If changes are proposed or made during the production process, require the builder document any additional costs before any work is performed (all change orders must include a cost and be approved by an authorized representative of the purchaser before work is performed). What may seem to be a simple and benign change can result in unforeseen engineering and design costs.

INSPECTING THE AMBULANCE

Your ambulance specifications should include language to require both a preconstruction conference and an on-site inspection of the vehicle at least twice during the production process. At the **prebuild conference**, the inspection team should review (with your salesperson and a knowledgeable representative from the production facility) the entire scope of the project. This includes a detailed review of your specifications document from front to back. Most ambulance manufacturers will develop and use an order or build document to price the vehicle with all the options and equipment that have been specified. The manufacturer should provide a copy of this document at the preconstruction conference so that the procurement team can account for each and every detail on your vehicle. This process can often be time consuming, but it is a wise investment to ensure that no detail is left unaddressed prior to the first piece of metal or wood being cut.

The manufacturer should also provide initial drawings for its construction. This will provide your team with at least a two-dimensional rendering of what is being proposed to meet your specifications. From these drawings you can confirm the cabinetry and compartmentalization

design, affirm that lights are in the locations intended, and that any customization requested has been addressed.

This conference is also a good opportunity to ask the manufacturer if it has noted anything that could be added to enhance the functionality or practicality of the vehicle, or any design features that it considers unwise. Experienced ambulance manufacturers have seen many ambulances in production. There may be a concept that another buyer has developed that will meet a specific need of yours in a more efficient manner.

The first inspection of the vehicle is best scheduled around the time the first cabinets are installed in the module (Figure 9.17). At this point in production, the module will have been framed, had the external sheeting installed, been mounted on the chassis, and had some of the electrical wiring installed. This inspection will allow you to examine the workmanship of the welding and metal fabrication, visually examine the work to ensure that the required insulation has been properly installed in the vehicle, and see the cabinetry (both partially installed and awaiting

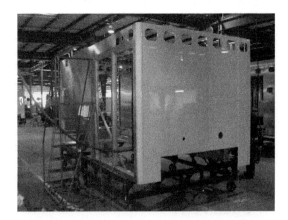

FIGURE 9.17 ■ Viewing the construction of an ambulance near the midpoint will allow you to see the various construction methods and how things are put together. *Courtesy of the Author*

installation). This visit will also give your team the opportunity to see other vehicles at various stages of production and the different processes involved in constructing a completed vehicle.

At the **final inspection**, your objective is to ensure that the vehicle is built completely to specifications prior to leaving the production facility. This responsibility should not be taken lightly. It is best to go into this process with a game plan and checklists, ensuring that no detail is left unattended.

This final inspection should be more than just kicking the tires and admiring the warning lights. A sound methodology is to start at the front of the vehicle and work your way through to the back doors. The operation of each piece of equipment installed by the chassis manufacturer and the ambulance builder should be tested to ensure that it functions exactly as intended. You would hate to get a completed vehicle delivered only to find, for example, that the windshield wipers were inadvertently disconnected while a wiring harness was installed. This process should include testing the charging system of the vehicle with a shoreline, checking the functionality of each power outlet in the vehicle, and running the heating and air conditioning systems at length to ensure that they function properly. The final inspection should also include driving the vehicle to ensure that it runs and shifts smoothly, there are no rattles or creaks, and it rides comfortably.

The final inspection should also focus heavily on the fit and finish of the vehicle. The paint on the ambulance should not be accepted if flaws, including blemishes, debris, or inconsistency to the finish, are noted. If the graphics were applied at the factory, they should be exactly as you specified them to be. Ensure that vinyl material has properly adhered to the body, is free from bubbles, and is appropriately trimmed around seams and door jambs. Check the wheel wells and doorjambs for overspray,

both of the paint and the undercoating. Each door should open and close easily and quietly. Check the edges of all metalwork inside cabinets for sharp edges or burrs and ensure that all shelves are secured in place.

In the interior of the module, inspect to see that all seams in the wall covering are sealed thoroughly, including the linings in the cabinets. Visually inspect to ensure that the flooring and surfaces are damage free and installed to your specifications. Pull on the handles, open and shut the doors and drawers, adjust the seats, test a stretcher in the mount, and perform any other function that is liable to be found to be faulty or defective when the vehicle is placed into service. If you have specified the installation of conduit or coaxial cable, ensure that it is in the correct location and that pull wires have been properly installed. This is your opportunity to verify that *everything* that you have asked for is present and functions as intended (Figure 9.18).

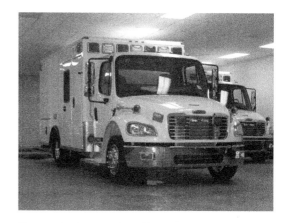

FIGURE 9.18 ■ Performing a thorough final inspection at the manufacturer's facility will permit any small details to be addressed prior to delivery and will afford you the opportunity for training on new equipment by those who performed the installation. *Courtesy of the Author.*

Best Practice

Midlife Fleet Rehabilitation, Wake County, North Carolina

It's been a common practice for many EMS agencies to remount ambulance modules onto new chassis to extend the initial investment in the vehicle. The cost to do this can vary greatly based on the degree of refurbishment and upgrades done to the remounted vehicle. Oftentimes, remounts occur when the chassis is deemed mechanically unreliable and the cost of the remount is advantageous to the cost of maintaining the old ambulance. But what about ambulances purchased using medium-duty chassis that are designed for much higher mileage than we anticipate from ambulances using lighter-duty chassis?

Wake County EMS is using a program referred to as a "midlife rehabilitation" to extend the usable life of the truck prior to getting into the remount process. Ambulances will naturally be subject to wear and tear during daily use. In an ambulance that is intended to have a life of 300,000 miles or more, this wear and tear can result in a less-than-appealing ambulance, impacting its professional appearance and being demoralizing to the employees.

The midlife rehabilitation is focused specifically on addressing these items. When a vehicle has been on the road for about 150,000 miles, it will be pulled out of service for rehabilitation. In the process, all exterior surfaces are repaired to like-new condition. Painted surfaces are polished to remove scratches and repainted where required. Any damaged vinyl on the graphics package is replaced. Aluminum treadplate is polished to like-new condition. All interior surfaces are cleaned and repaired, including upholstered seats in the cabs and cracked transparent plastic in the module. Electronics installed on the vehicle receive a thorough preventive maintenance and recalibration, and all mechanical systems are subject to a thorough review to ensure they are restored to like-new condition. By implementing this process, the overall life of the vehicle is not necessarily extended, but the agency has an older vehicle that does not necessarily look like an older vehicle.

CHAPTER REVIEW

Summary

The task of developing specifications for the purchase of an ambulance requires planning, research, and attention to detail. Ambulances are not cheap and often represent a significant financial investment for an ambulance service. Procurement is a process that cannot afford to be given anything less than a maximum effort. The delivery and placing into service of a vehicle that does not meet the specific needs of an agency can result in decreased productivity, unnecessary downtime, and potential jeopardy for paramedics, patients, and others. By careful planning, seeking the input of the users on improvements, and carefully reviewing all stages of the process, a new ambulance can be an asset to any organization and community.

WHAT WOULD YOU DO? Reflection

You have identified the stakeholders in your organization—paramedics of varying levels of credentials, fleet service technicians (mechanics), and logistics specialists. With a committee of eight, including yourself, you have researched the state and local regulations governing the requirements for ambulances to be licensed in your jurisdiction. You have surveyed your workforce, both informally and using an Internet survey instrument. You've measured every station you operate from, facilities that you frequently serve (those nursing home overhangs are killers!), and the shop where your ambulances are serviced. You've also visited several other ambulance services within your region and examined the unique features that they have built into their ambulances. You've also obtained, from several sources, the specifications that those organizations used to purchase their last rounds of ambulances. Armed with this information, you meet, discuss, and start writing.

Review Questions

1. List three requirements of the process of procuring an ambulance.
2. Define and discuss the needs and the wants that must be considered in the ambulance procurement process.
3. Discuss the limitations that may be placed on an ambulance procurement process.
4. Describe the advantages and disadvantages of aluminum ambulance cabinetry over cabinets made of wood.
5. What are two concepts that should be considered when addressing the design of ambulance shorelines?
6. What topics should be addressed when considering the subject of vehicle markings and conspicuity?

References

Levick, N. (2008, October). "Rig Safety 911." *Journal of Emergency Medical Services* 66–67.

National Fire Protection Association. (2009). "NFPA 1901: Standard for Automotive Fire Apparatus." See the organization website.

State of New Jersey (2005). New Jersey Statutes Annotated, General Statute 39:3-54:Mounting and Use of Emergency Warning Lights.

State of North Carolina (2010). General Statute 20-130.1: Use of Red and Blue Light on Vehicles Prohibited; Exceptions.

U.S. Fire Administration. (2009, August). "Emergency Vehicle Visibility and Conspicuity Study." See the organization website.

U.S. General Services Administration. (2007, July 1). "Federal Specification for the Star-of-Life Ambulance KKK-A-1822F." See the organization website.

Whelen. (2010). "Lightheads." See the Whelen website.

Key Terms

applicable requirements and regulations Govern ambulance design, construction, and equipment in a particular jurisdiction or specified in a particular contract for service.

angle of departure Angle between the ground and a line running from the rear of the rear tire (where the tire meets the ground) to the lowest hanging vehicular component to the rear of that point. The angle of departure addresses the ability of a vehicle to drive off of a ramp, curve, and so on without the further-to-the-rear component impacting the ground.

final inspection Performed by representatives of the ambulance service prior to the ambulance leaving the production facility to ensure that the vehicle is built completely to specification. This inspection should utilize checklists to ensure that that every vehicle system and feature is functional before the vehicle is accepted by the buyer.

gross vehicle weight rating (GVWR) Maximum operating weight of a vehicle, as specified by the manufacturer. The weight of an ambulance, including equipment, fuel, crew, patients, and so on may not safely exceed the GVWR.

prebuild conference Meeting between the ambulance service representative(s), ambulance vendor, and ambulance manufacturer, during which a complete review of the buyer's specifications is conducted, and during which any questions about any vehicle details are resolved, prior to beginning construction of the ambulance.

Patient Care Reporting Documentation and Documentation Systems

Kevin M. Sullivan, M.S., NREMT-P

Objectives

After reading this chapter, the student should be able to:

10.1 Describe and discuss the functions and importance of the patient care report.

10.2 Demonstrate the basic requirements for adequate patient care report writing.

10.3 Discuss the legal and regulatory requirements related to patient care reporting.

10.4 Describe the impact that patient care report documentation has on billing and collection efforts.

10.5 Discuss the various policies and procedures that are required for patient care report administration.

10.6 Discuss the emergence of electronic patient care reporting systems and the benefits that these systems bring to the EMS services that utilize them.

10.7 List the elements necessary for the successful procurement and implementation of electronic patient care reporting systems.

10.8 Discuss storage and data security in the administration of patient care reporting systems.

10.9 Discuss developments that will impact patient care report reporting and EMS documentation in the future.

Overview

Ambulance services in the United States range in size from one ambulance operated by volunteers and managed by a community board of directors to large governmental agencies and even larger, private, for-profit corporations. This text presents information that the manager of an ambulance service, large or small, needs in order to keep the business solvent and provide clinically excellent service to the community.

Key Terms

business logic

chief complaint

   call disposition

computer-aided

   dispatch (CAD)

   system

data element

False Claims Act

health information

   exchange (HIE)

Health Insurance

   Portability and

Accountability Act

   (HIPAA)

National EMS

   Information System

   (NEMSIS Version 3)

negligence

patient care report

   (PCR)

PCR narrative

scripting validation

WHAT WOULD YOU DO?

You are the newly promoted administrator of a municipal EMS department. As you take the helm of your organization, you begin to realize the serious toll that declining reimbursements and increasing costs are having on your department. As you begin to look at your expenses, you are surprised to find that so many of your largest expenses are related to documentation and billing/collections. You pay what think of as a small fortune for billing and collection services, including a per chart fee for data entry to turn a copy of each **patient care report (PCR)** into a billing entry. You have dedicated, secure fax lines at each station to transmit those PCRs to the billing company. You have a courier who goes from station to station to collect the PCRs and another employee who spends a good deal of her time processing medical records requests. You pay a printer to create the three-ply PCR forms that you use. There is a storage

fee for the company that houses your records and transfer fees every time you need to access those stored records. On top of all this, you still seem to have hundreds of the pink "Quality Assurance" copies floating around the administrative offices. You have heard colleagues at other services talk about all the benefits of "going electronic." Given all that goes into your paper system, you can imagine that there might be some benefit, but how do you decide?

1. What are the financial implications for your organization if you decide to make the switch from paper to electronic?
2. What impact will switching from paper to electronic have on your agency's operations?
3. If you do move forward on this, what steps should you take, and what do you need to think about or plan for as part of the transition?

INTRODUCTION

The PCR is a fundamental and undervalued aspect of the EMS encounter. It is something we use on every call, for every individual patient. It is frequently used by others (attorneys, insurance companies, nurses, physicians, etc.) who are seeking to understand what happened with a patient from the onset of an event through transportation to a hospital. In the aggregate, it is used to determine the quality of an organization's overall care. It serves more functions than any other item we carry and it follows us indefinitely after a patient encounter ends.

Despite the broad applications of a PCR, we spend relatively little time focused on it. The initial education of EMTs and paramedics frequently neglects the fundamentals of this vital skill; it is often covered in a single lecture along with multiple other topics. It is not tested as part of skills stations during licensing and exams. Most organizations do not assess an applicant's ability to formulate a well-written PCR prior to hiring, and they take little action to enhance the abilities of providers who document poorly.

This chapter will focus on the various aspects of patient care reporting. By the end of this chapter, you will gain an understanding of the core aspects of PCR writing and the systems used to document them. You will better understand the choice you have as an EMS manager when it comes to contracting for electronic patient care reporting (ePCR) systems and some of the important considerations you will need to make related to their implementation.

THE IMPORTANCE OF THE PATIENT CARE REPORT

The PCR has numerous functions. These functions are related both directly to the patient care encounter documented on the report and to the larger system. A few of the direct functions of the PCR are as follows:

1. The fundamental function of the PCR is to serve as a record of all information gained and actions taken during a clinical patient encounter. This includes the patient's complaint(s), all of the assessment findings, subjective and objective information gained through patient questioning, and treatment actions. It also includes information about the providers who were assigned to the call, the response itself, and additional pieces of reference information such as the call number and response times. At a minimum, at least 81 data points are collected about a patient encounter on a standard PCR; most reports have double or triple that number of data points.

2. The PCR serves as the permanent record of the encounter. It becomes both an immediate reference for everything that happened during a patient encounter and a permanent record for the care provided during the call. It is the document that you will refer back to if questions arise about the encounter.

3. The PCR informs future providers. Paramedics are often unaware of the varied uses of the EMS PCR later in the patient's care. We incorrectly presume that no one cares about the prehospital report and that its completion is not a matter of concern for the nurses and physicians who will also treat the patient. This could not be more misguided thinking. EMS managers frequently field phone calls from surgeons, emergency physicians, cardiac and stroke nurses, researchers, police officers, medical examiners, organ donation groups, and others who are seeking information about a patient. In fact, hospital oversight and accreditation agencies frequently require that prehospital care reports be included in a patient's hospital record because they are seen as an essential part of the patient's record of care.

4. The PCR also documents information that is important to billing and collection efforts. This

information includes the patient's full legal name, Social Security number, date of birth, sex, legal address, and insurance coverage (if any). The PCR also is utilized to classify the level of care provided for billing and reimbursement purposes.

5. The PCR can also assist with ensuring compliance with certain regulatory and billing requirements. For instance, Medicare requires an authorization signature (authorizing the ambulance service to bill Medicare on behalf of the patient) from a patient as part of anti-fraud measures; that authorization signature is often the last part of the patient's PCR. Others organizations imbed checklists into the PCR to ensure that providers follow strictly established protocols and document them correctly.

The preceding are just a few of the core functions of the PCR that relate directly to a specific patient encounter. The document also serves a number of systemwide functions:

1. *Systemwide data collection.* The PCR is one of the two main systems for collecting data within an EMS operation. (The other system is the **computer-aided dispatch (CAD) system**.) As each individual data point is documented in the PCR, it becomes part of a massive data set that can be used for many important purposes. As EMS systems have moved to document PCRs electronically, it has become increasingly easy for systems to use this massive amount of system data for organizational purposes.

2. *State and national data collection efforts.* The data collected at the service level does not simply sit in a database for the service's exclusive use. Some of the data collected are transmitted to statewide databases; some of those data are then transferred to a national database. This flow of information allows EMS researchers to more easily analyze a significant amount of EMS data.

3. *Quality management.* Review of PCRs is the primary method by which ambulance services and other EMS system components conduct quality management efforts. Quality management programs often review individuals PCRs for individual performance review. Information gained from individuals PCRs is often summarized, categorized, and trended to follow the performance of the group as a whole. The impact of ePCR systems on quality management programs has been profound and will be discussed later in this chapter.

4. *Internal and external research efforts.* Data collected from PCRs is also the primary source of data for most EMS research. Retrospective review of PCRs is the most common way that EMS researchers utilize the PCR data. This is another area that has expanded dramatically with the introduction of the ePCR systems.

5. *Supply usage and inventory management.* Many ambulance services have developed approaches to managing inventory that involve either direct or indirect use of PCR data. In many cases, systems include a "supplies used" section in a PCR and later translate that section into a materials management report, used to restock vehicles or stations.

Given the numerous functions of the PCR, it is hard to fathom how it could be neglected. Yet every day, providers downplay the importance of the PCR and ambulance services turn a blind eye to systematic documentations problems. The consequences of this neglect are profound and affect the organization in numerous ways, including these:

1. Unknown or unreportable quality of patient care
2. Suboptimal collection of revenue needed to sustain the service
3. Increased liability, as poor or missing records limit the service's ability to defend itself against complaints, lawsuits, or compliance audits
4. Inability to perform beneficial research or quality management processes

PATIENT CARE REPORT WRITING

The PCR is currently evolving from its traditional, written format, which has existed for more than a generation, to the electronic format of the future. As the PCR undergoes this change, it will grow dramatically beyond the simple one-page written format that was utilized between 1960 and 2000. Regardless of the format or the medium utilized, a few basic elements will remain as the foundation of every well-written PCR (Figure 10.1).

All PCRs must be comprehensive, accurate, legible, understandable, and consistent:

* *Comprehensive.* It is often said that the PCR should paint a picture of the scene and the care provided. The goal is to document the encounter in such a way that anyone who comes behind the provider may understand the patient's condition and the provider's action by reading the report alone.
* *Accurate.* It is just as important for PCRs to be accurate. Reports that convey incorrect information threaten the health of the patient and ruin the credibility of the provider.
* *Legible.* If the report is handwritten, the provider must monitor his penmanship and ensure that others will be able to easily read the written report.
* *Understandable.* As PCRs have transitioned from handwritten to electronic documents, concerns about legibility have been replaced by difficulty understanding many reports as they have been written. Some of these problems are related to serious grammatical errors that leave the reader confused about the intended message. In other cases, providers adopt their own unique shorthand with associated abbreviations that lead to misinterpretations by readers not familiar with the shorthand.
* *Consistent.* As with any form that contains a significant amount of data, it is always possible

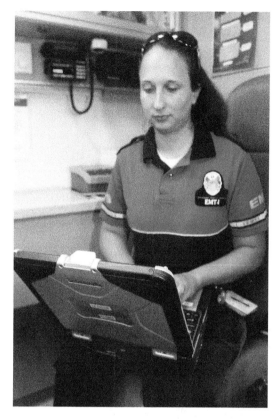

FIGURE 10.1 ■ The patient care report should record an accurate verbal picture of the scene, the patient's condition, and the care provided. Here, an EMT uses a ruggedized laptop computer to record a patient encounter. *Source: Official Wake County EMS Photo by Mike Legeros, used by permission.*

that a piece of information in one part of the form may contradict information in another part. This is especially true in most PCRs, where the large free-text narrative portion of the form offers the documenter the ability to convey a lot of information that has already been conveyed in another way on another part of the form. The EMS provider must be especially careful when documenting a PCR to ensure that the information reported is consistent and factually correct through the document.

Side Bar

Did You Do It?

Remember this old adage: "If you did not document it, you did not do it."

Two special challenges exist in this area: First, if more than one EMS unit responds to a call and completes a PCR, the information in each PCR should mirror the information in the other PCR. Second, when dealing with ePCR systems that utilize default answers to certain questions, the provider must ensure that all fields are accurately entered; skipping a default-answered question can mean inaccurate information in your PCR.

As a general rule, providers should remember that each PCR is written for an extremely large audience. It is not inconceivable that, in the normal course of business, a PCR may be read by six or more people within the EMS organization and twelve or more people at the receiving hospital. Each of these readers has a use for the report that is valuable to the patient and the patient's interests. Therefore, a well-written report should be seen as an important treatment element in the care of every patient.

Side Bar

The Role of Reports

Ambulance medics often do not believe that their reports are important to patient care. They turn the PCR over to a busy emergency nurse or other staff member who does not immediately refer to the written document. However, that document is important to many downstream providers, who must have accurate information about the patient's condition at the time of onset of symptoms, what medications have been administered, and so on.

DATA ELEMENTS

Comprehensive PCRs and the systems in which they exist have one thing in common: a clearly defined, consistent set of data elements. A **data element** is each question or piece of information gathered on the PCR. These data elements ensure complete and comprehensive reporting by organizing the information provided and allowing consistent answers to frequently asked questions.

A recent review of a fairly simple PCR system found that the report contained 166 data elements. The **National EMS Information System (NEMSIS Version 3)** (2005) data set has identified 292 elements. These data sets have been developed incrementally, often by various efforts to collect better data on one particular area or another. One of the first data sets to be developed for EMS was published by the American Heart Association in "Recommended Guidelines for Uniform Reporting of Data from Out of Hospital Cardiac Arrest: The Utstein Style" (Cummins et al., 1991)." NHTSA followed with the publication of a national consensus document that detailed eighty-one elements necessary for a prehospital report data set (National EMS Information System, 1993).

PCR NARRATIVE

Depending on one's perspective, it is easy to imagine someone concluding that the narrative section found in most PCRs is the most problematic data element in the report. As a large, free-form text field, the **PCR narrative** can be fraught with problems for both the provider and the administrator. As the most flexible and versatile field, information is collected in it in a way that is often difficult and cumbersome to search through. And yet, for the provider it offers the best opportunity to really describe what happened on a call.

The best way to avoid problems with the narrative is to ensure that all providers within an organization follow a logical, organized manner of narrative documentation. There are several time-tested methods of writing patient care PCR narratives:

1. The SOAP format characterizes information derived from the patient as *s*ubjective (information told to the provider by others), *o*bjective (information observed by the provider), an *a*ssessment (a working diagnosis of the patient's condition), and a *p*lan (or course of treatment). Care must be taken in using the SOAP format, in that it was designed for use in long-term-care facilities where physician visits are infrequent and long-term-care plans are developed. Incorrect classification of information as subjective or objective can detract from the credibility of the writer.
2. The CHART narrative format is used to report the **chief complaint**, *h*istory, *a*ssessment, *R*x (treatment), and *t*ransportation information.
3. An older physician-style note, involving narrative reporting of the history, physical exam, impression, and treatments prescribed or rendered, is also still in use.

As electronic PCRs (ePCRs) have developed, more and more information is captured in data fields, with the narrative portion of the report used only to report those items that are not recorded elsewhere in the chart (e.g., all treatments will be recorded in a flowchart with time-stamped data points). It is important to ensure that narrative information does not conflict with data elements in the flowchart. The best way to avoid data conflicts is for the author to avoid repeating in the narrative what has already been captured as a data point.

Whichever method or methods are chosen, the organization should promulgate that to staff members and ensure that the organization's orientation and field training programs provide concrete instruction on how the organization wants narrative reports to be written.

OTHER IMPORTANT ELEMENTS OF THE PCR

Several other elements of the PCR are vital to the process of documentation.

Chief Complaint

The chief complaint is the reason that the patient (or someone else) summoned the ambulance. Health care personnel are often taught that the chief complaint should be recorded in the patient's own words. However, many ePCR systems require the provider to classify the chief complaint as a standard data element (e.g., the patient might say "It feels like someone is standing on my chest;" the provider would record the chief complaint as the data element "chest pain/pressure" in the ePCR).

Two implications immediately result from poorly documented chief complaints. The first and most serious is the potential impact on patient care. If an EMS provider incorrectly records a chief complaint, he may inadvertently lead other health care providers to under-triage the patient and thereby delay time-sensitive care. The second implication of this poorly documented chief complaint impacts billing and reimbursement efforts. A low-acuity chief complaint can lead to the event being billed at a lower level of reimbursement than might have been otherwise justified by a more appropriate chief complaint.

Pertinent Negatives

The pertinent negative(s) document assesses findings (both physical exam and history) that one might expect if a patient were experiencing a certain type of acute illness, but that were not present in the patient at the time of assessment. Just as a good assessment requires that the provider investigate a broad array of possible problems, adequate documentation demands that both the things one finds and the things one does *not* find be included in the PCR. As some organizations transition to

PCR systems that diminish the importance of the narrative, finding a way to include pertinent negatives in other parts of the PCR is extremely important. Good-quality ePCR systems will allow for complete documentation of both positives and negatives. Losing the ability to document a pertinent negative is not only a blow to an organization's ability to depict the care provided, but it may actually expose the organization to a claim of **negligence**; one such case is detailed in this chapter.

Call Dispositions

The NEMSIS data set introduces ten possible incident or patient dispositions:

1. Canceled
2. Dead at Scene
3. No Patient Found
4. No Treatment Required
5. Patient Refused Care
6. Treated and Released
7. Treated, Transferred Care
8. Treated, Transported by EMS
9. Treated, Transported by Law Enforcement
10. Treated, Transported by Private Vehicle

For some, it is difficult to see the differences between some of these expanded disposition choices when they consider the choices in light of the circumstances. For instance, does the patient need to sign a Refusal of Transport form with a **call disposition** of "no treatment required." If the patient does sign a refusal, should he then be classified as "patient refused care"? As providers develop their own interpretation of these ten outcomes, their choices can make quality management and statistic gathering efforts more difficult. To overcome this challenge, organizations need to develop a universal understanding of these definitions and how they will be used in the field. This understanding must be conveyed consistently and clearly to staff members. NEMSIS documents provide clear, detailed data point definitions that should be part of the training of every ePCR user.

Reporting of Medical Errors

It is widely believed that medical errors are underreported in all medical settings (Levinson, 2012). An Institute of Medicine white paper entitled "To Err Is Human" estimated that as many as one million patient injuries and 100,000 patient deaths occur each year as a result of medical errors (Institute of Medicine, 1999). One research study specific to the prehospital setting suggests that as many as half of the recognized errors committed in the EMS setting go unreported (Hobgood, Bowen, Brice, Overby, and Tamayo-Sarver, 2006). Though the Joint Commission implemented a requirement for sentinel event reporting in 1996, few EMS oversight organizations have adopted any form of sentinel event reporting for EMS providers.

Side Bar

E.V.E.N.T.

National EMS organizations in the United States, including the National Association of EMTs and the National EMS Management Association, have recently developed and released the EMS Voluntary Event Notification Tool (E.V.E.N.T.). E.V.E.N.T. is a tool designed to improve the safety, quality, and consistent delivery of EMS. It collects data submitted anonymously by EMS practitioners. The data collected will be used to develop policies, procedures, and training programs to improve the safe delivery of EMS. Any individual who encounters or recognizes a situation in which an EMS safety event occurred, or could have occurred, is strongly encouraged to submit a report by completing the appropriate E.V.E.N.T. Voluntary Event Notification Tool, at http://event.clirems.org. The confidentiality and anonymity of this reporting tool is designed to encourage EMS practitioners to readily report EMS safety events without fear of repercussion.

The reporting of errors in the PCR is complementary to fundamental requirements for complete and accurate PCRs. Providers should never omit relevant information from a report, even if that information may be seen as less than flattering of the provider or care provided.

Documenting Refusals of Care or Non-Transport

One general presumption in the world of EMS is that most patients we counter will be transported to the hospital. If that presumption is not realized, we must take very special care to document the circumstances surrounding that non-transport. This documentation is necessary to explain to any future reader of the report exactly what happened on that non-transport and what actions the provider took or attempted to take related to that non-transport. In addition to all of the regular elements of a quality PCR, this report must clearly contain an indication that the provider did the following:

1. Assessed the decision-making capacity of the patient and found that the patient did in fact demonstrate the capacity to understand the decisions he was being asked to make, and the consequences of those decisions. Confirmed that the patient was an adult, if that status is not absolutely certain.

2. Advised the patient of the potential consequences of his refusal of treatment and/or transportation to the hospital. The provider should also include all efforts he made to convince the patient to be transported, including the identities of other persons involved in the discussion.

3. Documented that he advised the patient that, should his condition worsen, he may call back at any time.

▓ LEGAL ASPECTS OF PATIENT CARE REPORTING ——————————

This chapter is not about the legal aspects of EMS, but it would be incomplete if it did not at least touch on some of the legal aspects of PCR writing. As a general disclaimer, the reader should understand that this section is meant to serve as a brief overview of these topics. It should not be considered to be comprehensive, and readers should take time to investigate and understand the legal requirements that apply to their particular organization and jurisdiction.

Legal issues abound concerning the PCR. One of the most obvious concerns relates to how the PCR may be used in legal proceedings. When discussing documentation, many instructors present the concepts surrounding quality documentation as primarily necessary to protect the provider from an overly litigious society. The term *CYA* ("cover your ass") abounds.

Just as those who fail to document medical errors do a disservice to both the patient and the organization, the provider who documents only to protect himself from liability is likely to fail to be comprehensive and accurate in his PCR writing. These individuals often believe in a modified version of the "less is better" philosophy, which should be rejected as detrimental to the best interests of the patient, the ambulance service, and the profession.

Complete, well-written reports can prevent litigation before it begins. A patient who is dissatisfied with the outcome of a particular clinical event (often involving first responders, ambulance services, emergency departments, and hospital inpatient services) may contact an attorney. Prior to filing a lawsuit, the attorney will review the records and determine if there appear to be grounds for litigation. Since most plaintiffs' attorneys are compensated through contingency arrangements (where the attorney gets paid only if money damages are paid), they are reluctant to invest hours in a case that is not winnable. If the attorney reviews the PCR, perhaps consulting with someone considered to be an expert witness in the process, and finds that the care rendered is complete, completely documented, and meets the standard of care, then the involved people may never be named in the event a lawsuit is initiated.

NEGLIGENCE IN DOCUMENTATION

Providers and managers should understand that appropriate documentation is part of the standard of care for EMS. A deviation from the standard (i.e., poor documentation that fails to adequately document the assessment findings and care of a patient) is not just unprofessional, but it also may also be considered negligence.

For example, look no further than the case of *De Tarquino vs. Jersey City*.[1] In this case, Jersey City EMS paramedics were found to be liable for negligence when they failed to appropriately document a patient's nausea and vomiting. The plaintiff held that hospital staff relied on EMS documentation to make decisions about whether or not the patient needed more in-depth assessment and diagnostic testing (such as a CT scan). By leaving critical symptoms of a more serious problem out of the PCR, EMS providers were negligent, and their care ultimately contributed to the death of the patient. The court agreed, finding that the EMS providers' failure to document constituted negligence in and of itself, without any accusation of a failure to appropriately assess or treat the patient. Similar cases in Washington, D.C., and Louisiana have demonstrated that failure to completely document a patient care encounter, including the failure to document that providers informed the patient of the severity of his illness and the consequences of his refusal to accept transport to an appropriate facility, can be considered as grounds for a claim of

malpractice.[2] Other cases have established clearly that good documentation of a patient's informed (though not very wise) refusal of treatment and transport can prevent ambulance personnel from being held liable, even in the case of a very bad outcome.[3]

FEDERAL AND STATE LAWS THAT IMPACT EMS DOCUMENTATION

The following laws, some more commonly recognized than others, exert tremendous influence on EMS documentation.

Health Insurance Portability and Accountability Act

The **Health Insurance Portability and Accountability Act (HIPAA)** was signed into law in 1996. The statute and its implementing regulations are intended to increase the efficiency of the health care system by creating standards related to the use, storage, and transfer of medical records. This provision also includes the Privacy Rule and the Security Rule, which have very direct implications on the sharing and storage of EMS PCRs.[4]

Patient Privacy Laws

Patient privacy laws often exist at the state level and may supplement or strengthen requirements for patient privacy. These laws are different in each state and various administrative regulations will likely shape the provisions of the law into practical applications. Managers will need to be aware of the applicable laws in

---

[1]*Francesca C.V. De Tarquino v. The City of Jersey City*, 352 N.J. Super. 450, 800 A.2d 255 (decided June 28, 2002).

[2]*Weber v. City Council*, 2001 WL 109196 (Ohio App. 2. Dist.). EMTs avoided malpractice liability only because of statutory immunity, despite deviation from the standard of care.

[3]*Kyser v. Metro Ambulance*, 764 So.2d 215 (La. App. 2000).

[4]Health Insurance Portability and Accountability Act of 1996 (HIPAA), 42 U.S.C. §§ 300gg et seq., P.L. 104-191, and 45 C.F.R. parts 160, 162, and 164.

their state and would do well to make their providers aware of the practical implications of these laws.

CMS Regulations

The Centers for Medicare and Medicaid Services has a tremendous number of rules, regulations, interpretations, and clarifications that govern billing for ambulance services. These billing rules have a direct impact on our documentation practices.

False Claims Act

The federal **False Claims Act** of 1986[5] was designed to combat fraud against the government and governmental programs. The act allows individuals to file suit on behalf of the government against others who are defrauding the government. These lawsuits are called *qui tam* or *whistle-blower* suits. This provision of the law allows the individual filing suit to receive a portion of the money that the government recovers from the perpetrators of the fraud. In the ambulance industry, a number of these suits have resulted in substantial judgments against EMS organizations.

Record Retention Laws

Each state has different record retention laws as they relate to medical records. These laws and regulations establish a minimum time frame for which records must be retained and often differ even within the health care industry. Many of these laws do not specifically mention ambulance services and may require the ambulance service manager to seek guidance from the regulators. Typical record retention timelines are about 7 years, but they vary extremely widely from state to state.[6]

---

[5]31 U.S.C. §§ 3729–3733 as amended.
[6]See, for example, North Carolina General Statutes Sections 121 and 132.

FDA Equipment Failure Reporting

The U.S. Food and Drug Administration (FDA) requires that users of medical equipment report suspected medical device failure to the manufacturer and the FDA if that device failure is related to the death of a patient. If the malfunction or failure results in serious injury, it is only reported to the FDA if the manufacturer is unknown. Manufacturers, in turn, are required to report these deaths, serious injuries, and certain other types of malfunctions to the FDA.

This reporting occurs through the Medical Device Reporting (MDR) program, which has an online mechanism for reporting, a toll-free hotline, and a paper-based option (titled MEDWATCH 3500A) for submission. Organizations (users) who experience a medical equipment failure that contributes to the death of a patient are also required to submit an annual report to the FDA summarizing their reported equipment failures (Form FDA 3419). It is important for ambulance service managers to realize that they have a responsibility beyond their organization to report device failures.

ADMINISTRATIVE ISSUES IN PATIENT CARE REPORT WRITING

Determining when a PCR should be completed is often a matter of controversy. Some feel that a PCR is completed only when patient contact has occurred. Those who take this approach are then required to define what constitutes a patient contact. The definitions created to define the patient contact can leave the organization vulnerable if providers do not share a universal understanding of the definition and its practical interpretation. Additional liability accrues for both the provider and the organization if the definition used is not broad enough to capture all those who might have a claim that a patient-provider relationship has been developed. Many agencies have adopted an "any time the wheels turn" approach to PCR generation. This practice allows the agency to utilize the ePCR database as a source of information on every response, which can be very helpful to daily operations management. It also allows paramedics to document, via brief narrative, what they observe if their response is canceled by another agency after arriving on scene.

Managers should remember that the PCR is not just a vessel for capturing patient care information when treatment or transport is provided. Having documentation about responses that were canceled and why that response was canceled can be invaluable if questions arise about that canceled response or if the organization wants to conduct research into call dispositions.

The best practice in this area is to complete a PCR for each and every dispatch (sometimes described as "every time the wheels roll"). This ensures that no legitimate patient contact can happen without the procedural requirement of a PCR that provides at least a tertiary explanation of the encounter. It does not necessarily ensure that the encounter is documented completely, but it does provide a starting point. Since the EMS PCR has a functional place in helping the organization track certain statistics, having a PCR for every response offers administrative value. Organizations that utilize computer-aided dispatch (CAD) systems usually perform a daily CAD-ePCR reconciliation, which ensures that there is a CAD record for every ePCR, and an ePCR for every CAD event.

If an organization determines that it will not complete a PCR for every dispatch or response, the organization will need to craft a definition to determine when a report is needed. In this case, tying the requirement to a patient contact is the standard practice.

Patient contact is often defined when any one of three criteria is met:

1. Any time an individual requests an evaluation or requests that someone else be evaluated.
2. Any time an individual voices a complaint or symptom that indicated a need for further assessment or treatment. This includes instances in which a third party gives voice to the complaints on behalf of the patient, regardless of whether or not the patient may be seeking the assessment himself.
3. Any time a provider observes injuries, or a mechanism of injury, or a symptomatic pattern that indicates a need for assessment or treatment.

If an organization decides to utilize an approach that relies on a defined patient contact to trigger the requirement for a PCR, it is essential that everyone in the organization shares the same understanding and interpretation of the criteria being used. Individual variations in interpretation on this kind of policy often render the policy itself useless. Anything less than "every time the wheels turn" can lead to missing information about significant events. Ambulance services should make every effort to simplify this process, such that a person writing a report on a canceled call does not have to fill out dozens of fields to which the answer is "n/a."

SPECIAL CIRCUMSTANCES REGARDING PCR COMPLETION

Two frequently encountered special circumstances require organizations to take a different approach to when to document and what type of documentation they require.

Mass Casualty Incidents

In a mass casualty incident (MCI), it is often impractical to expect a provider to complete a PCR immediately or conjunction with each patient. In such circumstances, organizations should preplan a policy that speaks to the level of documentation a provider should complete on a given patient during an MCI. This policy must address the system's particular MCI capabilities (MCI buses, etc.) and the requirements for providers playing different roles.

The best practice in MCI documentation requires the incident commander or his delegate to maintain a basic, but adequate, record of each patient encountered and each patient's disposition. This may be as simple as keeping a list of each patient's name (or description), triage level, transport destination, and transporting unit. Some systems also require that the transporting unit maintain part of a treatment tag or a copy of the same for documentation purposes. It is common for organizations to ask providers who transported patients to fill out a PCR after completion of the incident, knowing that the provider may have limited recall of individual patient information. In such cases, supplemental information (such as information from the patient's triage tag) may allow the provider to more completely document demographic information about the patient.

Public Health Screenings

The second circumstance that warrants a possible deviation from standard PCR practices occurs when EMS organizations perform public health screens of various sorts. These screenings may include blood pressure checks, blood sugar checks, or similar activities aimed at giving the patient an understanding of his health status. Such events may be organized at a public venue or may take the form of some kind of continuous opportunity that is always available to members of the public if they come to a certain place (e.g., blood pressure checkpoints at stations).

Public health screenings are an excellent way to provide an added service to the public, but requiring a standard PCR for each

participant would turn the screening into a burden. In these cases, it is necessary for the organization to develop a policy that addresses when an individual screening participant transitions into a "patient" (based on some voiced complaint or screening finding). At a minimum, a log of each screening contact should be maintained.

ACCOUNTABILITY FOR PCRS

Regardless of the type of PCR system in use, it is important for an organization to have a method of ensuring that the number of completed PCRs matches the number of PCRs expected. Few things are more problematic than finding that your organization does not have a PCR for a patient you have treated or evaluated.

One of the easiest ways to ensure that all PCRs are completed in an appropriate and timely manner is to frequently compare your PCRs with CAD system data. The best practice in this area calls for a comparison at least once per shift or before any given crew ends its shift for the evening. Organizations using ePCR systems may find that this reconciliation can be completed in an extremely expedited manner if the ePCR system has been integrated with the CAD system.

PATIENT CARE REPORT VERSUS INCIDENT REPORT

Many ambulance services utilize an incident report (IR) or unusual event report (UER) to document happenings that do not involve the assessment and treatment of a particular patient. An IR typically serves a nonclinical purpose and its focus is not patient care related. Even though there may be overlap between details that are appropriate to include in a PCR and details that should be included in an IR, providers should understand that these are two distinctly separate types of documents. The PCR is about the assessment, treatment, and transport of the patient. Details that fall outside of that limited scope may not be appropriate for inclusion in the PCR but should be reserved for an IR. For example, if an accident with a stretcher occurred during a call, the PCR should include details about any assessment or injuries to the patient as a result of that accident, although an IR should separately document the non-clinical details of that accident (who was holding the stretcher, what caused the accident, if the supervisor was notified, etc.).

Recently, the EMS community embraced the concept of *near miss* reporting so that individuals not involved in potentially serious events can share their stories, thereby contributing to the overall knowledge of the community. The EMS Voluntary Event Notification Tool (E.V.E.N.T.) is designed to improve the safety, quality and consistent delivery of EMS (http://event.clirems.org). It collects data submitted anonymously by EMS practitioners. The data collected will be used to develop policies, procedures, and training programs to improve the safe delivery of EMS. A similar system used by airline pilots has led to important airline system improvements based on pilot-reported near-miss situations and errors. Any individual who encounters or recognizes a situation in which an EMS safety event occurred, or could have occurred, is strongly encouraged to submit a report by completing the appropriate E.V.E.N.T. The confidentiality and anonymity of this reporting tool is designed to encourage EMS practitioners to readily report EMS safety events without fear of repercussion.

■ ELECTRONIC PATIENT CARE REPORTING SYSTEMS———

Without question, ePCR systems are the way of the future. Over the course of the last 10 years, ePCR technology has changed and

advanced substantially. What was initially a tool that captured basic information about a patient in a format that was meant to be easier to read and easier to use has developed into complex systems that store past patient information, interact with numerous other databases, link to clinical protocols, calculate drug doses, and perform numerous other tasks that make the work of providers and managers infinitely easier.

EMS organizations that began using ePCR systems more than 10 years ago were on the leading edge of this technology. Today, organizations that have yet to adopt some version of ePCR technology are behind the curve and may even be seen as failing to meet the standard of care in their area.

ADVANTAGES OF EPCR

An ePCR system offers tremendous value to systems that utilize the technology to its fullest capabilities. These values cross a number of operational, clinical, and administrative areas.

PCR Documentation

Use of ePCRs can lead to improvements in documentation. These systems eliminate common problems related to the legibility of handwriting. Some allow providers to follow predetermined narrative templates when entering data, providing supplemental structure to the individual provider's narrative. Data validation rules (discussed later in this chapter) allow system administrators to mandate that certain fields be filled out completely and draw a provider's attention to the fields that he has left blank. Supplemental questions/fields can be added to collect additional information based on certain data elements imputed into the basic PCR. All this ensures more comprehensive documentation.

Patient Care

Current-generation ePCR systems offer a number of enhancements that add concrete and immediate value for a paramedic as he is treating a patient. One feature that is extremely helpful is the ability to see past EMS PCR data related to a particular patient once that patient has been identified. Another feature common among ePCR systems is the option to either insert or link to clinical protocols in real time as treatment is being rendered.

Quality Management and Research Abilities

The way systems conduct quality management and research efforts has been revolutionized by ePCR systems. In a paper-based EMS PCR system, these efforts are arduous and daunting. In an electronic system, data are available in a wide variety of very easily queried formats as soon as they are uploaded to the system's servers. Quality control managers can utilize queries and system search engines to quickly sort through records that match desired criteria, thereby improving productivity and offering potential improvement to overall efforts.

Billing and Collections

The value most likely to convince stakeholders outside the EMS organization about the value of the ePCR system is its ability to streamline and enhance billing and collections processes. An ePCR system can cut days off the interval between time of service and the issuance of a bill for service. The system may also be capable of using logic trees to code the PCR and determine its appropriate level of service automatically. This can mean significant improvements in both revenue processing and the amounts collected.

Regulatory Compliance

State and federal regulations require that certain information be collected on each response and that each patient care encounter be recorded appropriately. Data validation functions can be used to ensure compliance with required fields and reduce an organization's exposure to regulatory compliance issues. Audit trail records within the ePCR can provide required records for whoever has accessed and/or changed data. Transmission functions can ensure that completed reports are always transmitted to the appropriate hospitals and databases. Electronic security measures can protect against HIPAA violations and reduce the potential for violations of patient privacy expectations. Some systems even have functions that monitor paramedic certification and licensure status.

Record Storage

Storage of paper records can present serious logistical challenges for an EMS organization. Depending on the particulars of state record retention laws, organizations may be faced with a requirement to retain a copy of a paper record indefinitely. With an ePCR system, record retention and retrieval are significantly simplified. The job of retrieving records and processing records requests can be simplified to an online request submission, verified by the agency and then delivered electronically.

PROCUREMENT CONSIDERATIONS

To reap the benefits of an ePCR system, one of the first steps an organization takes is to select an ePCR system that meets the system's needs and abilities. Municipal and governmental systems may be required to select a system based on a competitive bid process. Nongovernmental systems may be able to utilize a less structured process to determine which system they would like you to use. If done properly, either selection method can be structured to empower the system to select the most appropriate system for its own needs and uses.

There are two important aspects to a procurement process for an EMS ePCR system. First, you must develop an appropriately representative stakeholder group to evaluate the various options. At a minimum, this group should consist of paramedics, EMS managers, quality assurance personnel, the medical director, and IT personnel. The best practice in this area is to involve multiple field users who have a variety of skill levels with computers. By selecting only the most interested, technically savvy providers to participate in the selection process, an organization risks a potentially detrimental selection bias that could have profound consequences when the system is implemented at the field level.

The second step in the procurement process is to determine the needs that the ePCR system will fulfill for the organization and to develop from those needs a general set of variables for evaluating systems. It may be helpful to stratify various needs according to the strength of the system's need for them. Absolutely mandatory variables can be used in a binary manner for initial screening of potential systems. For instance, if state government requires that organization use software that is NEMSIS Gold Compliant, that criterion can be used to screen out systems that would not be feasible if selected.

In general, some variables are more important than all others in the selection process. Some of the most important variables are ease of use, platform of delivery, major functionalities, cost, and ability to interface.

Ease of Use

If field providers cannot navigate an ePCR system, it will be nearly impossible for an organization to gain all the benefits of a high-performing ePCR system. This makes ease of use one of the single most important criteria in selecting an ePCR system.

Evaluating the ease of use of a device is not necessarily easy. The first step may be you and your organization working with a select group of end users, but it may also be helpful to poll other organizations that have recently implemented a particular vendor's system. It may be helpful to know the initial frustrations expressed by field users and how quickly field crews adapted to the use of the system.

One particular ease of use consideration that may be easy for people who are not familiar with the system to evaluate is the types of fields used in various data elements and the way the user moves from one field to another. Can the user tab through fields? Is it easier to have a drop-down menu or a check box when documenting the patient's sex or race? Is the user able to scroll down through one continuous form as he fills out the ePCR, or does he have to move through multiple pages? These types of considerations can significantly affect the user's speed and ability to smoothly move through a PCR.

Platform of Delivery

Increasingly important in the selection of an ePCR system is the type of platform used to deliver the electronic record system. For years, all ePCR systems involved the installation of some type of software solution onto a computer. Today's options have expanded to include Internet browser-based solutions (i.e., website completion of an ePCR) and iPad-compliant applications.

Major Functionalities

The term *major functionalities* refers to the major functional components of the ePCR system. The particular desires of an organization may shape which major functional aspects of the system are more important in the selection process. Some of the most common major functions include the following:

* *Patient information database.* These databases may come in the form of a past patient database that stores information from previous

ePCRs completed for that particular patient, or it may come in the form of universal record databases of individual (nonhealth) information based on the patient's Social Security number. Organizations should evaluate how easy it is for users to utilize and recall these data, select partial record data, or refine the stored information.

- *Physical exam findings documentation.* Increasingly common in ePCR systems is the ability to use pictorial methods to document assessment findings. For example, by pointing at the left arm and checking a box for "Deformity," the provider might be able to document assessment findings in a non-narrative format.
- *Narrative generation.* Some systems offer the ability to autogenerate a narrative based on information provided in other parts of the PCR; other offer a semi-autogenerated narrative or a number of different predefined narrative outlines. More than one system has no narrative at all.
- ***Scripting validation** rules.* Also known as closed call rules, this function allows the organization and/or the ePCR system to mandate the completion of certain fields before the record can be closed and exported. Each system has a slightly different approach to how a user can identify the mandatory and desired fields and different methods for reviewing those fields before the record is closed.
- *System **business logic**.* Similar to scripting validation rules, business logic links one data element in a report to others in a way that makes it easier for the user to fill out the report. For example, if a user selects the "No patient found" value in the Incident Disposition data element, the system's business logic rules may make the patient demographic, treatment, and vital sections all unavailable or even unseen. Business logic tools make it easier for the user to fill out a report and can decrease the user's ability to create inconsistent reports; advanced business logic may even recognize inconsistent information and point it out to the user.

- *CAD-PCR reconciliation process.* In the era of electronic PCRs, the best practice has become that each CAD record have an associated ePCR record. Different ePCR vendors have different methods of conducting reconciliation between these two systems.
- *Incomplete report identification.* One problem that ePCR system users can face is the ability to identify and recapture incomplete records. An ePCR system that offers the ability to easily or automatically identify these outstanding records makes it easier to manage the system.
- *Record search functions.* Every ePCR system stores records electronically, but not every electronic search function is as easy to use as the user might like it to be. During the evaluation process, EMS managers should explore how easy it is to use these search functions given the sometimes limited information with which the manager may have to locate a record. Using the kind of difficult search terms that sometimes come with customer service complaints made by hospital staff members or members of the public is sometimes helpful.
- *Quality management tools.* Like the record search function, each vendor has a suite of back-end products and tools that lend tremendous value to their system. As you evaluate various vendors, you should pay close attention to the differences among their quality management tools. Does the system have a number of easy-to-use reports built on metrics important to system performance? Does the vendor's system require you to create your own reports, purchase additional functions to get access to their reports, or learn how to use computer database search tools (such as Chrystal Reports) to get at your data? These factors have a significant impact on how easily you will be able to use the plethora of new information that your system has at its fingertips.
- *Dashboard functions.* Similar to the quality management functions, many systems offer

the ability to build "dashboard" metrics that allow various users to see important information or statistics at a glance. This type of function can prompt users to direct their attention to critical information immediately.

♦ *Billing system.* Another major feature of some systems is the ability to access and utilize a suite of billing tools that may allow an organization to utilize a single system for both related operations. For organizations that perform in-house billing, this type of functionality may save the organization a significant amount of money and may offer enhancements related to centralized storage of information. Other ambulance services may wish to provide for the daily electronic transfer of billing data to their billing contractor or service.

Cost

The cost of an ePCR system may be the foremost consideration for an organization. System price varies depending on vendor, size of the organization, and a number of other market factors.

Ability to Interface

Interfacing with other technology gives the ePCR system and the EMS organization a competitive advantage in numerous operational and business aspects of operations. It has the potential to streamline, maximize, and exponentially increase the benefits that each of these individual systems offers its users. The major interfaces that an ePCR system may make are with the CAD system, billing systems, hospital record systems, cardiac monitoring devices, and employee scheduling systems.

Organizations commonly define the cost of an ePCR system as the only variable that matters. This is a mistake that can have profound, long-lasting consequences. Finances may be a limiting factor in ePCR system

selection, but it cannot be the only factor. A free ePCR system that does not meet the needs of an organization will not help the organization reach its full potential. It will cost that organization more money than if it had paid for a system that was more suited to the organization. The same is true for the major functionalities of a system; if end users cannot effectively navigate the system, it does not really matter what the system can do with the data that the provider inputs.

Beyond the preceding variables listed, a number of other variables should be considered when selecting an ePCR system. In no particular order, these are some of those variables:

♦ *Technical support.* Does the company have live support available 24 hours per day, 7 days per week? How quickly will service requests be handled? How does the system update its software? What is the longest system outage that the vendor has experienced, and what solutions does the vendor offer for documentation during system downtime?

♦ *Size of the service provider.* Is the vendor large enough to support an organization of your size? Is the vendor so large that an organization your size will not get the attention that it needs?

♦ *Setup and go-live support.* Does the system have other system implementations or organizations that will be going live at the same time your system is going live? Will the vendor send a company representative to assist you in the launch of your system? Is there an added cost for doing so? How will your staff members be trained on how to use the system?

♦ *Tertiary functionalities.* Does the system have any other value-added functions that are important or interesting for you? Some systems have tools that manage records requests, track provider certifications, store separate IRs, and provide messaging tools to employees.

♦ *Hardware.* What type of hardware will you use to run this system? Organizations have a number of choices to select from, including ruggedized laptop computers, fixed workstations, handheld devices, and tablet computers. Other hardware needed to run the system may include printers, charging stations or power cord installations, modems, and more.

* *Data transfer.* Structuring your system in such a way that it optimizes the ePCR system's ability to stay connected to the Internet is extremely important for most ePCR systems. Depending on the reliability of the data carriers available to the organization, it may be prudent to utilize two different data carriers. Hardware configurations that make a ePCR device the wireless gateway are usually preferred to configurations that rely on wireless networks established in ambulances, hospitals, and stations. Maximum data transfer should be encouraged, as incorporation of physiologic data and treatment markers from cardiac monitors can improve both the speed and the accuracy of PCR generation. Electronic attachment of the electrocardiogram or other physiologic data to the ePCR is a current best practice.

* *Workflow considerations.* As part of your procurement effort, you should consider how your various users will work this new technology into their daily workflow. At the field and supervisory levels, it may be helpful to follow a field provider through a call or part of a shift to determine how the ePCR system affects the provider's work habits. Using a real device in some version of test mode, test the system. How long will the battery last? How will reports go from the computer into the hands of the ED staff? Where will the computer be stored? All these considerations and more may play a role in the system you select and how you configure that system.

* *Ability to customize.* Some organizations have a strong desire to customize certain aspects of the ePCR system. Some ePCR systems have very little flexibility in this area; if this is important to an organization, it may be helpful to identify that up front.

SYSTEM IMPLEMENTATION

Once an organization has completed its selection process, efforts will turn to implementing the selected system. As for every project, the implementation of this system will depend on numerous factors that may be outside the control of the ambulance service manager. Once the contracting and purchasing phases are completed, an organization can begin working with its selected vendor to begin implementation planning in earnest. This effort will largely

Best Practice

Bundling of Information and Billing Services

Ambulance services have numerous information technology needs—ePCR systems being the largest. Others include scheduling systems, learning management systems, inventory systems, fleet management systems, and IR/UER systems. In 2010, the Wake County EMS system took a unique approach to system procurement. Instead of procuring each system separately and struggling to integrate them, a procurement process was designed that utilized prospective billing companies as system integrators. A request for proposals (RFP) was developed that required a prospective billing contractor to assemble, integrate, and deliver each of these systems as part of the contract for billing services. As a result, the EMS system enjoys a single point of contact for technology services, and realized significant improvements in pricing over multiple procurements.

be guided by the vendor, but some universal lessons are available.

Timeline

Implementation timelines are difficult to estimate. The timetable is often deeply affected by numerous stakeholders outside the ambulance service, and these stakeholders often have a very different set of priorities. Ambulance service managers who have a strong and effective mandate to implement the system expeditiously are the lucky few. Those who have less control are encouraged to develop a realistic timetable and include additional buffer time at critical junctures.

Generally speaking, ambulance service managers should plan for the following phases, at a minimum:

1. Procurement and selection
2. Contracting with vendor
3. Purchasing (Equipment availability, build times, and shipping may all impact this phase.)
4. Equipment setup and installation (Include planning for setup of PCR delivery methods to hospitals, etc.)
5. Field testing with select users, including workflow modifications
6. Special user trainings (for supervisors, quality management staff members, etc.)
7. General staff training
8. "Go live" period
9. Assessment and modification

Hardware Considerations

As an ambulance service implements an ePCR system, it will begin to understand the significant role that the hardware selected will play in the operation of the system. It is wise to make the hardware purchasing aspect of the decision a thoughtful one. As the agency prepare to go live with its system, those responsible will need to give serious consideration to how this hardware will be managed,

stored, maintained, and repaired. The ambulance service should ensure that it has an adequate number of reserve pieces to manage equipment breakdowns without impacting the system. The agency should develop a Plan B for documentation should part or all of the hardware or software system become unavailable. Staff will need to think through how and when crews will charge their mobile hardware devices (and they will need to charge them during the course of their shift); the best practice in this area is to provide a source of hardwired electricity within the ambulance. Project managers will want to consider the value of commercially available anti-theft devices or GPS tracking of hardware. Staff will also need to consider how the hardware devices will be stored or used in the ambulance (Figure 10.2), giving due consideration to safety standards for personnel in ambulances (a ruggedized laptop computer becomes an 8-pound missile if left unsecured during a vehicle collision).

Human Resources

The amount of staff time the agency will have to dedicate to this project will vary during each phase of implementation. Peak staffing needs will occur during the go live period, which may last for more than a week depending on shift schedules and training. During this period, it is recommended that a number of expert or power users be available throughout the service to assist users with problems or questions. These expert users are best developed by having a select group of technically proficient providers field test the system prior to training general staff members. When the entire organization begins using the system, these users will be available to assist supervisors and managers in the transition.

During the go live period, managers may want to consider small additions to their normal staffing plan, if possible. During the user's initial orientation to the system, he will typically

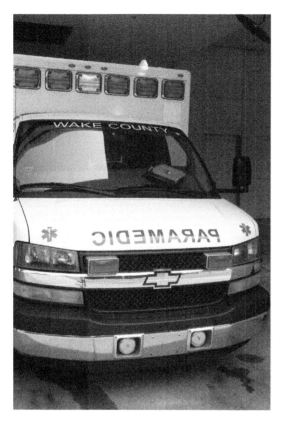

FIGURE 10.2 ▓ An improperly secured portable computer can become a dangerous projectile in a collision. The dashboard of an ambulance is one of the worst possible places to store a laptop, however briefly. *Source: Official Wake County EMS Photo by Mike Legeros, used by permission.*

require extra time to learn to navigate it appropriately. Having additional unit hours deployed

will assist the overall system in managing these slight increases in call times.

Workflow Considerations

As part of field testing, testers and managers need to give serious consideration to how they will incorporate this new technology into the workflow of field staff and other users. Depending on the approach of the providers, it may not be practical or valuable to expect the user to utilize the electronic solution in the same way he utilizes a paper-based report. Managers will need to take these changes into account and ensure that the user continues to have all the tools that he needs to meet the demands of patient care and capture needed information during the call.

It is best to try to determine what habits or practices should be changed or adopted to most efficiently use this new technology before general staff training occurs. Likewise, it is recommended that system implementers make special efforts to reach out to and understand the impact that this new technology will have on providers who are not extremely technically savvy.

Training

EMS managers will need to work collaboratively with vendors to design the appropriate training programs for various types of staff members who will use the system. Training a select group of users to the expert level and giving them an opportunity to test the system

Best Practice

Expert Users

When Grady EMS implemented an EPCR system in 2009, managers made an intentional effort to train expert users who worked shifts outside of normal

business hours. This gave the organization the ability to handle technical problems and answer user questions after IT staff and training officers had gone home for the evening.

will help guide the training efforts for the remaining field staff. Likewise, it is helpful to train frontline supervisors and staff trainers to become expert users from both a field level and from their own supervisory perspective.

Having created a deep bench of expert users, the service can now move to train the remaining field staff members. When developing a training program for field staff members, consider subdividing training sessions for computer savvy staff members or designated special training sessions for users who self-identify as less then technically proficient. This will assist both types of users in getting the most out of your training efforts. It is best to plan general staff training to dates as close to the go live date as possible. Simple flow-charts and one-page instruction handouts may also be valuable.

Some managers are tempted to short-change staff training programs or try to fit 4 hours of training into 2 hours of budgeted overtime. This is a dangerous move that may undermine success. This rushed and inadequate training will result in staff deficiencies that will require training personnel and deficient staff members to spend more time on remedial retraining than they would have on comprehensive initial training. It will also result in widespread underutilization of the system, which can diminish the value of this time of technical advancement.

■ ADMINISTRATIVE ISSUES IN PATIENT CARE REPORTING SYSTEMS———

Two key administrative issues in PCR systems are data security and data storage.

DATA SECURITY

When dealing with protected health information (PHI) and other sensitive personal information, security is a major concern. No one wants the local newspaper running a headline that reads, "County EMS Agency Loses Patient Data." Likewise, no one wants to be fined for HIPAA violations or to be cited for other violations of patient privacy.

Data Security in Paper-Based Systems

The primary concern in paper-based systems relates to maintaining control of each individual paper report. The prevailing sentiment is that, if you have physical control of the paper report, you have done everything you need to do to secure patient data. Organizational policies are focused on requirements to drop reports in the secure location, accessing and transferring the reports, and long-term storage.

Organizations using paper-based reports must expand beyond this point of view. It is important to consider a number of other factors when talking about the security of patient information. A well-written policy for data and record security in a paper-based system should include the following elements.

Pre-Lockbox Control of PCR. Employees do not always have the opportunity to transfer completed reports to a lockbox or drop-box immediately. In many systems, providers will complete multiple reports before they have an opportunity to properly transfer PCRs to the appropriate place or person. Without thinking about it, providers may leave PCRs on the dashboard of their ambulance or inside an open patient care compartment while they are at a local hospital. This leaves PHI vulnerable to theft and other inappropriate access. To prevent this type of loss, organizations should address how and where providers should store these reports between the time they are completed and the time they are properly transferred.

Handling and Destruction of Scrap Paper. When using both paper-based and electronic PCRs, users frequently keep notes and record initial patient information on notepads, scrap paper, gloves, tape, and other surfaces. These notes are later transcribed onto the formal PCR. Managers should keep in mind that these notes often contain Social Security numbers, names, and other PHI. Organizational policy that tried to prohibit this form of note taking is foolhardy; instead, organizations should instruct employees that these scrap papers contain PHI and should be destroyed promptly after use in an appropriate manner.

Hand-Off Reports, Face Sheets, and Other Records. In addition to various pieces of scrap paper that might be collected, providers may receive paper hand-off reports from first responders and other providers. They may also receive a patient information summary commonly referred to as a face sheet at a hospital, other medical records from other providers, 12-lead ECGs obtained in the field, and numerous other valuable pieces of tertiary information. Unlike scrap paper, the organization may want to retain this supplemental information. Ambulance service managers should collaborate with field providers to determine the types of supplemental information they receive and craft a policy to determine the best way to deal with that information.

Additional Copies of Reports. One of the biggest vulnerabilities of both paper and electronic reports is the ease with which reports are copied or printed. Frequently, organizations require that a copy of a PCR accompany certain training records, for pharmacy or materials management purposes (e.g., with narcotics usage logs or with broken equipment), and with IRs. Organizations should contemplate the acceptable reasons for creating an additional copy of a PCR and the handling of that additional record. It may be appropriate to take steps to redesign processes to eliminate the need for a duplicate PCR in order to ensure the protection of PHI.

Record Storage Areas. In many organizations, record storage may fall into three separate categories: short-term storage, intermediate storage, and long-term storage. The short-term storage location will likely be in a lockbox or dropbox; the service may have a number of different short-term storage solutions to provide an accessible area for crews to drop off reports at the end of their shift. Once reports are collected from the primary drop point, those records may be moved to any number of other places. It is very likely that these PCRs will be delivered to at least one administrative location for quality management, billing, or other administrative purposes. It is often in this intermediate location that record storage and security procedures are the most lax. Consider how many times you have seen a number of PCRs sitting on a desk in an unsecured office or left out overnight. At this intermediate location, you will need to develop a secure method of storing and protecting PCRs and the PHI they contain. Once all administrative work has been completed with these PCRs, they will likely be moved to a long-term storage area. In this final location, records will remain available for record requests and other inquiries, but they will not be accessed on a daily basis. The main considerations for long-term storage locations are the need to limit access to the records and the need to protect the records from damage.

Access to Records. In all cases, you will need to limit access to records to only those employees who have a need to review PCRs and only for the time that they will need to review them.

Data Security in ePCR Systems

Data security in an ePCR system often seems more complex than data security in a paper-based system. *Hacking, encryption, server*, and other terms outside the EMS vernacular can be confusing and intimidating. To evaluate these risks, ambulance service managers should utilize technical experts to ensure that data security measures are appropriate to the system and functioning.

Beyond the technical details, the manager may be called on to make a number of security policy decisions that will affect how providers use an ePCR system. These policy decisions may be made as part of vendor selection/software development, or they may be made during the implementation process. They fall into three broad categories: user settings, hardware/software capabilities and settings, and data storage.

User Settings.

1. *Usernames.* A username will identify each user within a system. Usernames are often straightforward and easy for the user to remember. The common pitfall that occurs with usernames is seen when systems issue usernames that are not tied to individual employees. Generic usernames and passwords undermine system security.
2. *Passwords.* The ePCR systems will require some kind of password to access the system. System administrators will need to decide the parameters of the passwords and how frequently the password should be changed. "Weak" passwords (default passwords, series of consecutive numbers or letters, etc.) should be prohibited, and passwords should be changed at least once per quarter.
3. *Access privileges.* Within ePCR systems, there are often more than a few levels of user access. Service managers will have to decide which employees need which type of access. Access to anything beyond the ability to create and edit

reports should be restricted to as few members as is necessary to accomplish required tasks.

Hardware/Software Capabilities.

1. *IP address restrictions.* Most ePCR systems give the system administrator the option of limiting the number of IP addresses from which employees can log into the system. This can restrict users from logging into the ePCR system from locations outside the workplace, or it can be used to require users to utilize a specific set of computers from which to access the system. A number of technical considerations must be weighed when making this choice, not least of which is the method by which field users will connect to the Internet. It is often impractical for systems to strictly limit the IP addresses from which users can access the system without first reconfiguring how wireless devices access the Internet.
2. *Auto-log out features.* This common security feature logs out a user after a certain period of inactivity. System administrators should use this feature to ensure that the ePCR system is not accessed by unauthorized individuals when an employee walks away from his computer. Field users and computers in public locations (including computers in vehicles) should auto-log out quickly (5 minutes or less of inactivity) to prevent intrusion into the system.
3. *System protection (antivirus).* Three general types of software protection are available for deployed computers:
   - Standard antivirus software can be installed and run on computers; these systems will require regular updates and may interfere with other software applications on the computer.
   - Browser-restriction software can be used to limit the website that can be visited by users. Typically, users' access is restricted to one or two sites, such as the ePCR site and the organization's intranet site. This restricts use of the computers to particular

work functions only and is a good security protection that may not interfere with required software applications.

- Steady-state software can be used to erase any and all changes made to the computer each time the computer is turned off. At the end of use or if any problem is encountered, a simple reboot will return the system to its original configurations.

4. *Device tracking with GPS.* Another common security feature for ePCR systems offers an organization the ability to track system hardware with a GPS locator. This is often offered for an additional price and may be manufacturer and device specific. Since mobile computers are at much higher risk for loss and theft and can be very expensive, many organizations determine that having the ability to track a device via GPS is worth the expense.

5. *Remote access capabilities.* In some cases, organizations are less interested in recovering the computer itself than they are in ensuring that data on the computer cannot be accessed. To meet this need, many software vendors have created a feature that allows the system to automatically erase all information on the computer's hard drive the next time the computer connects to the software's server.

Data Storage.

1. *Frequency and method of uploading data.* One of the most effective methods of protecting data security is to (securely) hand off the data to someone else. The best practice in this area is to automatically upload data to a secure server at a frequent interval. Data uploads that occur every few seconds are preferred over data uploads that happen at intervals of more than a minute. Systems that wait until a call is completed to upload data do so at the peril of losing a significant amount of data if a technical problem develops during the call.

Systems that upload data automatically have an advantage over systems that require a user action to initiate an upload. These automatic uploads ensure that data are transferred to the server in a seamless and reliable way. User-initiated uploads introduce an additional failure point if users forget to upload data or upload the same data multiple times.

The frequency of data uploading is not always determined by the type of software being used. To upload data, a user must have the Internet connectivity required to connect the local computer with the server or device that stores system data. The way the system is designed will determine how readily a connection is available. The best practice in this area is to design the system in such a way that each device used for data entry in the field has its own independent ability to connect to the Internet. Because these devices are highly mobile, this is usually accomplished with an aircard or similar wireless modem that connects the user to the Internet via a cellular service. Although not foolproof, the reliability of these systems has expanded dramatically as consumer demand for mobile Internet access has surged. Other alternatives involve the development of wireless hotspots and the installation of upload cables at access points.

2. *Local storage vs. server storage.* A question faced less frequently with ePCR systems available today is where the data will be stored. Some organizations choose to store data on a local computer. This method of data storage is fraught with problems and not recommended. It carries the significant risk of data loss and opens the service to a number of information security compliance issues.

3. *Server location.* One consideration that is available related to data housing is where the server housing the system's ePCR data is located. Systems can be configured to allow a local agency to house data in a server within the organization's IT infrastructure. More commonly, a software vendor will host data from all of its customers in one central, secure location. Data servers hosted by a software

vendor are typically a better option for ambulance services; they not only reduce the organization's liability but also make it easier for the vendor to provide system updates and other technical support. The ambulance service should require the vendor to provide a local copy of all ePCR data at specified intervals.

4. *Server backups.* Regardless of where a server is located, it should have at least one independent backup. This redundancy protects data in the event that the primary server suffers a catastrophic failure or is rendered unavailable.

5. *Encryption.* Much like storage of system data on a remote server, encryption of system data is an essential element of data security measures. Encryption technology is constantly evolving, so ePCR system administrators should consult with their IT advisors and vendors to ensure that the system in use meets the current standard for data protection. Electronic PCR systems that store PHI (any patient records) or personal information about providers (certification numbers) on portable-device hard drives (laptops or tablets) should be avoided; if that is not possible, continuous whole-disc encryption should be utilized. Unnecessary ports (e.g., USB ports) that might allow for unauthorized data transfer should be disabled.

In addition to these basic technical considerations regarding electronic security, organizations should be aware of state and federal regulations that may impact data security measures. For instance, state EMS regulations may require that EMS systems utilize a NEMSIS-compliant software program. Since there are two levels of NEMSIS compliance (Gold and Silver), organizations should take care to understand the full scope of any regulatory requirements in their area and ensure that whatever software they utilize meets state regulations. Likewise, organizations should investigate their obligations to meet data security requirements related to HIPAA, CMS regulations, and other

federal regulations. These regulations are complex and may require the assistance of an IT professional and/or legal advisor with a health care background.

■ THE FUTURE OF PATIENT CARE REPORTING

There is no question that the PCR of the future will move from paper to electronic. It could easily be argued that the standard of care has shifted so far in this direction already that it threatens to leave others behind. For those organizations that have not yet made the transition, the recent introduction of inexpensive tablet computers with inexpensive data plans from major carriers will likely make what was previously a prohibitively expensive transition into an affordable one.

EMS will also continue to benefit from the development of health care technology. Electronic medical record standardization will give us the ability to share an unparalleled amount of patient information in ways that may give us an opportunity to transform the way we provide EMS care. Combined with the development of the Advanced Practice Paramedic and Community Paramedic models, it is reasonable to foresee paramedics providing health care services to the community in a way that no longer restricts EMS to a transport-only model but, rather, gives paramedics a comprehensive view of the patient's past medical records instantly. Imagine how care for cardiac patients could be improved if a paramedic could instantly access and review a patient's most recent 12-lead ECG prior to making treatment and transport decisions.

OUTCOME SHARING BETWEEN HOSPITALS AND EMS

Every time EMS providers transfer a patient to a hospital emergency department, the providers share all of the details we know about the patient. If you categorize these details into the broad category of outcome data, you will recognize that there has always been a very one-way flow of these data from the field into the hospital. Over the past few years, some leaders in EMS have discussed the value of transforming that one-way data path into a two-way flow of information. By sharing the eventual diagnosis reached in the hospital, leaders hope to improve the assessment abilities of EMS providers and broaden their perspective on the condition and treatment of the patient.

In 2010, Dr. Craig Newgard and his colleagues in the Center for Policy and Research in Emergency Medicine at the Oregon Health & Science University demonstrated that EMS is not as far from this data-sharing opportunity as one might think (Newgard, Zive, Malveau, Leopold, Worrall, and Sahni, 2011). In a statewide demonstration project, Newgard and his team attempted to connect data from every EMS encounter that occurred in a single month to outcome records stored in various statewide patient outcome databases.

This effort involved the mapping of NEMSIS fields in EMS records to databases such as the Oregon Trauma Registry. Though the research team did not connect every patient encounter with a record in a statewide database, they were successful at connecting enough records to show us that this type of outcome feedback could be more than just a theoretical desire. The implications of this are extraordinary for EMS providers.

HEALTH CARE INFORMATION EXCHANGE

Though still in its relative infancy, leaders in health care technology (including stakeholders in EMS) have looked to further advance the ability to share medical records beyond the walls of individual health care institutions. This effort, known as the **health information exchange** (HIE), will standardize fields and streamline the ability of systems to automatically connect one record type with others from the same patient. For EMS, this could mean that an electronic PCR and its associated data could transition seamlessly into a hospital database and be connected to the

Best Practice

Bidirectional Data Exchange

It is important for ambulance services and other EMS system components to know what happened to the patient after arrival at the hospital. Was the field diagnosis consistent with what was found in the emergency department? Were treatments available in the prehospital arena provided shortly after arrival at the hospital? Did the patient with suspected STEMI go directly to the cardiac catheterization laboratory, or was the field interpretation of the 12-lead ECG incorrect? It is possible to answer these questions, and many more, with an electronic

exchange of data between the ambulance service and the hospital. Instead of printing an ePCR to paper, the ePCR data can be uploaded directly into the patient's electronic hospital record, for immediate use by receiving physicians and nurses. When the patient is discharged from the ED, or discharged from the hospital, information about ED and discharge diagnoses, treatments, and outcome status can be electronically passed back to the ambulance service and made available for QI and performance reporting.

patient's medical record at the receiving facility with the click of a button.

NEMSIS

In 2001, the National Association of State EMS Officials in conjunction with the National Highway Traffic Safety Administration (NHTSA) Office of Emergency Medical Services' EMS and Trauma/EMS Systems program (within a program administered by the Department of Health and Human Services' Health Resources and Services Administration [HRSA] Maternal Child Health Bureau [MCHB]) began to work collaboratively to develop the National EMS Information System. By 2005, these efforts had led to two very important developments for EMS: First, industry leaders developed the EMS Uniform Prehospital Dataset with an associated data dictionary (defining the terms in the data set) and a standard language for the conveyance of those terms (XML). This development represented a long-needed standardization of the data language that we use and began to make it possible to collect comparable data on a large scale. Second, various federal agencies, led by NHTSA's Office of EMS, created funding to provide a pilot phase for a Technical Assistance Center (TAC). This center, located at the University of Utah School of Medicine, would begin the work of collecting this Uniform Prehospital Dataset from participating states and making it available for researchers across the United States.

The development of the NEMSIS program and the support provided by the TAC has had a substantial impact on EMS research. In less than 10 years of work, the TAC is already collecting data from thirty states and providing researchers access to over 18 million EMS records. State EMS leaders can use one of three reporting tools to analyze their own data; researchers have access to two public databases from which they can draw information. The information that both groups are able to harness has already started to change the way EMS is practiced.

One of the efforts that will have both an immediate and enduring effect on EMS documentation relates to the creation and revision of the NEMSIS data set. This data set improves EMS documentation by creating consistency among the data elements and values within those elements used by electronic PCR systems. This standardization is reflected in virtually every vendor's ePCR offerings; by virtue of that, it impacts every end user of ePCR systems. By improving the data collected by our ePCR systems, the NEMSIS data sets are improving our actual documentation.

CHAPTER REVIEW

Summary

By now, the reader should have no doubts about the importance of the PCR or the value of the systems and policies that support the writing of PCRs. This chapter has presented some of the fundamental concepts that surround the writing of a quality PCR. It has also presented some of the key considerations related to the selection, implementation, and use of electronic PCR systems. For many of these topics, this chapter is little more than a primer. Deeper research may be needed into many topics, especially on topics such as EMS finance, the legal aspects of EMS documentation, and the quality management implications of ePCR systems. Whole chapters and books have been written on these topics.

There are three fundamental take-away points that the reader should take to heart above all others in this chapter:

1. Quality documentation is a hallmark of a good EMS system. Without quality documentation, the providers, patients, and system will fail to thrive.
2. The ePCR system is not only the wave of the future but also the next standard of care in documentation and quality management. Early adopters have pioneered the way for the rest of the profession, and recent advances in technology have made these applications available to users with a limited budget. If your organization has not adopted an ePCR system, you should begin the work to do so.
3. Field-level providers need to have a much deeper understanding of the concepts of documentation, the implications of poor documentation, and developments in the world of EMS information systems. Providers should know how poor documentation limits reimbursement and hampers the success of their system. Providers also should be aware that technology is driving many improvements and changes at the EMS system level. Their participation and assistance are valuable to the entire profession.

The world of EMS documentation will continue to advance. These advancements offer the opportunity to expand and improve our care, expand our knowledge, and create better EMS systems for the communities we serve. With any luck, these improvements will positively impact the careers and lives of EMS professionals across the United States.

WHAT WOULD YOU DO? Reflection

After a few hours on the phone with friends at other EMS services, you were easily convinced that improving your organization's documentation skills and abilities would be a valuable use of your time. Developing an RFP for an ePCR system was probably the most time-consuming part of your effort. Your staff members enjoyed participating in the selection process, even though it took longer that you would have liked. The challenge that stands before you is the implementation phase. You'll need to gather representatives from the local public safety access point (PSAP), the IT department, and the various hospitals to fully coordinate a comprehensive implementation. Staff training will require a great deal of effort, but you only have a few people with limited computer skills; hopefully, that will make things a little bit easier for you.

One of the biggest challenges you faced in the process was the cost of the system. An ePCR system certainly requires some up-front investment, but you were able to demonstrate a clear reduction in overall expenses in the first year. You hope that the organization will realize even greater cost reductions than your estimates indicate, and you know that your staff will now have more time to handle other tasks that have been neglected.

Your quality management efforts will probably be impacted the most by the change. By going electronic, you are giving your quality management staff the ability to view and use your clinical data in a whole new way. It will now be much easier to report on key metrics, review high-risk calls, and track skill proficiency by individual provider. With any luck, these improvements in documentation will also help you process patient billing in a faster and more accurate way.

Review Questions

1. Define the term *chief complaint* and explain its function in the context of the PCR.
2. What is a data element? How many are there in the NEMSIS Version 3 data set?
3. What are scripting validation rules? How do they impact EPCR documentation?
4. What are some of the problems that an EMS organization will face if it neglects the importance of patient care reporting?

5. What special challenges exist in documenting an accurate and consistent PCR when multiple agencies or units have responded to the same call?
6. Explain how HIE efforts will improve information exchanges between EMS providers and hospitals.

References

City of Fort Lauderdale. (2011, March). "EMS Ambulance Billing and Electronic Patient Care Reporting Services—Rebid." See the organization website.

Cummins, R. O., D. A. Chamberlain, N. S. Abramson, M. Allen, P. J. Baskett, et al. "Recommended Guidelines for Uniform Reporting of Data from Out-of-Hospital Cardiac Arrest: The Utstein Style. A Statement for Health Professionals from a Task Force of the American Heart Association, the European Resuscitation Council, the Heart and Stroke Foundation of Canada, and the Australian Resuscitation Council." *Circulation 84*(2), 960–975.

Hobgood, C., J. B. Bowen, J. H. Brice, B. Overby, and J. H. Tamayo-Sarver. (2006). "Do EMS Personnel Identify, Report and Disclose Medical Errors?" *Prehospital Emergency Care 10*(1), 21–27.

Institute of Medicine. (1999, November). "To Err Is Human: Building a Safer Health System." See the organization website.

Levinson, D. (2012, January). "Hospital Incident Reporting Systems Do Not Capture Most Patient Harm." Inspector General, Department of Health and Human Services. See the organization website.

Manatee County, Florida. (2010, November). "Request for Proposals: Electronic Patient Care Reporting for EMS." See the organization website.

Mattera, C. (1995). "Principles of EMS Documentation for Mobile Intensive Care Nurses." *Journal of Emergency Nursing 21*(3), 231–237.

Mears, G., J. P. Ornato, and D. E. Dawson. (2002). "Emergency Medical Services Information Systems and a Future EMS National Database." *Prehospital Emergency Care 6*(1), 123–130.

Meislin, H., D. W. Spaite, C. Conroy, M. Detwiler, and T. D Valenzuela. (1999, January–March). "Development of an Electronic Emergency Medical Services Patient Care Record." *Prehospital Emergency Care 3*(1), 54–59.

NASEMSO and NAEMSP. (2006, December). "Emergency Medical Services Performance Measures Project: Recommended Attributes and Indicators for System/Service Performance." See the organization website.

National EMS Information System. (1993). "Uniform EMS Data Element Dictionary Format." See the organization website.

National EMS Information System. (2005). "NEMSIS Version 3." See the organization website.

Newgard, C. D., D. Zive, S. Malveau, R. Leopold, W. Worrall, and R. Sahni. (2011). "Developing a Statewide Emergency Medical Services Database Linked to Hospital Outcomes: A Feasibility Study." *Prehospital Emergency Care 15*(3), 303–319.

New York State Department of Health, Bureau of EMS. (2002, October 29). "Policy Statements on Pre Hospital Care Reports." See the organization website.

NHTSA, Office of EMS. (2006, September). "A Closer Look." *EMS Update*. See the organization website.

Snyder, J. (2007). *EMS Documentation*. Upper Saddle River, NJ: Prentice Hall

Wang, H.E., R. M. Domeier, D. F. Kupas, M. J. Greenwood, R. E. O'Connor, and National Association of EMS Physicians. (2004, January–March). "Recommended Guidelines for Uniform Reporting of Data from Out-of-Hospital Airway Management: Position Statement of the National Association of EMS Physicians." *Prehospital Emergency Care 8*(1), 58–72.

Key Terms

business logic Coding with a particular ePCR program that recognizes the relationship between certain data elements within an ePCR document and adjusts the document based on input in certain key data elements. For example, if the "no patient found" call disposition is selected, the name and other demographic fields may become disabled in that form.

chief complaint A very brief summary of the most serious aspect of the patient's assessment, usually in five words or less. It should reflect the patient's condition more than the patient's verbally stated complaint.

call disposition The outcome of a call for service or an individual response.

computer-aided dispatch (CAD) system A computer system that manages information related to each call for service in a dispatching center and assists dispatch personnel in the assignment and management of system resources.

data element An individual piece of data collected on a form or in a report, typically in the form of a question or a field that must be filled in by a provider.

False Claims Act A federal law designed to combat fraud against the government and governmental programs.

health information exchange (HIE) An effort to standardize elements of patient electronic health records.

Health Insurance Portability and Accountability Act (HIPAA) A federal law dealing with patient privacy and the handling of medical records that has particular implications for EMS services and their documentation practices.

National EMS Information Systems (NEMSIS Version 3) A program developed by the federal government to advance information collection within EMS, thereby creating a single national database of EMS information for the purpose of EMS research and system development.

negligence Conduct that falls below the standard of behavior established by law or industry for the protection of others against unreasonable risk of harm.

patient care report (PCR) Document that is currently evolving from its traditional, written format, which has existed for more than a generation, to the electronic format of the future.

PCR narrative A free-form, paragraph-style aspect of the PCR that often serves as the primary summary and explanation of the events of the patient encounter.

scripting validation Commonly known as closed call rules, these parameters define what data elements in a PCR must be completed before that report can be considered complete.

Marketing, Media, and Community Relations

Tom Tornstrom, M.B.A., EMT-P, and Keith Griffiths

Objectives

After reading this chapter, the student will be able to:

11.1 Identify and define the various categories of organizational stakeholders.

11.2 Describe the importance of utilizing technology as part of effective ambulance marketing.

11.3 Identify the various types and methods of available marketing technology.

11.4 Describe various types of traditional marketing mediums.

11.5 Describe how to work with the press to get your message out and to provide community outreach.

11.6 Identify the benefits of ongoing community outreach in positioning your organization.

Overview

Ambulance services in the United States range in size from one ambulance operated by volunteers and managed by a community board of directors to large governmental agencies and even larger, private, for-profit corporations. This text presents information that the manager of an ambulance service, large or small, needs in order to keep the business solvent and provide clinically excellent service to the community.

Key Terms

business intelligence	intranet	stakeholder	virtual meeting
data dashboard	social media	traditional media	Web presence
Internet			

WHAT WOULD YOU DO?

In your new role as operations manager, you have been tasked with the mission of preparing to enter the competitive bidding process. You and three other ambulance services will be vying for your current service area. Although you are a nonprofit organization that has been providing excellent service for many years, a local political entity has decided that your rates are too high and believes you are taking advantage of their citizens. A big part of your plan is to create a marketing campaign that will help the stakeholders in your community understand how you operate and why your ambulance rates are set as they are.

1. What can ambulance suppliers do to help prevent public objection over service fee increases?
2. Discuss some pros and cons regarding contracting for ambulance services.
3. Discuss the public's perception of for-profit, nonprofit, and government-based ambulance services.

■ INTRODUCTION

Whether an ambulance service is in the public or private sector, the importance of ongoing, persistent, and effective communication with a diverse group of community stakeholders should not be underestimated. An organization's communication may take many forms, from traditional advertising, to visible outreach in the community, to the organization's website. As a result of the advent of e-mail and the **Internet**, most people, including **stakeholders**, expect information to be delivered to them quickly and in an easy-to-comprehend format. It is unlikely that all stakeholders with decision-making authority will take the time or put in the effort to seek out the information needed to make a well-informed decision. Because of

this, when two or more ambulance providers are vying for a service area, it is often the organization that holds a stronger relationship with the decision-making stakeholders that will hold the competitive edge.

It is also important to note that an organization's reputation in the community isn't going to be determined by a good marketing campaign. Public communications and marketing strategy help an agency to *articulate* the story—but the story is *who you are*, and you can't fake that. You can help make the case that your agency is an integral part of the community through outreach programs such as injury prevention education, blood pressure screenings, and so on; through the professionalism and friendliness of your crews; and through sincere and visible efforts to enhance safety, awareness, and education.

Best Practice

How Three Agencies Have Provided Innovative Community Outreach

By Jenifer Goodwin

It's always rewarding to be highly regarded, whether it's by customers, co-workers, or your community. This is especially true for EMS. How patients, community leaders, and elected officials regard an EMS agency can impact the level of support—financial and otherwise—an organization receives. That's no small matter during times when difficult spending decisions are made.

"If the population loves the EMS system, they are going to stand up and make sure it gets the needed funding," says Janna Binder, director of marketing and public relations for Professional Research Consultants (PRC), a survey and market research company in Omaha, Neb. that specializes in health care-related clients, including EMS.

The question for EMS is: How do you build a better reputation?

The most obvious answer is: Provide excellent patient care.

Indeed, according to a 2008 survey of 1,000 patients who'd recently been transported by one of 20 EMS agencies nationwide, PRC found that those who perceived their paramedics as highly knowledgeable and skilled were more likely to be very satisfied with their treatment and level of care during their EMS encounter.

Yes, skill and knowledge matter, but those weren't the most important factors driving patient perceptions. The top two? Teamwork among EMS personnel and offering clear explanations for treatment or tests being done were highest, according to the survey. Both factors measure how well EMS crews are communicating to one another and to patients, a critical aspect of patient care, says Brooks Dameier, PRC's EMS project manager.

That means always remembering to tell patients and their families what you're doing and why in language they can understand. It means making sure to show compassion and kindness in your words and body language, Dameier says.

In PRC surveys, patients who rated their experience with EMS as "outstanding" were over five times more likely to recommend the EMS agency or speak positively about it to others than patients who marked merely "very good." "It's those 'wow' experiences where you build loyalty," Dameier says. "That's how you create community ambassadors who can generate goodwill and help spread those perceptions."

Yet patients aren't the only ones that EMS agencies need to focus on to ensure effective communications. Many EMS leaders from well respected organizations say establishing community and programs that improve the health and safety of residents—some who may never need to dial 911—builds ties that benefit both the community and EMS.

That strategy is working for the Edina (Minn.) Fire Department. Chief Marty Scheerer appears at civic groups, women's clubs, schools, and senior organizations to talk about the services his firefighter/paramedics offer. That includes visiting homes of the elderly to change batteries in fire alarms, organizing holiday toy and food collection drives, and offering drop-in blood pressure checks in their stations.

"We don't want to just react to fires," Scheerer says. "We want to be proactive. It's the right thing to do. But as a side benefit, it helps our organization and lets people know we're not sitting there waiting for something to happen. We are being efficient with money and looking for ways to expand our responsibilities in the community."

Jeff Dumermuth, chief of West Des Moines (Iowa) EMS, agrees. Community outreach is certainly one aspect of building a sense of connectedness between EMS and the community. Yet in difficult economic times, EMS has to make sure it's not only efficient with money—but also making sure the community knows it.

Nine years ago, Dumermuth's third service EMS agency cut costs by sharing some administrative and billing staff with the county. More recently, West Des Moines EMS was chosen to provide ambulance transport to Iowa Health Des Moines, a four-hospital system. In return, the hospital system agreed to cover 30 percent of administrative costs for West Des Moines EMS, to hire eight new full-time paramedics and EMTs, and purchase three ambulances. The hospital system is planning to add a fourth ambulance soon, Dumermuth says.

In 2009, that arrangement saved the city of West Des Moines taxpayers $200,000 in administrative costs. And doing specialty transports for the city also gave paramedics and EMTs more experience in transporting neonatal and pediatric patients, groups they would not normally often encounter.

"While our city continues to struggle with budgets, we have been able to maintain service by being creative with partnerships and outside revenue sources," Dumermuth says.

Although maintaining an already strong reputation requires careful attention, altering perceptions is even tougher. That was the challenge faced by Bruce Baxter, CEO of New Britain (Conn.) EMS, which serves a city of about 70,000. Fourteen years ago, the city's common council (city council) lost faith in the organization and withdrew some $500,000 a year in funding, Baxter says. Turning that shop around was a painstaking process that included overhauling the agency's financial management, forming new strategic partnerships and reaching out to the community.

"Your reputation is everything in your community," Baxter says. "If your community doesn't believe in you, they are not going to support you."

Paramedics and EMTs provide numerous injury prevention and emergency preparedness education programs, including free child safety seat installation and inspections, and serving as an American Heart Association Community Training Center for CPR. The organization is also helping seniors and others sign up for Invisible Bracelet, a new, Internet-based medic-alert system that enables people to sign up, receive a personal ID number and store important medical information that can be easily accessed by EMS and physicians, as well enabling EMS to instantly generate text, email or phone messages to family members in case of emergency.

In an area of high unemployment, New Britain EMS is also offering job training. This includes partnering with the local high school to offer students emergency medical responder training programs, and joining forces with a local social services agency to offer summer internships through a federal grant. Both programs are designed to teach disadvantaged kids life skills and work habits to help them succeed after graduating.

Recently, the agency also opened the New Britain Emergency Medical Services Academy at Central Connecticut State University's Institute of Technology and Business Development. The center, which offers continuing education and new certifications for EMTs and paramedics, and AHA courses, served 3,000 students in its first year. Any profits generated will go back into supporting the city's emergency medical services.

"By binding yourself to the community, you start changing the way people think of you from being just an ambulance service to being a team player that is vested in the overall health and wellness of the community," Baxter says.

Source: Reprinted by permission from EMS Best Practices

▦ DEFINE YOUR TARGET AUDIENCE ─────────

A stakeholder is a person or group of people with an interest or concern in an ambulance service due to direct or indirect involvement. The ambulance industry, like most public safety sectors, has a sizable and diverse group of stakeholders. Political bodies, hospitals, patients, the general public, employees, and other public safety organizations are but a few examples of the stakeholders who are affected by the decisions and performance that an ambulance service may produce.

Because of this "stake" in the functionality and viability of the ambulance service, it is extremely important to communicate with the various stakeholders on a regular basis. Since not all ambulance provider stakeholders are interested in the same information, it's also important to categorize the groups of stakeholders and then identify which information is most important to each group. An effective way to categorize stakeholders is to classify them each in one or more of the following stakeholder types (Marsh, 1998):

1. *Core stakeholders.* People essential to the organization or process. This group could include employees, managers, and medical directors.
2. *Customers.* People who receive the service. This group should include patients, skilled nursing facilities, hospitals, or other entities receiving service from ambulance providers.
3. *Controllers.* People who define, regulate, and influence the ambulance provider. City or town councils, EMS commissions, parent organizations, owners, and state EMS departments can all be considered controllers.
4. *Partners.* People or groups of people through whom part or all of an EMS system is delivered. This should include other public safety agencies such as first responder squads, fire departments, police departments, dispatch centers, and emergency management offices.

PREPARING STAKEHOLDER INFORMATION

Once the stakeholders are identified and categorized by type of interest, a decision should be made to outline what kind of information and what level of detail should be shared with each respective stakeholder type.

When communicating with core stakeholders, such as employees, it will often depend on the culture of the ambulance organization to determine exactly what information and what level of detail should be shared. It is also important to realize and understand that frequent and effective communication with employees can play a significant role in employee job satisfaction (Ming-Ten, Shuang-Shii, and Ping, 2009).

A marketing piece to customer stakeholders, which is made up primarily of potential patients, should typically focus on high-level information, such as ambulance driving safety, levels of service offered (e.g., ALS, BLS, or critical care), and generally what each level offers. In addition, it would be useful to include employee or service accomplishments and items that have generated positive media attention. Keep the tone informational and positive.

When communicating and marketing to controller stakeholders, such as city councils, county boards, or EMS-specific decision makers, it is extremely important that the marketing information be nonsensationalized and limited to factual reporting. Political decision makers may be turned off by a sensationalized piece that lacks substance. A detailed report that highlights any regulated proficiencies or performance indicators, such as response times, is best produced with an easy-to-understand explanation of the various measures. It's imperative that controller stakeholders understand the basic concepts of your performance measures and why they are or are not important.

The ability to effectively and readily communicate to and with partner stakeholders, such as first responder squads and fire departments, can have a profound impact on not only the relationship between ambulance provider employees and the partner employees but also patient outcomes. Information that should be shared and proactively marketed to partners can include new employee introductions, veteran employee biographies, introduction of new medical procedures or medications, and changes to protocols. Keeping partners informed through marketing while maintaining open lines of communication is typically considered a best practice that will result in increased positive outcomes for patients.

■ COMMUNICATION MEDIUMS: CHOOSING THE RIGHT APPROACH

Once the various stakeholders have been identified and their respective marketing information defined, the ambulance organization should be aware and have some understanding of the numerous marketing venues available. In the past 10 to 15 years, the communications industry has seen tremendous change as various forms of Internet-based marketing and communication have become affordable and readily available. Countless blogging services and Internet websites, such as Facebook and Twitter, have empowered users to be content providers, a role that was once only available to traditional media outlets. Although this chapter focuses heavily on the use of modern communications technology, **traditional media**, such as television, radio, print, and direct mail, should not be overlooked, especially when communicating to customer stakeholders.

COMMUNICATING THROUGH TECHNOLOGY

This technological revolution has had a profound impact on many of the aspects involved with running an ambulance service. One of the areas impacted the most is the increase in available forms of electronic media that can be used to communicate with ambulance service stakeholders. The most common types of electronic marketing include website publishing, **intranet**, e-mail, Internet marketing, **virtual meeting**, social media, text messaging, instant messaging, stakeholder **data dashboards**. Marketing through technology can be very valuable by allowing for specific stakeholder targeting while remaining cost effective.

Public Website

With billions of individual Web pages and over 100 million websites in existence, and with stakeholders expecting to be able to quickly access information, an ambulance organization that does not have a **Web presence** may be missing out on one of the most affordable and responsive forms of marketing available. An attractive, intuitive, informational, and user-friendly website should be the primary goal of any organization wanting to have an effective Web presence (Figure 11.1). Research has shown that the overall usability of websites can be directly correlated to the site visitor's level of satisfaction with the site.[1]

Although website design and creation are typically best left to marketing professionals and graphic designers, it is extremely important that an ambulance organization be actively involved in the original website content. Through its look and feel, photos selected, positioning of key messages, and

---

[1]According to a study by Fu and Salvendy (2002), "in all Web page designs, inherent usability was the main factor contributing to user's satisfaction."

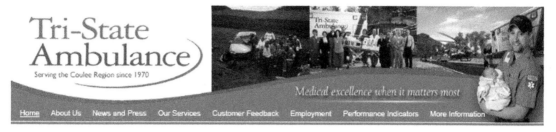

Tri-State
Ambulance
Serving the Coulee Region since 1970

Medical excellence when it matters most

Home   About Us   News and Press   Our Services   Customer Feedback   Employment   Performance Indicators   More Information

Welcome to Tri-State Ambulance

 Search

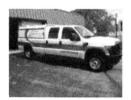

Since 1970, Tri-State Ambulance, a non-profit organization, has served as the sole 911 advanced life support provider for the greater Coulee Region. Covering nearly 2,200 square miles and serving a population of approximately 150,000, Tri-State Ambulance offers its residents and visitors alike unsurpassed pre-hospital care.

AED Loaner Program

Tri-State Ambulance is proud to announce the inception and creation of a valuable program that will aid our community in the treatment and survival of sudden cardiac arrest victims.

Click here to find out more!

Tri-State Ambulance Responds to Tornado in La Crosse

On May 22nd an EF1-EF2 tornado struck the south side of La Crosse causing widespread damage along its path. Fortunately for residents, the storm caused few minor injuries and no deaths. Tri-State Ambulance responded with 13 ambulances, multiple supervisors and managers with response vehicles, and over 40 total staff. Several mutual aid ambulances also assisted with disaster response as well as system-wide coverage of EMS requests. For detailed information on the response, see the Tri-State Ambulance Tornado Report.

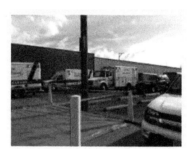

Tri-State Ambulances and other emergency vehicles stage during tornado response.

Freedom Honor Flight

FREEDOM HONOR FLIGHT

Since 2008, Tri-State Ambulance has provided fully equipped and experienced paramedics to accompany groups of U.S. veterans to Washington, D.C. In 2010, Tri-State Ambulance paramedics accompanied three additional flights. The Freedom Honor Flight has assisted hundreds of area veterans in visiting their memorial.

Tri-State Ambulance is honored to contribute our skilled paramedics to these important events. Please visit the Freedom Honor Flight website and join us in supporting this valuable program.

Tri-State Ambulance Vehicle Improvements

Tri-State Ambulance adds two new vehicles increasing safety and reducing cost. See news reports from WKBT and WXOW.

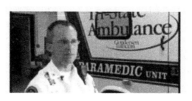

FIGURE 11.1   An example of a friendly, publicly accessible website. *Source: Reprinted by permission from Tri-State Ambulance, Lacrosse, Wisconsin.*

other content, your website represents who you are and what you value. Once a website is designed and goes live, it is also imperative that the site be kept fresh through frequent updates and original content. Because a public website is freely accessible by all stakeholders, special attention should be paid to ensure that the website content offers information applicable to each group. Keep in mind that a poorly designed or difficult-to-use website may actually reflect more negatively on an organization than not having a Web presence at all.

Website creation costs can range from a few hundred dollars to thousands or tens of thousands of dollars, depending on the amount and type of content, whether a design template is used or the site is created from scratch, whether the site is to be used for e-commerce, and the experience of the design vendor. Ongoing costs for content changes and server space can range from less than a hundred to thousands of dollars per month. Most ambulance services should be able to start up a reasonably usable and content-rich website relatively inexpensively, although it is necessary to consider the hidden costs of EMS staff time in identifying, writing, and editing original content.

Intranet Website

An effective and dynamic way to market and communicate with core stakeholders is to develop and maintain an internal website. An intranet is typically accessible only by employees and other closely connected stakeholders, such as a board of directors. Since an intranet website is secure and accessible only by this limited group, the information shared can be of a more confidential or "employee only" nature. Many ambulance services use intranet websites for such tasks as vehicle issue tracking, incident reporting, employee or manager announcements, and intraorganizational polls or surveys.

An intranet website can be an affordable and effective tool for marketing and communicating with core stakeholders. Many vendors offer hosted intranet solutions as well as server software that can be hosted by the individual ambulance service.

To be used as an effective marketing tool for core stakeholders, it's important that an intranet website not be passive. In other words, an intranet website will be most effective if employees are required to log in and visit as part of their daily duties. The usability of an intranet website can be ensured by posting required information such as a daily reporting tool or by setting the company home page to the intranet on all computers, as shown in Figure 11.2.

E-mail

It seems as though almost everyone in modern society has an e-mail address. Certainly the four stakeholder groups will have a very high percentage of e-mail literate members. Although e-mail marketing can be an affordable strategy, caution should be taken as to its effectiveness. E-mail marketing should only be used for those who have opted in or have actually given their consent to receive the e-mails. Purchasing of mass e-mail lists or targeted e-mail lists without the recipient's permission is considered spam and bad business practice, and it may be illegal in some states.

Much thought should go into developing a plan for an e-mail marketing campaign. Some basic questions to consider can include these: What is the purpose of the campaign, and who will be the stakeholder group(s) receiving the e-mail? Is the campaign intended only to disseminate information such as performance reports, or is the campaign part of a multifaceted marketing plan aimed at garnering new business? Other considerations should include the relative importance of the e-mail campaign. It would be unwise to mass-e-mail an

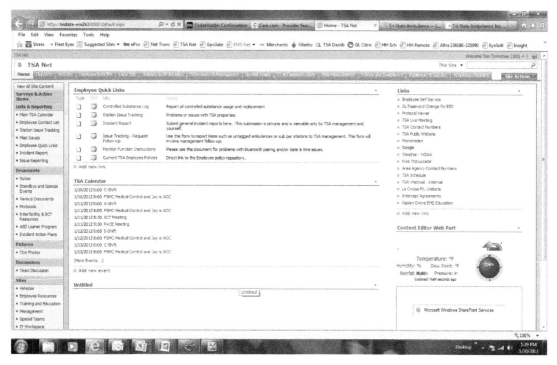

FIGURE 11.2 An example of a company intranet website. *Source: Reprinted by permission from Tri-State Ambulance, Lacrosse, Wisconsin.*

important document or report to partner or controller stakeholders without a co-marketing strategy, such as regular mail.

Countless commercial e-mail marketing vendors offer an option to track the effectiveness of an e-mail campaign. In addition, most of these vendors offer the important requirement for subscribers to opt-in or unsubscribe at their leisure. When choosing an e-mail marketing vendor, make certain that they offer, at a minimum, the following reporting features:

- *Deliverability.* How many of your e-mail messages will actually reach the recipient inboxes? With spam and junk mail filters, the likelihood of actual delivery can be around 70 percent to 80 percent.
- *Open rate.* Of the recipients who received the e-mail, how many actually opened or read it?

This number can fluctuate greatly based on the recipient's interest in the e-mail and sender, the subject line of the e-mail, and how much time the recipient has available to open and read it. Keep in mind that opening an e-mail requires some effort on the recipient's part. This perceived effort by the recipient should be rewarded by e-mail content that contains worthy information and an expression of gratitude by the sender.

- *Click-through rate.* The click-through rate is another traceable action performed by the recipient. An ambulance service may rightfully decide that e-mailing a month's worth of performance reports as attachments may alienate recipients and overload their mailboxes. Because of this, the ambulance service instead may choose to insert into the body of the e-mail a hyperlink that takes the recipient to the organization's public website where the reports can be viewed, downloaded, or printed. By clicking on the hyperlink, a click-through is tracked, allowing the sender to have an idea of how many recipients are actually interested enough or have time enough to view its reports. Typical costs of e-mail marketing services can range from a few dollars per month for the sending and tracking service to several hundred or thousands of dollars for a full-service campaign.

Internet Marketing and Advertising

An increasingly common form of electronic advertising is the placement of banner advertisements or highlighted text boxes on websites based on keyword searches. Keyword searches use single words or short phrases chosen by an advertiser that will trigger the display of a banner ad or a prominent link to its website. Services such as Google AdWords, Microsoft adCenter, and Facebook offer the option, based on such keyword searches, to display banners or hyperlinks leading to your organization's website.

An ambulance service looking to attract paramedics may want the link to the recruitment portion of its website displayed prominently when a Google or MSN user types in the search term *paramedic jobs*. The cost for such advertising is typically based on click-throughs or the number of times a displayed link is followed. Charges can range from a few cents to more than a dollar per click-through.

The effectiveness of banner or link advertising is subject to much debate. A successful Internet marketing campaign should involve careful planning and an understanding of the numerous factors that can influence the campaign outcome. It should also be noted that at least one study found that "(banner) advertising is believed to be most effective when the ad content is compatible with the interests of those people exposed to the program with

which the ad is placed" (Cho, 2003, p. 209). In other words, this study determined that focusing banner advertising on websites that closely align with the service or products being promoted produces the best results.

Virtual Interactive Meetings and Communication

Throughout the past decade, the availability and technology for Internet-based virtual meetings have drastically improved. With these improvements have come increased competition and, in turn, lower costs. These virtual meeting services, often referred to as teleconferencing, video conferencing, Web meetings, and webinars, have typically been limited in usage to intraorganizational long-distance communication or training.

The potential for ambulance services to utilize virtual meeting services for marketing and communication should not be underestimated. All stakeholder groups have the potential to benefit from a well-planned and executed virtual meeting marketing campaign. Employees may find much value in being able to attend and interact with virtual meetings from home, a remote station, or even while sitting at post.

Virtual live or recorded presentations can be effective tools in communicating with stakeholders other than employees. Offering a busy city administrator the choice of meeting in person or meeting in an easy-to-use virtual environment may be an attractive option.

Many virtual meeting products and services are available, and each offers slightly different functionality. Microsoft Live Meeting, Webex, and GoToMeeeting are the virtual meeting offerings of three of the larger vendors. Prices for a virtual service typically depend on the number of simultaneous participants and can range anywhere from a few dollars to several thousand dollars per month. The future will bring new and innovative ways to meet in virtual space. Whether it's employee training meetings or patient telemedicine, ambulance services should plan on capitalizing on this increasingly popular marketing and communication option.

Social Media

The use of social networking as a form of communication with all types of stakeholders has tremendous potential. Social networking services such as Facebook, Twitter, and MySpace tend to focus on networking connections among friends and acquaintances but provide an option for businesses or special interest groups to host a Web page that can be linked to users' personal connections. Professional sites such as LinkedIn, JEMS Connection, and EMS Village typically focus on career- or industry-oriented topics and networking relationships.

Consider that Facebook has more than 500 million users worldwide and that 50 percent of those users log on at least once daily. In addition, the average user has 130 friend connections and follows 80 community pages, groups, or events (Facebook, 2011). The primary advantage to realize when considering stakeholder communication through **social media** sites, such as Facebook, is that the communication is instant, compounding, and extremely effective in relaying critical information. For example, think of your service area experiencing a sudden outbreak of influenza and thereby increasing your ambulance run volume to unprecedented levels. Although the vast majority of these influenza cases are not life threatening, the symptoms are severe and cause emergency department and ambulance response overloads. Since you already have a Facebook page with 200 followers, you have chosen to work with your medical director to create and pass along a brief press release highlighting what signs and symptoms to expect and when to call an ambulance. Considering that on average each of your 200

followers has 130 friends, you have the potential to reach 26,000 first-level relationships within hours and in turn remove some of the burden on your EMS system.

Use of social media and networking seems to be continually increasing. Ambulance services should understand and embrace this technology.

Text and Instant Messaging

Text messaging and instant messaging are often thought of as forms of nonbusiness social networking. Although this may often be the case, ambulance services should give consideration to the affordability and immediate marketing ability that text and instant messaging can offer. Stakeholders such as mayors, city administrators, and county board members may derive a great deal of value from receiving an occasional text message alerting them to an exceptional event such as an multiple casualty incident (MCI) or multiple-victim fire. A number of the computer-aided dispatch vendors offer automated texting based on preset criteria that can be defined to be pertinent for individual recipients.

Instant messaging can be a helpful form of marketing to patients or other core stakeholders when it is incorporated into the organizational website. Allowing a patient or other website visitor the ability to instant-message and chat live with a customer service or billing representative can reflect positively on an organization. In addition, incorporating a messaging system into an electronic patient care report or vehicle routing system can give dispatchers and supervisors the ability to send important but private information to crews. This ability can be viewed positively by employees and dispatchers.

Stakeholder Data Dashboards

A data dashboard is a visual representation of past, present, and projected financial, operational, or clinical information. Often in the form of charts and graphs, this information is typically displayed on a computer or television monitor. Dashboards can be organized in such a way that individual stakeholder groups have access only to the information that is pertinent to them. Dashboards have been gaining much popularity in recent years and can be a very effective marketing and communication tool for ambulance services.

Placing a dashboard view at an ambulance headquarters or linked from an ambulance's mobile data terminal can give managers the ability to instantly communicate to employees. This immediate communication can create better-informed employees and can be used for internal safety and employee satisfaction marketing. Employee dashboard views can display such operational items as current system status, units out of compliance with activation or response requirements, or daily operating conditions such as shown in Figures 11.3, 11.4, and 11.5. In addition, company announcements, upcoming training, weather conditions, traffic reports, and words of employee encouragement and support can be incorporated into a dashboard.

In addition to employee dashboards, ambulance services are also beginning to see the value in transparency by allowing controller and partner stakeholders access to dashboard

Tri-State Ambulance

Tri-State Operational Dashboards

SSM Level: 4

Active Vehicles

Unit	Vehicle	Status	Location	Zone	Address	City
T-301	2937	Available	5 - Central	LaCrosse	221 BUCHNER PL	LA CROSSE
T-302	1580	Available	2 - Station 2	LaCrosse	2827 26TH ST S	LA CROSSE
T-303	2478	Available	5 - Central	LaCrosse	221 BUCHNER PL	LA CROSSE
T-304	1579	EnR Post	4 - Station 5	LaCrosse	9TH AVE S & LA CROSSE ST	ONALASKA
T-305	2936	Busy		LaCrosse	3075 S KINNEY COULEE RD	ONALASKA
T-306	28	TSA NEXT UP	9 - Station 4	Viroqua	126 W JEFFERSON ST	VIROQUA
T-307	5512	Available	9 - Station 4	Viroqua	126 W JEFFERSON ST	VIROQUA
T-500	T-500	Available	TSA Management	LaCrosse	221 BUCHNER PL	LA CROSSE

Last Update: 2012-01-10 13:51:25

Active Trips

Unit	Vehicle	Status	Crew Member 1	Crew Member 2	Run Number	Nature of Call	Initial Priority	Response Zone	Activation Time	Response Time	At Scene Time	Clearing Time
T-305	2936	At Scene	Cessford, Bryan	Goettel, Jeffrey	422	Chest Pain	P1	Onalaska City	00:01:11	00:09:01		

Completed Trips - last 48 hours

Unit	Vehicle	Dispatch Date	Status	Crew Members	Run Number	Nature of Call	Initial Priority	Response Zone	Activation Time	Response Time	At Scene Time	Clearing Time
T-304	1579	01/10/2012 13:28:10	Canceled At Scene	Johnson, Jeff / Groebner, Brian	421	Unknown Medical	P1	Onalaska City	00:00:02	00:06:11	00:11:52	
T-303	2478	01/10/2012 12:49:48	Complete	Mcdonald, Cindy / Watson, Michael	420	Chest Pain	P1	La Crescent City	00:00:01	00:06:39	00:19:39	00:15:47
T-303	2478	01/10/2012 12:41:41	Canceled At Scene	Mcdonald, Cindy / Watson, Michael	419	Medical Alert	P2	La Crosse City	00:00:01	00:05:20	00:02:02	
T-302	1580	01/10/2012 11:48:02	Canceled At Scene	Kulas, Jennifer / Heiser, Maria	418	Traffic Accident (MVC)	P2	La Crosse City	00:00:25	00:04:12	00:04:36	
T-302	1580	01/10/2012 11:12:43	Canceled At Scene	Kulas, Jennifer / Heiser, Maria	417	Fall	P2	La Crosse City	00:00:37	00:09:58	00:09:09	
T-303	2478	01/10/2012 10:46:03	Complete	Mcdonald, Cindy / Watson, Michael	415	Medical	P1	La Crescent City	00:00:01	00:08:13	00:20:17	00:06:41
T-305	2936	01/10/2012 10:41:55	Complete	Cessford, Bryan / Goettel, Jeffrey	414	Chest Pain	P1	Onalaska City	00:00:36	00:07:09	00:20:31	00:06:32
T-304	1579	01/10/2012 10:33:11	Complete	Johnson, Jeff / Groebner, Brian	413	Pediatrics - Medical	P1	Onalaska City	00:00:37	00:03:50	00:15:38	00:16:37

FIGURE 11.3 ■ A custom dashboard screenshot. *Source: Reprinted by permission from Tri-State Ambulance, Lacrosse, Wisconsin.*

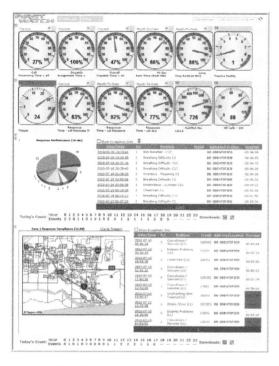

FIGURE 11.4 ■ A comprehensive dashboard.
Source: Reprinted by permission from Tri-State Ambulance, Lacrosse, Wisconsin.

views. Giving an emergency department the ability to view an operational dashboard that is customized to its wants may be a very beneficial marketing tool. Emergency departments may be able to plan more efficiently by having a dashboard that displays the number of incoming ambulances, their mode of transport (e.g., lights and sirens or nonlights and sirens), and their arrival time. This information would be available in real-time to emergency departments and would allow them not to depend solely on the ambulance radio or telephone report for an estimated arrival time. In addition, dashboards that can display real-time clinical data to receiving hospitals can play a positive role in ultimate patient outcome by involving receiving doctors and nurses earlier. Some ambulance services offer political and governmental officials, such as those involved or

employed in public health departments, access to dashboards that can contain such information as current system status, trends in call types, and alerts to increases in predefined presenting symptoms.

An increasing number of dashboard and **business intelligence** vendors are specific to EMS and health care. Some of the well-known vendors include FirstWatch, Zoll, iDashboards, and Corda. It should be noted that although business intelligence is mentioned here, the actual value of business intelligence software stems from forward-looking projections and not necessarily the display of data. Figure 11.6 shows how the Los Angeles Fire Department's Communications Center has worked with FirstWatch to develop a comprehensive big-screen dashboard.

COMMUNICATING THROUGH TRADITIONAL MEDIA

Traditional media typically includes television, cable television, radio, newspaper, magazines (and their associated websites), and direct mail. Although these venues of communication are widely utilized by most types of businesses, traditional media usage by ambulance services has typically been limited to public service announcements or name-branding campaigns in times of contract negotiations. Although nonemergency ambulance providers may find some value in targeting skilled nursing facilities or other customer stakeholders, it can be difficult to reach a target audience while keeping the campaign cost effective. One thing all the traditional media have in common is the need for content. The free publicity your service can receive when featured in the media can be far more valuable than any paid advertising. Developing a good relationship with the press and understanding how to do something as fundamental as a press release is critical.

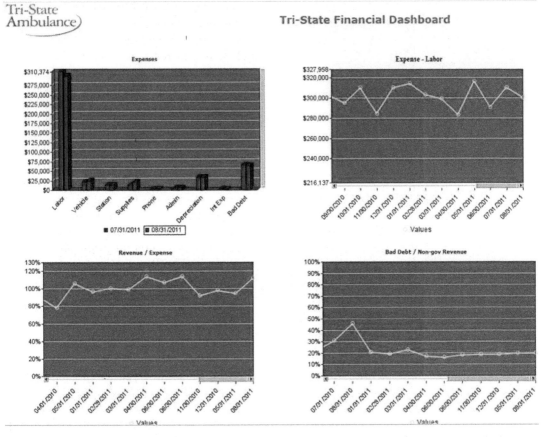

FIGURE 11.5 ■ Dashboards can be used to display numerous metrics and key performance indicators (KPIs). *Source: Reprinted by permission from First Watch Solutions, Inc.*

Side Bar

Seven Ways to Improve Media Relations

By Bob Davis

Media relations present challenges to Emergency Medical Services. Unfavorable news can hurt morale. Patient privacy must be protected. Reporters demand answers on very short deadlines, and sharing information quickly can lead to public relations missteps.

However, getting EMS messages out is good for everyone. EMS professionals deserve to be recognized publicly like other first responders and public safety agencies. EMS leaders can share potentially life-saving information with the public through the media, and transparency allows the public to better understand the resource needs of EMS.

From my perspective, the best way to navigate these challenges is to build trusting relationships with reporters—and bloggers—who express an interest in EMS.

Credibility comes first. During my 20 years as a newspaper reporter, my readers counted on me to judge the credibility of my sources. Honest brokers of information are the foundation of a meaningful story, especially health and public

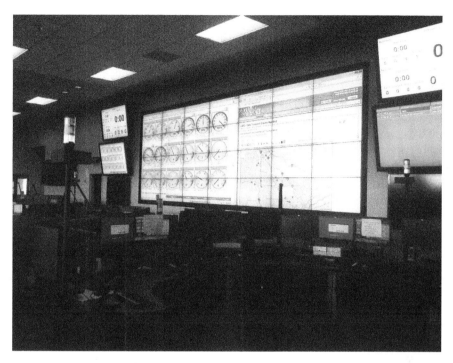

FIGURE 11.6 ■ The Los Angeles Fire Department's Communications Center uses integrated dashboard and GPS technology to provide situational and system status awareness. *Source: Tom Tornstrom, M.B.A., EMT-P.*

safety stories. When the story could save a life, provide education or promote awareness regarding emergency medical information, readers or viewers want to hear from only the most credible experts.

Trust is earned over time and a crisis is not the time to develop a relationship with members of the media. When I reported from the scene, I judged spokespersons almost instantaneously, as does the public. Those who earned my trust under fire were usually the people who demonstrated the courage to stand in front of the cameras and tell the unvarnished truth. They admitted when they did not have all the answers. They explained, with empathy, the details of mistakes. They were real. Human.

As a former paramedic, I could relate to the spokesperson who worked hard to find clarity in a complex and messy situation. I understood

what it was like to be over my head with lives on the line. I had felt the stress of having the lead without having all the answers.

Now that I work as a federal communications director, I see the media from the other side. I find myself asking the same questions I asked myself as a reporter. Can I trust this reporter? Are they going to work hard to get it right? Do they want to deliver accurate, credible information? When I trust the reporter, it's easy to share information with confidence.

EMS leaders would be wise to build trusting relationships with reporters before news is breaking—before that news deadline. Here are a few tips on how to build that trust:

1. Invite reporters to exercises and encourage them to play their role. Ask them to "ride along" so that they truly understand how

EMS operations work and let them get to know the medics behind the care rendered. Give them tours of your emergency operation center and briefings in your joint information center. Greater access leads to smarter reporting. Show what's behind the curtain.

2. Go visit the newsroom to see how tough the reporter's job is on deadline. Meeting editors and producers helps bring the whole newsgathering effort into perspective.

3. Discuss how they are getting their information and how you might serve their deadline needs better. Take the team approach to work together toward the same goal—a well-informed public.

4. Be transparent and accountable. If reporters know they can count on you to be candid they are more likely to believe you, even when you can't tell them everything on a tight deadline. Hold reporters accountable, too. An erroneous story is the reporter's responsibility first and foremost. Insist the newsroom be accountable.

5. Be open to the new breed of reporters. The media landscape continues to shift and some blogs and community websites are terrific information channels. Hold the new media "bloggers" to the same high standards of providing accurate, unbiased information if they are to be given the same access afforded to traditional reporters. Once they earn that trust, invite them in for briefings, exercises and ride-alongs and try to meet their specific needs. Their reports can be very helpful because they sometimes provide more details than traditional reporters.

6. Take crisis communication training. The best media spokespersons are those who get training and practice before facing the press. They may look like they are "winging it," just as a seasoned paramedic makes a resuscitation look effortless, but there are techniques that when learned and practiced bring out our best.

7. Identify and invest in a public information officer for your EMS system. This person is the "go to" person for EMS related news on a daily basis and during times of crisis. Their relationship with the local media will facilitate a productive working environment and benefit the citizens that are being served.

The bottom line: Both reporters and EMS providers work for the same people—the public. We both want to make sure people get the information that they need to protect themselves, their families, and their friends and neighbors. We all want them to know that they can trust what we are telling them—that they can trust us.

Source: Reprinted by permission from EMS Best Practices

Side Bar

Writing an Effective Press Release

By Jenifer Goodwin

When it comes to sharing news about your organization with the public, the most effective way to get your message out is through your local news media. But no matter how important your message is, it will not get covered unless you're able to clearly communicate to reporters, editors and producers—who may know nothing about EMS, or why it matters.

A concise, well-written press release provides the foot you need into the doors of the local media. The following are some tips and techniques for writing an interesting and newsworthy release, along with a few common pitfalls and how you can avoid them.

Pitching Your Story

The standard format for a press release includes a headline designed to grab the reader's attention, a subhead that provides further explanation, several paragraphs of text that explain the basics of the story—who, what, when, where and why—and contacts that reporters and other media representatives should call for more information or photo opportunities.

It's important to start strong, both in the headline and in your first sentence. Both will determine whether anyone will keep reading. Ask yourself the questions reporters will be asking themselves:

+ Why does this matter to my community?
+ What impact will it have?
+ How is this different from what's come before?

Here is an example of a bad headline:

Greenville Fire Department receives $50,000 State Grant

Subhead: Chief Ron Jones will hold a press conference on Tuesday to announce new program.

A better headline would be:

Greenville Fire Department Helps Seniors Stay in Their Homes

Subhead: New state grant enables firefighters to work with seniors to remove tripping hazards, replace light bulbs and install grab bars.

The intent of a press release is much different from an internal memo or company newsletter congratulating yourselves on a job well done. It's about grabbing the interest of a busy news outlet where the competition for ink and airtime is fierce.

When writing, avoid jargon as much as possible. If you must use it, don't take for granted that reporters will understand concepts or terms that you've used a thousand times. Spell out all acronyms. AED may roll off your tongue, but most reporters have never heard of it. When in doubt, define it.

What Is Newsworthy?

A press conference or announcement is not itself newsworthy, unless you're a major celebrity or sports star, or you are imparting news that everyone is sitting on the edges of their seats to hear. What matters to reporters is what you are announcing—make sure your press release makes clear why they should care. Factors that influence what gets covered include:

Timeliness It can help if you are able to connect your story to a current event, social issue or wider national story. For example, drowning in backyard pools dramatically goes up in many communities in April when the weather gets better. "April Pools Day" was actually created to frame this issue and March is the perfect time to pitch the local media about this timely story.

Novelty A new program, procedure or product that will have a substantial impact on patient care would fit well in this category. Make sure this topic or angle has not been covered before.

Controversy Pick up a newspaper and it's easy to see that conflict is news. Has your department found a new way to deal with a vexing issue? Explain the problem and describe how you're fixing it.

Human Interest Having a "real person" who was helped by EMS—such as a sudden cardiac arrest survivor—can pack an emotional wallop. For example, in the case of an elderly fall-prevention program, find one or two older people willing to talk to the media. Include a brief explanation of the people's stories in your release and let the media contact know they are available to speak further.

Sending Your Release

1. You can mail or fax a press release, but most are sent by email. Avoid sending multiple large photo files. If you're going to send a

photo, make it interesting. A clear, well-lit photo of a paramedic helping an older person tape down a floor mat is good. A shot of your fire chief or medical director standing at a podium is boring and would likely not be published.

2. Don't make the mistake of thinking that just because you sent a news release, it's been carefully considered or even read. TV stations and larger newspapers get hundreds of them every day. Cover your bases by sending your release to news editors, beat reporters who cover public safety and any reporters you have spoken to previously.

3. It's critical to follow up with a phone call and/or e-mail to ensure your contact has seen and read the press release. Re-send if necessary. A few days before your event, follow up with a media advisory (a brief, bullet-pointed version of your press release) and another phone call.

4. Don't send the release at the last minute. Media outlets have been besieged by cut-backs and layoffs in recent years and there are fewer people to do the work. That means ensuring reporters have at least a week's notice before your event.

Source: Reprinted by permission from EMS Best Practices

Television

Although often thought of as an expensive form of communication, positive television coverage for ambulance services can be accomplished at no cost. Through a proactive relationship with local station news departments, ambulance service managers often find that television stations are grateful for the opportunity to create stories focused around topics that the manager provides or suggests.

Common ambulance-centered news stories often revolve around abnormal situations such as extreme hot or cold weather, snow and ice storms, or large-crowd events where EMS plays a key role. Informational press releases about these types of situations or events can be key to establishing and maintaining a relationship with broadcast television stations.

Although cable television has less market reach than broadcast television, it is still present in 57.1 percent of U.S. households (National Cable and Telecommunications Association, 2008). Cable providers occasionally offer governmental and nonprofit organizations airtime for public service announcements that may be relative to their viewership. Cable television may be a great way to promote such public service topics as seat-belt use and bicycle safety. In addition, cable may be an affordable way to target stakeholders based on the type of programming that interests them.

Radio

Although broadcast radio is not typically associated with ambulance service marketing, there may be opportunities, especially with talk radio, to discuss important political or economic issues related to the provision of service. Keep in mind that ambulance service and emergency medical service in general are often mysterious topics to radio hosts. Because of this, the hosts may very well welcome an on-air discussion, which would have the potential to reach numerous stakeholders.

Newspaper

Although both the number of newspapers and circulation have been declining over the past 20 years, the typical circulation numbers are still very impressive. In 2009, there were 46 million Sunday subscribers to 911 different newspapers, resulting in average readership on Sundays of more than 50,000 (Newspaper Association of America, 2009). Since 64 percent of newspaper subscribers are over the age of forty-five, using newspaper as a communication tool to reach community stakeholders may be very effective.

Much like their television counterparts, newspaper reporters are often eager for news stories, and ambulance services by their very nature can provide interesting and dramatic stories while simultaneously spreading an important message. For example, what may seem like a straightforward treatment of a myocardial infarction patient for an ambulance provider could offer a newspaper writer a wealth of material for a human interest or health care–related article. These types of stories are a great venue through which to reach all stakeholders and build a positive image for the ambulance service.

Magazines

Magazines, much like newspapers, have experienced declining print circulation in recent years, but they tend to offer prominent and active websites to make up much of the readership loss. Although marketing and communication of an ambulance service through a national magazine may seem limited, positive national exposure can result in a positive impression on local stakeholders. In addition, magazines and professional journals are typically the most appropriate venue in which to publish research or industry innovations accomplished by an ambulance service.

CHAPTER REVIEW

Summary

Ambulance service managers should not underestimate the importance of understanding and utilizing the multiple forms of marketing. Proper identification of stakeholder groups along with creative marketing through the use of electronic or traditional media can have a profound impact on ambulance services credibility, level of transparency, and ultimately the bottom line.

WHAT WOULD YOU DO? Reflection

Now that you have a general idea of ways in which to market and promote your ambulance service, you should be better prepared to enter the competitive bidding process. Your core stakeholders, including your employees and board of directors, have been receiving regular e-mail to keep them updated on important happenings surrounding the process. In addition, data dashboards and your intranet website allow core stakeholders access to various performance measures and announcements that will help work toward a successful bid.

Your patients, potential patients, and customers receive marketing materials in print, as well as traditional media such as television and radio, that direct them to your public website. Your good works in the community, and your messages to the public about safety and injury prevention, are conveyed via positive press coverage. Once on your website, stakeholders find information about your organization that is easy to read and understand. Your website highlights your excellent operational and clinical performance and the reasons why your ambulance rates are justifiable.

You have been given permission by your individual controller stakeholders to e-mail them directly. You like this idea but aren't confident that they will take the time to read an e-mail. Because of this uncertainty, you choose to e-mail them a traceable link to a special area on your website that clearly explains your organization's position and reasons for the rates structures. You also complement the e-mail with a print mailing of the same information.

You realize that one of the most important pieces of support you will need will be your partner agencies. You choose to communicate with each of them via an e-mail newsletter and feature stories that they can relate to and appreciate; you even include a monthly feature in each newsletter about one of your partner agencies.

Although you're still very concerned about the upcoming bidding process, you rest easier knowing that your stakeholders will have a much clearer understanding of your organization.

Review Questions

1. Define *stakeholder*, and briefly discuss the four groups of stakeholders.
2. Explain why it's important to have a Web presence.
3. Define *intranet* and think of ways in which such a communication tool could serve your organization.
4. Discuss *open rate* and why knowing this percentage or number is so important.
5. Identify two to three popular social networking websites and briefly discuss how each could be used by ambulance services.
6. Discuss the use of data dashboards and think of ways in which your organization could use a dashboard.
7. Discuss the pros and cons of hosting virtual meetings in place of traditional face-to-face meetings.
8. Identify the four most common types of traditional media.

References

Cho, C. (2003). "Factors Influencing Clicking of Banner Ads on the WWW." *CyberPsychology & Behavior* 6(2), 201–215. doi:10.1089/109493103321640400.

Facebook. (2011). "Statistics." Facebook Newsroom. See the organization website.

Fu, L., and G. Salvendy. (2002, May). "The Contribution of Apparent and Inherent Usability to a User's Satisfaction in a Searching and Browsing Task on the Web." *Ergonomics* 45(6), 415–424. doi:10.1080/00140130110120033.

National Cable and Telecommunications Association. (2008). "Industry Data Statistics." See the organization website.

Newspaper Association of America. (2009). "Trends and Numbers." See the organization website.

Marsh, J. (1998). *A Stake in Tomorrow: World Class Lessons in Business Partnerships.* London: B.T. Batsford Limited.

Ming-Ten, T., C. Shuang-Shii, and H. Wei-Ping. (2009). "An Integrated Process Model of

Communication Satisfaction and Organizational Outcomes." *Social Behavior & Personality: An International Journal 37*(6), 825–834.

Key Terms

business intelligence The computerized collecting and analyzing of data in such a way that business decisions can be made. Business intelligence is most valuable when it can identify and trend otherwise seemingly useless data.

data dashboard Collection of data compiled into one or more visual representations that can be interpreted rapidly.

Internet A computer network consisting of a World Wide Web of connected computers sharing information.

intranet A computer network that is typically limited to sharing among employees in an individual organization.

social media Media designed to be shared through social interaction, typically via the Internet.

stakeholder A person or group of people who have an interest or concern in an ambulance service due to direct or indirect involvement.

traditional media Communication venues such as television, cable television, radio, newspaper, and magazines.

virtual meetings Any form of video face-to-face communication that allows individuals or groups communication greater than audio alone.

Web presence The impact or visibility that a particular organization may have on the Internet.

CHAPTER 12

Ambulance Service Dispatch and Radio Communications

BARRY FUREY

Objectives

After reading this chapter, the student will be able to:

12.1 Define key concepts and terms related to radio and telephone communications systems.

12.2 Identify key equipment utilized in ambulance communications centers.

12.3 Identify key components of a Public Safety Answering Point (PSAP).

12.4 Explain key differences between methodologies of call handling and dispatch.

12.5 Identify current issues regarding dispatch and radio communications, including staffing and technology.

Overview

Ambulance services in the United States range in size from one ambulance operated by volunteers and managed by a community board of directors to large governmental agencies and even larger, private, for-profit corporations. This text presents information that the manager of an ambulance service, large or small, needs in order to keep the business solvent and provide clinically excellent service to the community.

Key Terms

American Society for
  Testing and
  Materials (ASTM)
Association of
  Public-safety
  Communications
  Officials (APCO)
  International
automatic call
  distribution (ACD)

duplex
emergency
  medical dispatch
  (EMD)
Enhanced 9-1-1
  (E 9-1-1)
Federal
  Communications
  Commission (FCC)
interoperability

National Emergency
  Number Association
  (NENA)
National Fire
  Protection
  Association
  (NFPA)
Next Generation 9-1-1
  (Next Gen & NG
  9-1-1)

public switched
  telephone network
  (PSTN)
simplex
trunked
Voice over Internet
  Protocol (VoIP)

WHAT WOULD YOU DO?

You have been tasked with assessing and making recommendations for improvement of your agency's call receipt, dispatching, and communications needs. In order to do this, you must effectively analyze at minimum the existing state of your personnel, facility, technology, policies, and procedures. You must measure your current effectiveness as well as define goals and set a timetable for when improvements may be implemented (Figure 12.1). One important limitation to your assignment that cannot be overlooked is that no downtime is allowed. All services must continue to function throughout, and in the end they must meet both the needs and expectations of your agency and your customers as well as those of other emergency service, governmental, or private organizations with whom you must communicate on a daily basis and/or during disasters. These measures must also meet all applicable standards that are in place at the time. Further, all of these recommendations must take into account the increased level of financial scrutiny placed on governmental or quasi-governmental agencies during times of economic downturns.

1. Where do you start? Must you adhere to legal, operational, or financial constraints? How do you identify these?
2. Has your organization attempted a similar task in the past? How successful was it?
3. What roadblocks decreased its acceptance or efficiency?
4. Who, if anyone, within your agency can give testimony or advice?
5. Has any nearby local or regional service faced the same challenge recently? What lessons can be learned from that?
6. What types of technology are available to you? What are the relative merits of each?
7. What is the minimal level of service that must be provided, and how will this be measured? These, and many more questions, must be answered as you move ahead.

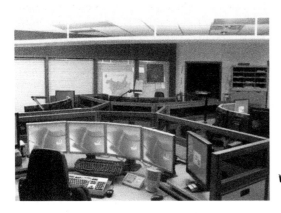

FIGURE 12.1 ■ Modern communications facilities employ a variety of people and technologies. Careful planning for the future is required. *Source: Raleigh-Wake Emergency Communications.*

■ INTRODUCTION

On any given incident, ambulance personnel may arrive to discover that the patient's symptoms do not match what the dispatcher communicated. The number of patients for transport may be different from what was initially reported by the caller. There may not even be a patient. Paramedics may or may not be called on to use an array of skills and equipment to manage a particular emergency. Almost every incident is different. However, one common thread ties them all together: communications.

On a majority of all assignments that will be faced by paramedics in their daily duties, the initial information will be received by telephone and then forwarded to them by radio and some form of data communications. Now, certainly, there are exceptions. Paramedics may actually witness a traffic accident happen, or a citizen may approach the ambulance and directly inform paramedics of the need for emergency medical services. But these are rare occurrences, indeed, when compared to

the more common practice of "responding to a call." But here too, vehicle and handheld devices typically rely on a radio-based network connection back to the communications center.

Although the basic dispatch process may have much in common from agency to agency, that is not to say that it is standardized. Nothing could be further from the truth. The number, qualifications, and skills of those involved can vary greatly among agencies, and facilities can range from shared use of a commercial answering service to a dedicated multimillion-dollar public safety answering point (PSAP). Just as communications procedures and facilities may vary, so too will there be a divergence in technology. Some organizations will have the minimal amount of equipment required to do the job. In many cases, this is nothing more than a telephone, a radio, a map book, and a collection of paper forms. Others operate only state-of-the-art devices that seemingly automate the entire call-taking and dispatch process. Regardless of the level of an ambulance service's current operation, changes in the consumer electronics, radio communications, and computer industries will have a significant effect on the tools that will be required tomorrow.

ASTM International, known until 2001 as the **American Society for Testing and Materials (ASTM)**, is an international standards organization that develops and publishes voluntary consensus technical standards for a wide range of materials, products, systems, and services. ASTM International recognizes EMS communications centers as having four functions:

* The receipt and processing of calls for assistance
* The dispatch and coordination of appropriate available resources
* The provision of information and prearrival instructions
* Coordination with other agencies and emergency services (ASTM, 2006)

This chapter will deal with what it takes to make these functions happen.

■ TELEPHONE OVERVIEW

The telephone remains the primary means of requesting ambulance services. Whether this call is made to a ten-digit number by a health care facility arranging for a transport, or from a citizen reporting an emergency to 9-1-1, this information will be carried, in part, over what is known as the **public switched telephone network (PSTN)**. Built on the interconnection of telephone company central offices and land lines into homes and businesses, it has evolved over time to accept input from wireless telephones, as well as **Voice Over Internet Protocol (VOIP)** devices. We will discuss the impact of these additions later in this chapter. For now, and as a point of clarification, remember that 9-1-1 traffic is carried on special circuits, independent of normal telephone lines. However, the same facilities that support the PSTN also support 9-1-1.

HISTORICAL CONTEXT

The 9-1-1 emergency number was first put to use in 1968 in the small town of Haleyville, Alabama (Alabama Chapter of NENA, 2011). It carried with it several advantages over the conventional ten-digit numbers typically in use at that time. Among these were that:

- it was easily remembered.
- it was a free call from pay phones.
- it was universal.

Keep in mind that Great Britain had a three-digit emergency number in service since the 1930s (9-9-9), and that initial press releases targeted 9-1-1 as a "police emergency number" (Dispatch Magazine On-line, 2011) Through time, it has morphed into what the **National Emergency Number Association (NENA)**, a group of public safety professionals dedicated to improving public safety access, terms "One Nation–One Number" (National Emergency Number Association, 2012–2013a). Through this transition, however, proposals have been made at times to dedicate other "N-1-1" numbers to fire and ambulance/EMS usage; however, all three-digit N-1-1 numbers have been officially assigned, and educating the public as to which number to call would have been problematic. For example, in the case of a personal injury auto accident that involved fire or extrication, which number would be appropriate to call? Should you call the police because they are in charge of accidents? Or perhaps EMS since someone is injured? Maybe you should call the fire department because the car is smoking? Obviously, all three services are needed, but three separate numbers would only add to the dilemma. A single emergency number for all classes of calls helps sort out the confusion.

It is also important to note what 9-1-1 is *not*. Although purists rightfully argue that the three digits refer only to the emergency telephone number, over time 9-1-1 has come to stand for rapid or emergency services. The three digits have even worked their way into text messaging as shorthand for "urgent." In the ambulance community, the term *9-1-1 service* is sometimes used to indicate advanced life support rather than basic life support response, or to differentiate an emergency call rather than a transport. For the purpose of this text, the discussion of 9-1-1 is limited to the emergency telephone number and notification processes.

The growth of 9-1-1 in North America can be traced on a decade-to-decade basis. Don't forget that North America is specified, since 9-1-1 is not universal; a host of other emergency numbers are supported around the globe.

- *1970s. Basic* 9-1-1 expands and planning moves ahead for **Enhanced 9-1-1 (E 9-1-1)**. To the basic features, E 9-1-1 adds Automatic Number

Identification (ANI), which provides the call taker with instant information on the caller's number, and Automatic Location Identification (ALI), which provides the caller's address.

Since telephones at the time were all land lines" and hard wired to a fixed location, installer records from the telephone company could be used to accurately pinpoint the source of any call. In large buildings or mixed occupancies, this included the floor and office number as well as the company name. This ability was diminished over time through the popularity of wireless and VoIP devices that have no fixed location assigned.

* *1980s*. Enhanced 9-1-1 is expanded and computer-aided dispatch (CAD) is expanded/introduced.
* *1990s*. Wireless/cellular calls are introduced.
  * *1996*. **Federal Communications Commission (FCC)** passes "Report and Order 94-102," which establishes guidelines for wireless 9-1-1 service.
  * *1998*. First "Phase 1" wireless 9-1-1 system becomes operational. Phase 1 systems pass only the location of the nearest cell tower, not the location of the cellular caller. Phase 1 systems also provide the telephone number of the receiving cell tower, but not the calling telephone number. This tower telephone number is often referred to as "Pseudo Automatic Number Information" (P-ANI).
  * *1999*. First "Phase II" enhanced wireless 9-1-1 system are activated. Phase II systems provide caller phone number and approximate location information. Typically, information provided by wireless telephones is not sufficient in and of itself to dispatch an ambulance. Additional questioning is required by the call taker to extract a street address. Data are received in a latitude/longitude format and do not contain, for example, information regarding altitude. So, in an urban setting with many closely packed high-rise structures, latitude/longitude data would probably be insufficient to locate the patient.

In 1999, 9-1-1 finally became recognized as the official emergency number of the United States, albeit three decades after its initial use.

With the start of the twenty-first century came the advent of VoIP devices that revolutionized the way that telephone calls were made. Some milestones with regard to public safety include the following:

* *2004*. VoIP providers begin service.
* *2007*. 9-1-1 Modernization & Public Safety Act is passed.
* *2008*. Net 9-1-1 Act is passed.
* *2010*. Federal Communications Commission opens public comment on **Next Generation 9-1-1 (NG 9-1-1)**.

The effect of all legislative efforts was to provide a level playing field for all providers of 9-1-1 services, and to establish a roadmap for transition to NG 9-1-1 solutions (National Emergency Number Association, 2012).

NEXT GENERATION 9-1-1

No discussion of ambulance communications would be complete without the inclusion of NG 9-1-1. According to the National Emergency Number Association, NG9-1-1 is the "next evolutionary step in the development of the 9-1-1 emergency communications system known as E9-1-1 that has been in place since the 1970s. NG9-1-1 is a system comprised of managed IP-based networks and elements that augment present-day E9-1-1 features and functions and add new capabilities. NG9-1-1 will eventually replace the present E9-1-1 system. NG9-1-1 is designed to provide access to emergency services from all sources, and to provide multimedia data capabilities for PSAPs and other emergency service organizations" (National Emergency Number Association, 2012–2013b).

Perhaps a more concise description is also provided by NENA, through its statement "EMERGENCY HELP; Anytime, anywhere, any device" (National Emergency Number Association, 2012–2013c). Whatever your definition, NG 9-1-1 is an attempt to bring emergency reporting technology into sync with consumer electronics. Much of the 9-1-1 technology currently in use today is based on designs drafted more than 40 years ago when the first 9-1-1 systems rolled out. It is analog in a decidedly digital world. To complete this upgrade, both the network and customer premise equipment (CPE, or phones at the answering point) will need to be modernized or replaced.

To this end, NG 9-1-1 has been called a "network of networks" (National Emergency Number Association, 2012) in that the architecture will resemble that of a computer system more so than a telephone. A series of digital loops from a variety of sources—including the public Internet—will interface and intermingle to provide seamless service to a host of consumer electronic devices and services. Among the capacities envisioned for NG 9-1-1 are these:

* The ability to text 9-1-1
* The ability to send movies and or still photos as part of a 9-1-1 "call"
* Universal transfer of data between answering points
* The acceptance of data directly from alarm companies or automatic devices such as Automatic Crash Notification (ACN) sensors mounted in automobiles and personal medical devices. Much of this telematic data will no longer have to be processed by a third party but, rather, will be directly routed to the responding agency. As of this writing, at least one automobile manufacturer already provides an interface between their vehicles and the driver's cellular telephone, enabling it to automatically dial 9-1-1 in the event of an emergency.

To many, NG 9-1-1 does not end with the call intake, and they may be right. The technology and data exchange involved mandate that a seamless interface be created between the public and public safety. This requires that information received at the dispatch center be shared in real time with units in the field. Hardware and software will need to be developed that allow for instantaneous relay of these photos, movies, and sensor data to the ambulances assigned (National Emergency Number Association, 2004, p. 8). Imagine being able to view real-time video of an emergency scene while still en route. What benefits would this provide? How would this impact size-up and preparation? What if the video were of an accident with injuries and carried with it a data stream of preincident vehicle activity and the ability to communicate directly with the victims? To some degree, video observation of patients is already being used as a tool in rural areas where doctors utilize this technology to assist with remote diagnosis (National Emergency Number Association, 2012–2013d).

But the interaction doesn't stop here. Public alerting of disasters and emergencies is an ever-changing concern. Where outside audible devices such as tornado sirens were once the norm, our connected lifestyles call for more modern measures. With the decline of conventional telephones, even the once tried-and-true reverse notification systems are becoming less effective due to their reliance on land-line databases. E-mails, texts, and Tweets are now finding their way into this arena, and work is well underway on establishing systems that will sense which cell phones are active in a given geographic area and automatically send them an emergency message regardless of carrier (National Association of State EMS Officials, 2009). Although notification responsibilities may not fall under the auspices of EMS, it is worthwhile to discuss this progression, because it is symbolic of the changes that all managers must face in the future.

Best Practice

The Horizon Award

In 2009 the Association of Public Safety Communications Officials (APCO) International began issuing the Horizon Award for public safety agencies that have proactively assessed and met the technological and operational needs of their center, employees, and service population (Association of Public Safety Communications Officials, 2009). The initial award for large organizations went to Fairfax County, Virginia, for the creation of the McConnell Public Safety and Transportation Operations Center. This facility combines communications and command-and-control operations from state and local public safety agencies with those of the Virginia Department of Transportation to create a unique model. Although interoperability is often thought of solely from the radio perspective of the first responder, information exchange at the call receipt and dispatch level coupled with traffic information allows for both economy of scale and immediate sharing of intelligence. In 2010, this honor was presented to the Raleigh-Wake North Carolina Emergency Communications Center for the use of commercially available software and social media to post event information real time on the World Wide Web (Figure 12.2). The leveraging of these free assets reduced nonemergency calls received by the center by more than 1,000 per week (Association of Public Safety Communications Officials, 2010a). These are prime examples of how alternate solutions can be used to successfully address ongoing problems in communications.

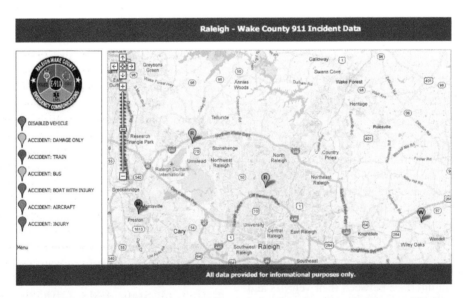

FIGURE 12.2 ■ Raleigh-Wake (NC) Emergency Communications uses Google Maps and Twitter to support the automatic release of traffic accidents locations to the media and public. *Source: Reprinted by permission from Raleigh-Wake Emergency Communications.*

PSAP TELEPHONE EQUIPMENT

Whether you are a provider with a single ambulance or a major fleet, some basic principles apply. Your telephone equipment must be:

- *Reliable.* There should be little or no down time.
- *Durable.* It must withstand heavy and constant operation without failure.
- *Fixable.* If it breaks, it must be able to be repaired quickly.

Standards for public safety telephone systems are provided by the National Emergency Number Association (2012–2013e), the **National Fire Protection Association (NFPA)** (2010), and other sources. Compliance with many of these standards is often voluntary, but these documents do highlight the critical need for redundancy, robustness, and backup for telephone systems that are used in life critical environments. Individual states may also impose standards on emergency telecommunications devices. Such standards may, or may not, apply to both public and private sector operations. Therefore, as is the case with any regulation discussed herein, it is incumbent on agencies to check with the appropriate regulatory bodies in their jurisdictions when seeking official guidance on such matters.

Regardless of your source for telephone standards, some common sense applies. Consideration must be given to a variety of features and functions that address the unique requirements of the public safety environment. Among these are the following:

- *Having sufficient telephone lines to prevent callers from receiving busy signals.* Supporting data may be provided by the incumbent telephone company, or independently through the use of industry-accepted formulae (National Fire Protection Association, 2010).
- *Having sufficient equipment and personnel to answer calls in a timely manner.*

- *Having high-reliability equipment that has no single point of failure and/or automatically compensates for failures, thereby ensuring a high degree of uptime.*
- *Having equipment powered by an alternate source of electricity such as batteries or generator.* Conventional telephones historically were energized by current on the telephone lines themselves. However, many modern systems—especially those that use computer telephony integration (CTI) have the same power requirements as other microprocessor-based devices.
- *Having both master and individual instant playback recording devices.* This provides for a historical archiving of all radio and telephone calls, while also allowing the telecommunicator the highly desirable ability to replay portions of audio that may be garbled or hard to understand. The term *recording devices* is used here in lieu of the past references to *tape recorders* since a significant number of agencies no longer rely on magnetic tape for this purpose. As is the case with consumer electronics, audio is frequently stored in a digital format such as a WAV file, MP3, or the like. Although tape recorders do still exist, it is more common to find audio being stored on disc, and the once daily chore of "changing the logging tape" has gone by the wayside.

Instant playback recorders are now often built into workstation hardware and run as an application on the terminal device rather than as a stand-alone unit. Some may be adjustable in terms of the duration of the audio recorded, and often they are coupled to both the telephone and the selected radio channel at an operating position. For public agencies, state law may address the retention period of master logging records. For nonpublic entities, retention may be dictated by good business practices or by standards set by licensing boards or other agencies.

- *Having the ability to accept a Telecommunications Device for the Deaf (TDD) call* (U.S.

Department of Justice, 1998). Since the telephone, in one form or another, remains the primary means of accessing emergency services, the federal government, through the U.S. Department of Justice, requires that all citizens have equal access. Although we often think of barrier-free design as providing ramps instead of stairs, the telephone itself does present a barrier to those with speech and/or hearing limitations. TDDs allow individuals to type, rather than talk, their emergency messages. Like playback recorders, TDDs are now often part of workstations rather than unique devices.

- *Having caller ID, ANI/ALI displays, CAD, geographically accurate digital mapping, and sufficient other tools and aids to allow for proper identification and recording of the location of all requests for service.* CAD systems are also critical in making the appropriate recommendations for dispatch, whether emergency or nonemergency incidents are involved. CAD systems can also be configured to recognize specialized addresses where unique responses are required.
- *Having a records management system (RMS) and/or a management information system (MIS) to maintain all required documentation and to provide data correlation on which to make critical decisions.* Some vendors may use these terms interchangeably, but oftentimes MIS refers to a limited software suite used for report writing on a particular application, whereas RMS may be a more robust application that contains not only records concerning responses but also a wide range of data that can include vehicle maintenance, personnel, asset inventory, and patient histories. Release of information from an RMS may be governed by a variety of regulations; however, these will not be discussed here.
- *Having the appropriate type of telephone system for your needs.* For example, many larger facilities may utilize an **automatic call distribution (ACD)** system to improve call answering

times. Such systems deliver incoming calls to available agents based on predetermined priorities. This methodology is of particular benefit for larger agencies because a pool of call takers is available, but provides little benefit in smaller agencies.

EOC emergency operations center.

■ PSAP CONFIGURATION———————

Regardless of whether or not the call is of an emergent nature, there must be some way of receiving and processing the information. In some cases, such as medical alert pendants and alarms, the request will be received electronically on a monitoring device, and the corresponding data will be used to place a verification call, make a dispatch, or take some other action specified by procedure. In some cases, an automatic telephone dialing device may also be used to report an emergency, but in most cases requests from service still come as a result of a human-to-human telephone call.

How and where these calls are received and processed is a matter of local choice. As previously referenced, a relatively small, low-volume ambulance provider—especially a rural BLS or transport service—may utilize a commercial answering service to field and forward its calls. Here, too, local regulation may differentiate between ALS and BLS requirements, and especially between private and public sector concerns. Although 9-1-1 may be the national emergency number, states exercise control over many factors of deployment and operation, and facilities that receive 9-1-1 calls may be subject to these rules (Association of Public Safety Communications Officials, 2010b).

TYPES OF PSAPS

By definition, a *primary* PSAP is one that receives 9-1-1 calls directly, whereas a *secondary*

PSAP receives transfers of 9-1-1 calls from a primary PSAP. Ambulance dispatching may be carried out from either type of facility. In a *consolidated* center, one or more jurisdictions or services share the operation.

According to APCO International's Communications Center Consolidated Checklist, there are numerous subsets of consolidation, including the following:

1. *Co-location only.* Multiple agencies share a common facility but maintain separate call taking/dispatch capability.
2. *Single discipline call taking.* Multiple agencies of common discipline (e.g., police only) share a common facility and consolidate call-taking operations.
3. *Single discipline dispatch.* Multiple agencies of common discipline (e.g., police only) share a common facility and consolidate dispatch operations.
4. *Consolidated call taking.* Multiple agencies share a common facility and consolidate call-taking operations for more than one discipline.
5. *Full consolidation.* Multiple agencies share a common facility and consolidate call-taking and dispatch operations across multiple disciplines.
6. *Virtual consolidation.* Variation of scenarios 2 through 5, wherein PSAP maintains separate physical locations but shares common call-taking and/or dispatch capabilities over a secure managed network.
7. *Dual mode consolidation.* Variation of scenarios 1 through 5, whereby both public safety and nonpublic safety agencies share a common facility and potentially a degree of shared technology (e.g., 9-1-1 and 3-1-1 sharing common facility and common CAD system). (Association of Public Safety Communications Officials, 2010b)

PSAP MANAGEMENT STRUCTURE

Consolidated PSAPs can function under a variety of management configurations. One user agency may serve as the main provider, with services essentially sold to other participants, or a joint powers board may be formed to manage by committee. In these latter cases, the PSAP and the employees are typically part of an independent agency designed specifically for the purpose of providing communications services. Charging fees based on calls for service is a common funding mechanism, but there are others, including the creation of a special taxing district. In examples across the United States, both private and public EMS providers have become active members of consolidated centers. Formalized service contracts often exist regardless of the organizational structure. Dispatch center responsibility is often measured by the time it takes to answer and process calls, although ambulance services may be held to response-time criteria for emergencies.

It is also not uncommon for an ambulance/EMS provider to operate as a secondary PSAP. An example of such an arrangement would be where the local law enforcement agency answers the 9-1-1 call but transfers or relays the ambulance request to another facility. This can be either a private or public sector entity.

In the *transfer* method, the physical call will be switched electronically from the original answering point to the provider. In the case of E 9-1-1 calls, this will include address and number data, if available. (However, due to limitations on legacy 9-1-1 systems, even when such data are available, they may not be transferred if the two PSAPs are served by different telephone companies.) In the *relay* method, all of the pertinent information will be gathered by the original answering point and then passed along to the secondary facility by telephone, radio, CAD, or other means (Association of Public Safety Communications Officials, 2010c). One of the potential drawbacks of secondary PSAPs is the time (and possibly information) lost during the transfer of responsibility from one facility to another. Although connectivity to a common

CAD system can lessen this exposure, it does not eliminate it. Proponents of secondary PSAPs often raise the issue of autonomy; this may be of special concern where a mix of private and public sectors exist. Depending on the community, there can be both political and financial considerations that can oftentimes overshadow the operational needs when PSAP configurations are established.

PSAP DESIGN

Obviously, a facility that is as critical as a 9-1-1 center must be designed with some forethought. The same is true for any location from which ambulances are dispatched or assigned. After all, for emergency calls to be received and processed, equipment must remain operational 24 × 7, and the telecommunicators must be able to work in a safe environment regardless of external influences. To this end, the reliability and levels of redundancy or backup on critical systems such as telephone, CAD, and radio must be significant. What suffices in a normal office environment does not come close to meeting public safety standards. Accordingly, in order to ensure continuous operation of all communications systems, the building itself must also be hardy.

Site Selection

When selecting a location for a dispatch center, hazards are a primary concern. Parcels that are close to railroads, interstates, or plants that store or manufacture hazardous materials are not preferred. Also problematic are sites that are prone to flooding or are difficult to reach in inclement weather. After all, water and electronics don't mix, and you must be able to ensure proper staffing even in the middle of a blizzard.

Security

Security against hazards of other sorts must also be provided. Bullet-resistant glass and locking vestibules are common features to keep out the unwanted, as are security cameras and card, fob, or biometric access readers. Fire protection is also another form of security, with sprinklers as well as specialized inert gas systems for use in electronics areas coming into play. Access to the property may also be restricted through the use of gates and fences, especially around key components such as radio towers and generator sets. The building may also be set back from the road and additionally protected by earthworks or bollards to lessen the potential of a vehicle assault. Utility and telephone lines should also be placed underground to prevent sabotage.

In today's world, security must also address unauthorized electronic access, with firewalls and antivirus protection being utilized. The sensitive nature of information—especially that stored on EMS and ambulance service computer systems—makes this precaution doubly important. In addition, as the industry transverses increasingly toward Internet-based and digital solutions, the more we are at risk from both intentional and unintentional infection.

Functionality

Of course, in order for all of the equipment to remain operational, electric power will be required. In addition to commercial electric service, critical facilities require an alternate source such as a generator. Although some agencies use natural gas engines, one school of thought suggests that since natural gas supply also can be interrupted, only fuels such as diesel or propane, which can be stored on site, truly provide a backup. Uninterruptable power supplies (UPS) both condition power and create another level of fallback should the generator fail. UPS capacity should be such so as to allow for sufficient time to transfer calls to another facility prior to the batteries going dead. In addition to the proven standbys, new technologies such as hydrogen fuel cells may also work their way into future use.

The size of the community as well as the call volume and number of user agencies will help to determine the size of the center. Again, similar factors will impact facilities that are built for private sector providers. There must be sufficient space for operational concerns, management functions, general building functions such as heating and cooling, and specialized communications and computer gear. Since the design needs to accommodate for $24 \times 7 \times 365$ occupancy in all types of weather, sufficient break and support areas should also be built in. Many facilities now include a quiet room in addition to the conventional break room, in order to provide telecommunicators with a place to unwind after a particularly stressful call. Many communities also choose to co-locate an emergency operations center (EOC) in the same building. This room (or suite of rooms) houses the command and control functions during major emergencies and can become an alternate seat of government. The addition of an EOC likely increases the need for more kitchen space, possibly more bunk space for protracted operations, and a larger parking lot to accommodate personnel assigned.

Regardless of the number and type of rooms contained within it, the structure should be laid out to accommodate both security and workflow. The dispatch center itself should consider the placement of related functions side by side, or at least in close proximity. There should be sufficient consoles to account for both daily workloads and full-scale emergencies. Accommodations should also be made for training positions as well as spares that can be used immediately should a primary console unexpectedly fail. Room for future growth must also be planned.

Overall construction type should address the hazards most frequently encountered locally, especially those that are weather related. Depending on location, the primary focus may be placed on hurricanes, tornadoes, floods, snowstorms, or earthquakes. Each one of these has a unique impact on building design.

Finally, enough emphasis cannot be placed on the human factor. Facilities of the past—especially those designed during the Cold War—were often underground bunkers. Although those had the potential to survive the perceived threat, they were often depressing, windowless environments that did little for employee alertness or morale. With the advent of "green" buildings and improvements in security products, focus has switched to making PSAPs more livable (Loomis, 2007; National Fire Protection Association, 2010).

■ CALL HANDLING

The receipt of initial information by the call taker consists of at least the basic information of an accurate location and problem. Additional data, such as the caller's name and number, are also typically requested. Obviously, this does not comprise much in the way of important facts. Therefore, many ambulance providers utilize **emergency medical dispatch (EMD)** protocols. These are a prescripted series of questions and instructions that follow a decision tree and may be read from a hard-copy flip card set or generated through a software program that interfaces with CAD.

EMD can normally be associated with the following benefits:

* Standardized call processing
* Medically approved and supervised questions
* Support of prearrival instruction
* Prioritization of calls to help manage resources
* Reduction in liability through use of proven guidelines

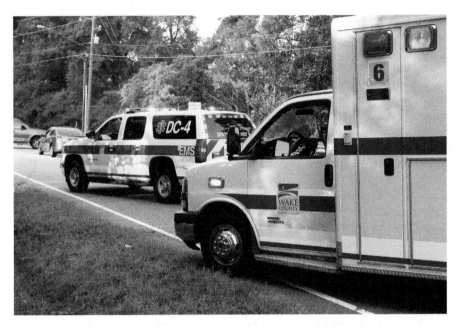

FIGURE 12.3 ■ EMD protocols assist in determining the priority of the response as well as the number and type of units assigned. *Source: Official Wake County EMS Photo by Mike Legeros, used by permission.*

♦ Associated quality assurance program to improve service (Legislative Program Review and Investigations Committee, 1999)

Regardless of whether or not a recognized EMD program is utilized, formal procedures for call handling and general operations should be in place (Figure 12.3).

In addition to protocols, how a telephone call is answered also has a bearing on processing. Smaller agencies may use the *single-stage* answering model, whereby the person who receives the call is also responsible for its dispatch. Larger volumes may dictate the use of *two-stage* or *dual-stage* processing, whereby dedicated call takers handle all telephone responsibilities and dispatchers control radio traffic. Some sort of record system—be it manual or CAD—is used to transfer the information from one person to another. In larger facilities with a number of call takers, devices known as Automatic Call Distributors (ACDs) may also be used. These have been previously mentioned in this chapter.

Ambulance services that also provide medical transport will likely have yet another set of protocols or standard operating procedures used to obtain the patient's billing or insurance information. In comparison to emergency call handling, both types of transport will need to know the current address requiring response; however, the medical transport agency will also need to know the address to which the patient is being transported. In the emergency world, these data are not typically gathered up front, as the extent of injuries and the location of the incident will have a part in making this decision. However, transport resources can be more efficiently scheduled by comparing the list of appointment times and locations against available resources.

◼ RADIO COMMUNICATIONS——

Once a request for service has been received, it obviously must be relayed to the appropriate unit or units in the field. Typically, this is done by radio, or by some technology driven by radio. Some services may even chose to use wireless telephones to transfer this information; however, it should be remembered that in actuality these, too, utilize radio signals to carry the call. Wireless telephone technology can also be used to support mobile data terminals (MDTs), which offer another option of information transfer.

FCC AND FREQUENCIES

A variety of systems as well as a number of frequencies can be used for radio communication. The Federal Communications Commission is responsible for establishing rules and regulations for these services (Federal Communications Commission, 2011).

The radio spectrum constitutes all available radio resources in terms of frequencies that can be used to broadcast, corresponding to the following categories:

* *Microwave.* Used for point-to-point fixed systems.
* *UHF.* Ultra high frequency.
* *VHF High.* Very high frequency.
* *VHF Low.* Very high frequency (low band).

The two latter frequency groups are often referred to as "high band" and "low band" without reference to "VHF." Public safety agencies have access to specified frequencies within these groups. Keep in mind that other services such as maritime, military, aviation, and commercial broadcast also have radio needs and are assigned their own unique frequencies. Commercial ambulance services may sometimes be licensed in the "business band" category, rather than in the public safety pool.

Side Bar

D-block

In 2012, Congress authorized the allocation of the so-called "D-block"—a 10 MHz block of radio spectrum—and provided $7 billion in funding for the build out of the next-generation public safety broadband communications network. This spectrum and the network to be built under it will enhance provider interoperability, and they will allow field and dispatch center use of video, high-speed data, and other twenty-first-century technologies for incident command and daily public safety operations.

In this section, care has been taken to use the word *frequency* rather than *channel*. Although sometimes synonymous, frequencies are an assigned piece of the bandwidth, and channels are technically only the name by which a frequency is known, or its position in a radio. For example, 46.18 MHz is a frequency, but it may also be called "Fire Dispatch" and "Channel One" in local parlance. That same frequency might be labeled differently in another jurisdiction.

TYPES OF SYSTEMS

Radio systems may also be categorized by the way in which they operate. The most common types are these:

* **Simplex**, whereby units transmit and receive on the same frequency and talk directly to each other without assistance
* **Duplex**, whereby units transmit and receive on different frequencies and communicate through a repeater which boosts their power
* **Trunked**, whereby intelligent radios talk through a computer-controlled device that assigns them an available frequency.

As is often the case, there are plusses and minuses to each of these configurations. Simplex, as the name suggests, is by far the simplest.

There are no intermediaries; therefore there are fewer points of failure. However, since there are limitations to the output power of radios, distance as well as human-made and natural barriers can affect communications. Low-band radios are traditionally simplex, but this portion of the spectrum is susceptible to a phenomenon known as skip, whereby transmission from distant stations on the same frequency may actually interfere with local exchanges if certain atmospheric conditions exist.

Duplex operation is normally associated with the higher frequencies, and it eliminates many of the deficiencies associated with simplex. However, again, because of the additional devices needed, it can be more expensive to operate and is reliant on repeaters. If a repeater fails, or if conversation is limited to a very small area, a talk-around feature is often employed that allows units to operate in a simplex mode and to talk around the repeater. Systems that cover large areas may have a number of repeated pairs of frequencies and may rely on the use of satellite receivers to capture messages from low-power mobile and portable radios. An additional device, called a voting comparator, may also be used to automatically select the best audio received from a number of satellite sites.

Trunked radios utilize a pool of frequencies coupled with intelligent radios to maximize resources. In conventional radio systems, users manually select a channel on which to operate. In a trunked system, a computer known as a controller searches for a quiet frequency and automatically assigns the units wishing to converse there. In trunked radio systems, the term *channel* is replaced by the term *talk group*, and units of related functions or departments typically are accordingly assigned.

Because all radios in trunked systems are intelligent, costs can be high. Also, the earliest models of trunked radio systems used proprietary technology, requiring that both units and infrastructure be purchased through the same vendor, thereby limiting options for replacement purchases. Trunked radio systems also often operate in the 800- or 700-MHz frequency zones, which have restrictions in terms of coverage and penetration into heavily constructed buildings such as hospitals and parking garages. This can obviously be of concern to public safety personnel who must operate freely throughout their service area.

Newer trunked radios are free of past proprietary limitations through a feature known as Common Air Interface (CAI), which allows for vendor neutrality and compatibility. These, and modern radios from all bands, are now moving toward digital audio, which in itself can cause issues. The fire service has been very active in working toward correcting what it considers to be deficiencies in the way that digital signals are processed in high-noise environments (Imel and Hart, 2003).

INTEROPERABILITY

Since September 11, 2001, a significant amount of attention has been given to the term **interoperability**, or the ability of public safety personnel to freely communicate with all other services involved in the same event. The following definitions come from Industry Canada's Consultation Paper on Public Safety Radio Interoperability Guidelines (2006) and cover several areas of operation.

Radio interoperability is the capability of a public safety agency to communicate by radio (either directly or via a network) with another public safety agency, on demand (planned and unplanned) and in real time.

The communications link may involve any combination of mobile radio terminals and fixed radio equipment (e.g., repeaters, dispatch positions, data resources). The points of communication are dependent on the specific needs of the situation and any operational procedures and policies that might exist among the involved agencies. The communications link may be classified as either of the following two types:

- *Infrastructure independent.* The communications link occurs between mobile radio terminals over a direct radio frequency path. An example is portable-to-portable tactical communications at the scene of an incident.
- *Infrastructure dependent.* The communications link requires the use of equipment, other than mobile radio terminals, for the establishment of the link and for complete operation. Some examples include a communications link in which a repeater station is deployed; a communications link that provides full system coverage for a visiting mobile radio terminal within a host-trunked radio system; and a communications link that provides interconnectivity between two or more otherwise incompatible radio systems by bridging the radio signals and/or appropriate signaling functions at some central point.

The communications link, whether infrastructure dependent or independent, must satisfy one or both of the following requirements:

- *Multijurisdictional.* Wireless communications involving agencies having different geographical areas of responsibility. Some examples include a fire agency from one city, communicating with a fire agency from another city; federal or provincial police forces communicating with a city police force; and the federal police force communicating within its divisional offices in another province, or with a police force in the United States.
- *Multidisciplinary.* Wireless communications involving two or more different agencies. Some examples include a police agency communicating with a fire agency and a parks agency communicating with an emergency medical services agency.

In addition to the multijurisdictional and multidisciplinary radio interoperability characteristics (Figure 12.4), different operating environments for public safety impose different requirements on the use of public safety

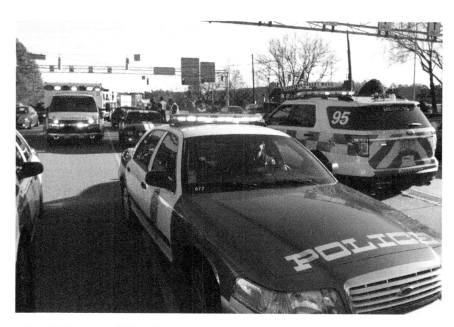

FIGURE 12.4 ■ Interoperability allows ambulance crews to communicate with other first responders such as law enforcement and fire. *Source: Mike Legeros.*

applications and therefore on the spectrum required. These operating environments include day-to-day operations, planned events, and large, unplanned events as well as disaster-relief operations.

This document goes on to discuss the ways in which interoperability is commonly provided, including the following:

- Agencies exchanging portable radios on scene
- Use of a patching or bridging mechanism to connect channels
- Use of regional preassigned mutual aid channels
- Stand-alone mutual aid radios (Industry Canada, 2006)

Another topic related to interoperability is the use of plain text. For years, public safety agencies have relied on a system of "10 codes" in order to shorten the time taken to send messages. Although some in law enforcement may have originally used codes in order to provide some level of security, codes such as "10-4" made their way into the common language a long time ago, and the preponderance of scanner listeners has certainly reduced the secrecy involved.

However, although the public may have been deciphering the 10 codes at their leisure, a problem exists in that there is no universal system of 10 codes. These vary from department to department and community to community. Imagine then the difficulties that can result when different agencies with different codes can suddenly communicate on the same channel. Obviously, confusion can ensue, and the end result can be less than desirable. Because of this, a significant effort is underway to turn to plain text messaging for all radio transmissions. There is less room for error when a unit is told to "respond to a cardiac arrest" than there is to respond to a 10 code, especially if that unit is not normally assigned to your agency and is temporarily filling in or assisting (SAFE-COM, n.d.).

■ STAFFING

It is apparent when a service has insufficient resources in the field. There are not enough ambulances for patients. Calls get backlogged. Crews must wait to summon additional help lifting a bariatric patient. The list goes on. However, staffing demands do not impact only mobile resources; they can be just as problematic in the dispatch center. In fact, if you search for the phrase "dispatcher shortage" online, you will get a response of "around 621 results."

The **Association of Public-safety Communications Officials (APCO) International** created Project RETAINS (2013) to study the issue of dispatch staffing, and created a formula that can be used to predict the staffing required in order to deal with a variety of commonly encountered variables. In addition, so-called *Erlang* formulae have been used for years in a variety of settings to determine the number of telephone lines and call takers needed to meet various levels of service (Westbay Engineers Limited, 2012). Both are excellent tools for the communications center manager. APCO also created the Professional Communications Human Resource Taskforce (*Pro-CHRT*) (Association of Public Safety Communications Officials, 2010b) as a follow-up to RETAINS to perform further study on the issues of telecommunicator training and retention. Among the findings were that only 3 percent of communicators remain on the job long enough to retire, which underlines the importance of improving candidate selection and support.

Detailed telecommunicator hiring standards, qualifications, training standards, and job descriptions are available from many sources including state law (Association of Public-safety Communications Officials, 2010c), National Fire Protection Association (2007), International Municipal Signal Association (1996, 2009), American Society for Testing and Materials (2006), and National Emergency Number Association (2006).

CHAPTER REVIEW

Summary

Emergency communications and emergency communications centers are the backbone of ambulance response, regardless of whether the call is a developing emergency or a prescheduled transport. A number of successful models of dispatching and call receipt are applicable in communities of varying sizes. More information is available to the EMS provider than ever before, and with the rapidly changing pace of technology even more will be available tomorrow.

Leaders of the future will have to carefully manage the mix of voluminous data, open architecture communications systems, and patients' rights and confidentiality concerns. In addition to dealing with technology, these same leaders must also weigh the human factors in the equation to install systems that are user friendly while ensuring that all aspects of the delivery mechanism are adequately staffed by trained, competent, and caring people.

WHAT WOULD YOU DO? Reflection

In the case study presented, a list of seven questions was included. The answers to these questions provide a good foundation for determining the best approach in finding a solution. Awareness of legal, procedural, and fiscal constraints is imperative, as is a careful examination of similar successful projects. Without this knowledge, a positive outcome is not likely. Understanding other key definitions within this chapter, as well as your relationships with technical systems and users with whom you must interface on a daily basis, will also be of great importance. Gathering this information will allow the establishment of a plan, budget, and timeline for the project.

In managing any undertaking of this magnitude, it is also critical to understand dependencies (in other words what has to happen first) as well as true total costs. For example, options must be examined for both their initial as well as long-term costs. What seems like a bargain up front may not be in the long run. The decision to integrate technologies discussed in this chapter, such as CAD, E 9-1-1, and the potential migration to NG 9-1-1, will obviously have a bearing on the model you choose, as will whether or not your agency functions as a primary or secondary PSAP. This, as well as answers to previously mentioned questions, will help to more clearly define your needs as well as limit the scope of acceptable solutions.

The qualification of no down time may be met in a number of ways, ranging from the installation of parallel systems to the position-by-position migration of existing technology. Keep in mind that there is no "one size fits all" answer to the problem posed, as subtleties among organizational needs will dictate similar subtleties for solutions. Of vast importance, however, is that proposed changes are carefully planned, researched, and documented, and that, in the true tradition of emergency services, alternate (backup) plans be in place for every step of the project.

Review Questions

1. Describe the differences between a primary and a secondary PSAP, and discuss the pros and cons of each configuration.
2. What radio systems are in use in your area? How can you communicate with other public safety agencies on a daily basis?
3. What other agencies might you need to talk to during a disaster? How can that be accomplished?
4. What are the current barriers to effective communication that exist in your area? How can these be removed?
5. What challenges will NG 9-1-1 systems present to ambulance providers? How can these issues best be addressed? How far along is your community/state in Next Generation planning?
6. What are the differences between two-stage and single-stage dispatching? When might they best be used?
7. What are the differences between a simplex, duplex, and trunked radio system?
8. Why are agencies moving toward the use of plain text?
9. What are three benefits associated with the use of EMD?
10. What is the purpose of a UPS device in a communications center?

References

Alabama Chapter of NENA. (2011). "World's First 9-1-1 Call." See the organization website.

Association of Public Safety Communications Officials (APCO). (2009). "APCO Announces Inaugural Horizon Award Winners." See the organization website.

Association of Public Safety Communications Officials. (2010a). "APCO Announces 2010 Aware Winners: Honoring Heroes." See the organization website.

Association of Public Safety Communications Officials (APCO). (2010b). "Interim Report on Challenges Facing Human Resources and Staffing in the 9-1-1 Public Safety Communications Center." Reported by APCO Pro-CHRT Professional Communications Human Resources Taskforce, Daytona Beach, FL.

Association of Public Safety Communications Officials (APCO). (2010c). "International Communications Center Consolidation Considerations," white paper.

Association of Public Safety Communications Officials (APCO). (2010d). "Project 33 Training Standards for Public Safety Telecommunicators." See the organization website.

Association of Public Safety Communications Officials (APCO). (2013). "Staffing and Retention Tool Kit for Public Safety Communications Center Managers." See the organization website.

American Society for Testing and Materials. (2006). "Standard Practice for Emergency Medical Dispatch, ASTM Standard F1258–95 ASTM International." See the organization website.

Dispatch Magazine On-line. (2011)."History of 911." See the organization website.

Federal Communications Commission. (2011). "About the FCC." See the organization website.

Imel, K. J., and J. W. Hart. (2003). "Understanding Wireless Communications in Public Safety: A Guidebook to Technology, Issues, Planning, and Management," 2nd ed. The National Law Enforcement and Corrections Technology Center (Rocky Mountain Region), A Program of the National Institute of Justice. See the organization website.

Industry Canada. (2006, June). "Consultation Paper on Public Safety Radio Interoperability Guidelines." See the organization website.

International Municipal Signal Association. (1996). "Telecommunicator Level II." See the organization website.

International Municipal Signal Association (IMSA). (2009). "Telecommunicator Level I." See the organization website.

Legislative Program Review and Investigations Committee. (1999). "Regulation of Emergency Medical Services. Phase 2. Chapter IV: Emergency Medical Dispatch (EMD)." See the Connecticut General Assembly website.

Loomis, S. E. (2007, Winter). "Ideals and Standards Affect 911 Center Design." *Newsletter of the Academy of Architecture for Justice.* See The American Institute of Architects website.

National Association of State EMS Officials. (2009, December). "Comments of the National Association of State Emergency Medical Services Officials – NBP Public Notice #17." See the organization website.

National Emergency Number Association, Future Models Working Group. (2004, June 1). "NENA Technical Information Document on Future 9-1-1 Models," NENA 07-501, Issue 11, p. 8. See the organization website.

National Emergency Number Association. (2006). "Hearing Standards for Telecommunicators." See the organization website.

National Emergency Number Association. (2012). "Master Glossary of 9-1-1 Terminology." See the organization website.

National Emergency Number Association. (2012–2013a). "Mission." See the organization website.

National Emergency Number Association. (2012–2013b). "NG9-1-1 Transition Planning Committee." See the organization website.

National Emergency Number Association. (2012–2013c). "NENA NG Partner Program." See the organization website.

National Emergency Number Association. (2012–2013d). "Functional & Interface Standards for NG9-1-1 (i3)." See the organization website.

National Emergency Number Association. (2012–2013e). "NENA Standards and Other Documents." See the organization website.

National Fire Protection Association. (2007). "NFPA 1601 Standard for Professional Qualifications for Public Safety Telecommunicator." See the organization website.

National Fire Protection Association. (2010). "NFPA 1221: Standard for the Installation, Maintenance, and Use of Emergency Services Communications Systems." See the organization website.

SAFECOM. (n.d.) "Making the Transition from Ten Codes to Plain Language." Safecomprogram.gov (Department of Homeland Security). See the organization website.

U.S. Department of Justice. (1998, July). "Americans with Disabilities Act: Access for 9-1-1 and Telephone Emergency Services." See the organization website.

Westbay Engineers Limited. (2012). "What Is an Erlang?" See the organization website.

Key Terms

American Society for Testing and Materials (ASTM) An international standards organization that develops and publishes voluntary consensus technical standards for a wide range of materials, products, systems, and services.

Association of Public-safety Communications Officials (APCO) International The world's largest association of communications professionals, providing professional development, technical assistance, outreach, and advocacy.

automatic call distribution (ACD) A device with which inbound calls are routed to specific persons based on a routine programmed into the telephone system.

duplex A radio system that uses a repeater to boost signals.

emergency medical dispatch (EMD) A scripted set of questions and prearrival instructions designed to categorize and assist EMS callers.

Enhanced 9-1-1 (E 9-1-1) A class of 9-1-1 service that delivers both the location and number of the calling party.

Federal Communications Commission (FCC) A government agency responsible for assigning radio licenses and promulgating rules for communications.

interoperability The ability of disparate users or systems to seamlessly communicate.

National Emergency Number Association (NENA) A professional organization solely focused on 9-1-1 policy, technology, operations, and education issues.

National Fire Protection Association (NFPA) An international nonprofit organization dedicated to reducing the worldwide burden of fire and other hazards on the quality of life by providing and advocating consensus codes and standards, research, training, and education.

Next Generation 9-1-1 (Next Gen & NG 9-1-1) The next level of 9-1-1 service that will include enhancements such as texting, video, and telematic data.

public switched telephone network (PSTN) Conventional wire line telephony; the system of trunks and switches that deliver calls.

simplex A radio system with which users talk radio to radio without a repeater.

trunked A radio system using smart radios that are assigned by computer to an open channel among a pool of frequencies.

Voice over Internet Protocol (VoIP) The transfer of telephony over the Internet.

Technology in Support of Ambulance Operations

13 CHAPTER

Skip Kirkwood, M.S., J.D., NREMT-P, EFO, CEMSO

Objectives

After reading this chapter, the student should be able to:

13.1 Identify eight technology tools that can be used to automate and enhance ambulance operations.

13.2 Discuss and describe the benefits that technology tools can bring to an ambulance service.

13.3 Identify the needs for operational support of an ambulance service, and select the proper technology to improve specific areas of performance.

Overview

Ambulance services in the United States range in size from one ambulance operated by volunteers and managed by a community board of directors to large governmental agencies and even larger, private, for-profit corporations. This text presents information that the manager of an ambulance service, large or small, needs in order to keep the business solvent and provide clinically excellent service to the community.

Key Terms

automatic vehicle
   location (AVL)
computer-aided
   dispatching (CAD)

deployment
   simulation
   software

global positioning
   system (GPS)
in-vehicle navigation
   (IVN)

mobile data computers (MDC)

syndromic surveillance (SS) systems

traffic preemption systems

vehicle-centered local area network (V-LAN)

vehicle on-board monitoring and driver feedback systems ("black boxes")

WHAT WOULD YOU DO?

You have recently been named operations manager for a municipal ambulance service in a town of 100,000 people. Your service is dispatched by the town police department, using the LAW-CAD Model 1980 system. Your medics use paper map books, and all communication is done by voice. You have 12-lead EKG monitors, but no ability to transmit your 12-lead to the regional heart (STEMI) center. The chief who appointed you, who has been there for 26 years, tells you that the service has grown so quickly that there is a young, inexperienced workforce, and that she "doesn't know where to begin" in getting a handle on current and future operational needs. She recently attended a national EMS conference, and came away with the impression that other ambulance services were using technology in a way that enhances their operations, and that their leadership seems to talk about being "data driven" in every area.

Her first challenge to you is "get a handle" on the service's response performance (which seems to be suffering), the deployment plan (which seems to be making the employees unhappy), and driver safety (which seems to be an increasing problem in the service). She also tells you that the budget is tight, and that any future requests for personnel or facilities will have to be supported by more than the usual "children will be dying in the streets" type of appeal. It will be 6 months before the next budget cycle begins, and she wants you to be ready with a plan to provide the manager and town council with a thorough appraisal of how the ambulance service can be made both more effective and more economical.

1. What elements will your plan contain?
2. Why will you prioritize them the way that you have?
3. Who, if anyone, will you partner with to improve your chances of success?

■ INTRODUCTION ——————

Technology is ubiquitous in the modern ambulance service. What began as a horizontal transportation service, locally operated by a funeral home, a towing company, a hospital or a fire department and offering the most basic of "first aid" services, has evolved into a medically advanced, often technologically sophisticated big business, involving publicly traded companies, large international businesses, coast-to-coast hospital-operated ambulance services, and huge municipal and county ambulance departments. Privately held services must deliver an acceptable level of service and a suitable profit margin, although publicly operated services must provide an acceptable level of service within an allocated budget. A responsible ambulance service manager must consider any tool that can help achieve those aims.

COMPUTER-AIDED DISPATCHING

In the early days of the modern EMS era (circa 1966), most ambulances were dispatched from central locations. A telephone request for ambulance service, received usually on a seven-digit telephone number, was recorded on paper. The dispatcher leaned out a window, shouted for an ambulance crew, and the unit was on its way. A copy, or a handmade duplicate, served as a dispatch record. As two-way radio communications became more widespread, ambulance crews reported their status back to the dispatch center, where manual entries, or time-clock stamps, recorded key events in the ambulance call—unit en route, arrived at scene, en route to the hospital, at the hospital, back in service, and so on. In large jurisdictions, complex arrangements of moving strings, clothespins, and punch cards were effective, though precarious, tools for monitoring the status and managing operations of EMS systems.

About this time, technology began to proliferate, and the first 9-1-1 systems began to emerge. Although the first 9-1-1 call is reported to have been made in 1968 in Hayleyville, Alabama, 9-1-1 systems were widely implemented across the country throughout the 1970s, 1980s, and 1990s (Bruckner, 2011).

As EMS systems began to develop and technology began to proliferate, there were greater demands for timely service, and the **computer-aided dispatching (CAD)** system became an important source of record-keeping data. In the late 1970s and early 1980s, driven by efforts to improve efficiency and productivity, some ambulance services and EMS systems began using computer-mediated dynamic deployment schemes that came to be known as system status management or SSM (Stout, 1989). In most communities, however, dispatching and the CAD systems were designed for, purchased by, and operated by law enforcement agencies, and lacked the capability to perform SSM functions, or even to capture data points unique to EMS, such as the time the ambulance unit left the scene en route to the hospital.

Over the years, CAD systems became more flexible, and with the advent of the consolidated dispatch center (where law enforcement, fire suppression, and ambulance service in a given community are dispatched from a central facility), ambulance dispatch capability was more often built into a "general purpose" CAD system. Several vendors entered the market with ambulance-specific CAD systems, utilizing software designed to optimize ambulance deployment and dispatching. As computers became more powerful, the emergency services community began to see CAD systems electronically attached (interfaced) to a variety of complimentary systems, including telephone systems with automatic number identification (ANI) and automatic location information (ALI), radio communication, alerting, and alphanumeric paging systems, **mobile data computers (MDC)**, and **automatic vehicle location (AVL)** and **in-vehicle navigation (IVN)** systems.

One of the greatest CAD developments was the advent of geo-verification of event locations, first based on the address provided by the caller using a cumbersome-to-maintain database, later simplified by the integration of ANI/ALI data and the incorporation of geographic information systems (GIS) capabilities in to the CAD system. Now, instead of requiring dispatchers to have an intimate knowledge of the geography, the call location can appear as a dot on a computer screen, allowing quick identification of nearby units.

■ MOBILE DATA COMPUTERS

Early mobile data terminals were custom products, relying on very slow point-to-point analog radio systems and a small number of buttons (video screens began to appear in the late 1980s and early 1990s) to communicate status changes and important messages. Commercial package delivery services, taxi services, and others continue to utilize custom (albeit sometimes very sophisticated) devices, while the emergency services community has migrated to general-purpose laptop computers, often in a ruggedized format. The MDC is used to duplicate and confirm voice dispatch information, provide specialized information (such as the existence of hazards at a particular address) contained in the CAD database, reduce voice radio traffic, and accurately record the incident status of the particular vehicle. Many MDC systems provide advanced features, including allowing officers, firefighters, and paramedics to chat and share incident and other appropriate information. The 4800-baud and 9600-baud radio modems have in large part been replaced by cellular digital data transmission, beginning with cellular digital packet data (CDPD) in the 1990s and evolving to today's 3G and 4G wireless Internet services.

■ AUTOMATIC VEHICLE LOCATION

In the late 1960s, Motorola Communications introduced the Metrocom system, using the radio signals of the Coast Guard's Long Range Radio Navigation (LORAN) system. Coverage was sparse, except on the East and West Coasts and on the Great Lakes. This was the first known commercial attempt at AVL.

The **global positioning system (GPS)** was activated by the U.S. Department of Defense in 1994. Since then, GPS equipment has become extremely cheap and highly reliable. In the emergency services community, specially configured GPS receivers interface with CAD systems, providing instantaneous and highly accurate location information. Now, instead of dispatching the ambulance that covers a particular city, town, or district, the CAD can select the closest available ambulance, thereby improving response performance throughout the system. More advanced CAD systems will display not only the incident location, but will allow dispatchers to observe the location and movement of EMS vehicles throughout the community, observing progress during travel, perhaps providing routing information, and generally improving response performance throughout the community.

■ IN-VEHICLE NAVIGATION

Since the inception of emergency services agencies, finding the location of the emergency has represented a challenge. Rookie police officers, firefighters, and ambulance medics spent their "spare" time learning their neighborhoods, often spending hours driving around undertaking "area familiarization." As agencies, systems, and communities became larger, operations became more flexible, the workforce became more mobile, and demands for efficiency and cost control increased, it became less and less likely that individual cops, firefighters, and medics would be assigned for a career (or even an extended period) to the same small geographic area. Map books became more extensive to keep current, and high levels of media scrutiny and concerns about liability made getting lost less and less of an option. The importance of accurate navigation was highlighted by the Court of Appeals of Minnesota in the case of *Blatz v. Allina Health*

System,[1] where a navigation error resulted in a multimillion dollar judgment against a 9-1-1 ambulance service.

In-vehicle navigation combines the power of the CAD system, geographic information systems (GIS), and location (GPS/AVL) data into a powerful tool for emergency responders and their agencies. Often thought of as "GPS on steroids," the system instantaneously performs the following functions:

* Call location information is obtained by the ANI/ALI from the 9-1-1 telephone system, confirmed by the call taker, and sent to the CAD system.
* The CAD system, using up-to-the-second vehicle location information, selects the closest appropriate response resource(s) based on AVL and vehicle status data.
* Using wireless data communication, the CAD transmits the incident location and information to the vehicle MDC, where it is interfaced with geographic routing information (a "map base") resident on the MDC. The IVN software picks up the location of the incident from the CAD, and its own location from the AVL, and calculates the most direct route to the call.
* The ambulance crew then pushes a button on the computer to inform the CAD that the unit is en route to the call. If traffic is heavy or construction delays require a re-route, the crew can vary from the prescribed route, identify an alternative, and push a button to ask the IVN to calculate a new route.

Where streets are closed for extended periods, a map change may be sent via wireless data communication to each MDC/IVN work station, ensuring that proper routing is instantly available. More sophisticated IVN systems allow dispatchers to instantly enter street delay data, and the most sophisticated are capable of hour-by-hour impedance-based routing,[2] providing different routes during rush hours of other times when traffic is routinely difficult in a particular area.

Side Bar

IS Commercial GPS/IVN Good Enough for EMS?

Paramedics working in technologically challenged ambulance services, where professional or public-safety-grade GPS, AVL, and IVN systems are not available, often ask whether or not it is acceptable to utilize personally owned systems (e.g., Garmin, TomTom) while on duty in the ambulance. A prudent ambulance executive will answer "Maybe." Here's why:

1. Personnel come to rely on devices, which may not be supplied with the latest maps or updated periodically. A medic who does not refer to the service's official map reference may be led astray. Delayed response due to poor navigation can result in costly liability judgments, as in *Blatz v. Allina Health System*.
2. Remote or rural areas are often poorly mapped and addressed. Coincidentally, these may be areas where public safety technology is limited. A service should not fall prey to "good enough" if professional alternatives are available. Partnering with other public safety, public works (highways), and public utilities, as well as the 9-1-1 center, may open doors where freestanding solutions are not possible.

---

[1]*Mary Blatz, et al., Respondents, vs. Allina Health System, d/b/a HealthSpan Transportation Services,* Appellant. C9-00-826, Court of Appeals. Published, February 6, 2001. Minnesota Court of Appeals C9-00-826.

[2]Impedance-based routing uses vehicle travel data to select routes based on historical actual speed data, rather than posted speed limits, to identify slowdowns that routinely occur in school zones, traffic jams, toll roads, and other locations where traffic speeds frequently don't coincide with posted limits.

3. Human-machine interfaces may not be optimized for emergency conditions. Remember the caution that pops up when you plug your commercial device into your vehicle—the one that says, "Don't be pushing buttons and trying to navigate while you are driving"? A paramedic driving an ambulance might move into dangerous territory trying to re-route to a different destination when things change en route to a call or a hospital.

Ambulance services should strive to provide professional-grade technology to staff, and if that is not possible, a well-considered policy should govern the use of personal devices.

■ TRAFFIC PREEMPTION SYSTEMS

Many people believe that the purpose of vehicle warning systems (lights, sirens, air horns, etc.) exist to allow ambulances and other emergency vehicles to speed to the scene of an emergency. Although this occasionally (and sometimes unfortunately) occurs, these systems are often most useful at lower speeds, allowing emergency vehicles to clear traffic that is moving at slow speeds, or that is stopped. It also permits (at least in the legal sense) emergency vehicles to pass through red lights or other traffic control devices.

Unfortunately, the legal authorization to exceed speed limits and to pass through traffic control devices does not ensure that either act can safely be accomplished. Current ambulance crash data suggest that a significant portion of ambulance collisions occur during daylight, in dry weather conditions, at intersections, while running emergency warning equipment (Kahn, Pirrallo, and Kuhn, 2001). Additional crashes occur when ambulances utilizing emergency warning equipment force nonemergency vehicles into intersections against traffic control devices.

For many years, **traffic preemption systems** such as Opticom, originally from 3-M Corporation and currently offered by Global Traffic Technologies, and Strobecom from Tomar Technologies, utilized specially timed strobe lights to change the red-green cycle of traffic lights such that approaching emergency vehicles enjoyed a green light, which kept traffic flowing and prevented clogging at intersections (Figure 13.1). Unfortunately, these systems were vulnerable to unauthorized use, with emitters being available from retail sources including eBay.

The current generation of traffic preemption devices relies on network-controlled traffic signals, GPS, secure communication, and sophisticated software to allow priority to emergency vehicles, and even to afford lower priority to mass transit vehicles (Advanced Traffic Products, 2013). A variety of studies have demonstrated improved response performance and traffic safety as a result of the implementation of traffic preemption systems (City of Surrey, 2003; U.S. Department of Transportation, 2006, 2008).

■ VEHICLE LOCAL-AREA NETWORKING

Today's ambulances are often a technology-rich environment. The MDC-AVL-IVN combination requires a wireless connection (either via a commercial wireless data carrier or proprietary radio) between vehicles and the CAD system. Modern physiologic monitoring systems, especially 12-lead electrocardiogram devices, collect digital data that often provide optimal patient care value if successfully transmitted to receiving facilities to facilitate early activation of interventional facilities (cardiac catheterization laboratories or neuroscience intervention facilities) for STEMI,

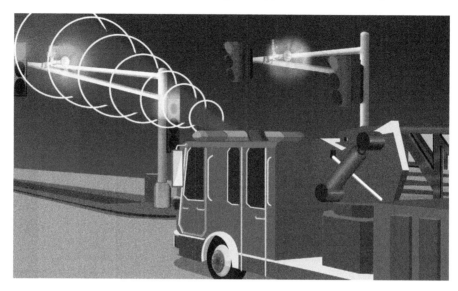

FIGURE 13.1 ▓ The Opticom system, from Global Transportation Technologies, may utilize light pulses, GPS data, or infrared technology to turn traffic lights green for emergency vehicles. *Source: Reprinted by permission from Global Traffic Technologies.*

stroke, and other high-risk patients. Electronic patient care reporting (ePCR) systems require data connections to transmit reports from mobile locations to receiving hospitals, ambulance headquarters, and billing companies. Some communities have experimented with video telemedicine capabilities for ambulance vehicles.

Using a separate radio modem or 3G/4G aircard for each of these functions can quickly increase costs. Commercial carriers typically charge monthly per-card fees that quickly multiply across a large ambulance fleet, and proprietary radio systems become costly as bandwidth demand increases.

Cost-conscious ambulance operators wishing to provide very reliable high-tech capabilities while limiting costs have recently looked to mobile wireless routers (often called onboard mobile gateways) to create a **vehicle-centered local area network (V-LAN)**, which integrates the data communication pathways from the ambulance through a single data stream to a variety of destinations via the Internet (Figure 13.2). These devices offer great flexibility, allowing data input from devices (computers, ECGs, etc.) using Bluetooth or WiFi technology, with output passing through the commercial wireless data system. Some manufacturers allow the integration of multiple data-out

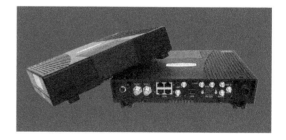

FIGURE 13.2 ▓ The In Motion Technology onBoard Mobile Gateway creates a local area network that can be accessed by computers, medical devices, and other onboard technology. *Source: In Motion Technology.*

capabilities, ensuring greater reliability in the event of data-carrier coverage issues and allowing in-building data communication to be handled by building-based Internet connections.

■ VEHICLE ONBOARD MONITORING AND DRIVER FEEDBACK SYSTEMS ─────────

The passenger aircraft industry has long utilized flight data recorders to capture aircraft data. Such data are most widely known for their post-incident value, allowing investigators to reconstruct events leading up to and at the time of an aircraft crash or collision. However, this same data (and more) are very useful to fleet managers, who are able to monitor the performance of vehicle systems, identifying worn and fatigued parts and managing subsystem life expectancies.

Similarly, **vehicle onboard monitoring systems** can monitor vehicle performance parameters, and in recent years they have been engineered to provide feedback (as well as recording) of operator performance. These systems monitor vehicle operations, tracking hard accelerations and decelerations, high-G turns, seat belt use, use of spotters for backing, and other vehicle telematics. Some systems record the use of vehicle warning systems and subsystems, so that (for example), either in real time or historically, vehicle speed, direction, and use of lights and sirens can be determined at any particular time and location. One well-known system (Figure 3.2) utilizes vehicle operations parameters to calculate servicewide and individual scores for each driver, allowing management to identify high-risk or high-maintenance-cost drivers whose driving habits are not conducive to achieving organizational goals.

Side Bar

"Black Boxes" Improve Driver Performance and Reduce Operating Costs

In 2003, a study was conducted at the Metro Emergency Medical Service (MEMS) in Little Rock, Arkansas, to determine if emergency vehicle driver behavior could be improved by installing an onboard computer-based monitoring device with real-time auditory feedback. Data from more than 1.9 million miles of vehicle operation were recorded. During a four-month period, seat belt violations dropped from 13,500 to 4. There was a 20 percent cost saving in vehicle maintenance within the first 6 months, with 10 percent to 20 percent less brake and tire wear and reduced oil consumption. There was no degradation of response performance during the study period.

Levick and Swanson (2005) conclude that improvement in driver performance has been dramatic and sustained in every measured area with the Zoll Rescue Net Road Safety onboard computer monitoring and feedback system.

■ DEPLOYMENT SIMULATION SYSTEMS ─────────

Unlike law enforcement and fire suppression services, most ambulance services are associated with a revenue stream. Private-sector ambulance services must demonstrate profitability to succeed, while public-sector ambulance services are pressed to efficiently deliver service within allocated budgetary constraints. Regardless of corporate pedigree, optimization of resources—having the right resources in the right place at the right hour of the day—is a fact of life for today's ambulance service manager.

Historically, decisions about deployment levels and locations have been made on a "best guess basis," with ambulance officers relying on personal knowledge of operations and the community they serve. In larger communities, and as organizations and services grow larger, the economic and health consequences of the "best guess" approach become significant. Budget officers and governing bodies are always seeking a more "scientific" or data-driven approach to resource allocation decisions.

Operations research (OR)—also referred to as operational research, decision science, or management science—is an interdisciplinary mathematical science that focuses on the effective use of technology by organizations. Practitioners of OR use mathematical modeling, statistical analysis, and game theory to analyze the potential of business decisions. The integration of computer technology with OR methods and techniques allow **deployment simulation software** to quickly and accurately test proposed deployment decisions, and answer questions such as the following:

- If we add a unit at 12th and Main Street from 0900 to 2100, what will be the effect on our compliance with the county-mandated response performance standard?
- If we close Medic 12 due to budgetary constraints, how busy will that cause adjoining units to be?

A variety of white papers published by the deployment simulation industry demonstrate that economies can be achieved and performance can be improved through the use of deployment simulation technology. Lee County, Florida, reported a 3 percent improvement in response performance using deployment simulation software from the Optima Corporation (Optima Corporation, 2010). The government of Denmark utilized this software to develop a firm statistical basis for issuing a tender (request for bids or proposals) (Optima Corporation, 2011). A number of fire and ambulance providers have successfully defended budgets, proposed station locations, and other administrative decisions in case studies provided by other vendors (Deccan International, 2006, 2008).

■ SYNDROMIC SURVEILLANCE SYSTEMS

Syndromic surveillance (SS) systems use individual and population health indicators that are available before confirmed diagnoses or laboratory confirmation to identify outbreaks or health events and monitor the health status of a community (Centers for Disease Control and Prevention, 2013). Although much of the effort in the area of syndromic surveillance has been directed toward monitoring laboratory results and hospital ED or hospital admission data, many in the EMS and public health communities believe that upswings in illnesses can best be detected by monitoring requests for ambulance service via the 9-1-1 system and/or ePCR data. Unusual spikes in activity can alert not only ambulance service operators but also other public health and safety authorities of newly begun epidemiologic events such as flu outbreaks, mass food poisonings, and even chemical and biological events.

First Watch, a product of Stout Solutions, Inc., is a product with a long track record of monitoring EMS dispatch and clinical data in near real time and alerting ambulance operators and others to significant public health events, including flu outbreaks, respiratory effects of wildfires, and other public health and public safety events (First Watch, 2004). A variety of case studies can be found on the company's website (First Watch, n.d.).

Ambulance operators wishing to be alerted automatically when there are unusual changes in the call mix, or who wish to be more tightly integrated with their community's public health and public safety enterprises, may wish to consider utilizing SS software as part of that effort.

CHAPTER REVIEW

Summary

A variety of technologies can be utilized by ambulance services to monitor and improve operational performance, including response-related communications, vehicle response, and vehicle safety. Ambulance service managers should strive to provide their services with those tools that will help them improve service to their community. In addition, constant scanning of the environment for emerging technologies is essential.

WHAT WOULD YOU DO? Reflection

After settling into your office and getting to know your staff, you close the door and contemplate your first major "project" assignment. Having recently visited with a former classmate at what is regarded as a "high-speed, low-drag" ambulance service, you realize that your service needs to make a quantum jump in technology to meet the operating and financial needs of the next decade. You've spent several months researching technology at other ambulance services, attending trade shows, and conversing with colleagues on the NEMSMA Listserv. You've concluded (and your chief agrees) that your service needs a multiyear performance improvement program to add technology that you think will be helpful. You've also spoken with the police department's officer in charge of the 9-1-1 and dispatch center, who tells you that service is badly in need of replacing the model 1980 CAD system, and would welcome the ambulance service to the CAD procurement process. Your plan begins to build out:

First Year. Work with the police technology staff to procure a CAD that has ambulance-specific capabilities, including capturing all of the NEMSIS time points, and with an MDC function. You will also upfit your vehicles with MDCs and AVL technology.

Second Year. Upgrade your vehicles to add IVN capability to the CAD system, and install onboard V-LAN gateways. Incorporate transmission of 12-lead ECGs to the STEMI center so that your patients can go directly to the cardiac catheterization laboratory if needed.

Third Year. Work with the regional EMS council to procure deployment simulation and syndromic surveillance software. Your colleagues are optimistic that federal grant monies can be obtained to support this effort.

Review Questions

1. What are some issues that arise when ambulance services are dispatched by centers using CAD systems not specifically designed for use by ambulance services?
2. What are some of the advantages of mobile data communication devices?
3. What is the primary advantage of AVL-based computer-aided dispatch systems?
4. How can in-vehicle navigation improve performance and reduce risk of an ambulance service?

5. Why might an ambulance service want to consider developing V-LANs aboard its ambulances?
6. How can deployment simulation software benefit an ambulance service? What decisions can it help management make more effectively?

Chapter Review continues on p. 298

References

Advanced Traffic Technologies. (2013). "Opticom GPS System." See the organization website.

Bruckner, J. (2011). "History of 911." *Dispatch Magazine On-Line.* See the organization website.

Centers for Disease Control and Prevention. (2010, June). "Public Health Surveillance Using Emergency Medical Service Logs—U.S.–Mexico Land Border, El Paso, Texas, 2009." *Morbidity and Morality Weekly Report (MMWR).* See the organization website.

Centers for Disease Control and Prevention. (2013). "Syndromic Surveillance (SS)." See the organization website.

City of Surrey, California. (2003, November). "Intersection Traffic Preemption System Expansion Proposal." See the organization website.

Deccan International. (2006). "Using ADAM to Defend Against Budget Limitations." See the organization website.

Deccan International. (2008). "Budget Defense Using CAD Analyst/ADAM: Chesapeake Fire Department, VA." See the organization website.

First Watch. (2004). "Early Warning of Flu Epidemic by Real-Time Monitoring of 9-1-1 Call Data, Richmond (Virginia), Oklahoma City and Tulsa (Oklahoma)." See the organization website.

Levick, N. R., and J. Swanson. (2005). "An Optimal Solution for Enhancing Ambulance Safety: Implementing a Driver Performance Feedback and Monitoring Device in Ground Emergency Medical Service Vehicles." *Annual Proceedings of the Association for the Advancement of Automotive Medicine 49,* 35–50.

Optima Corporation. (2010). "Case Study: Emergency Medical Services Provider Lee County Avoids More Than USD $750,000 in Unnecessary Costs, Sees Faster Response with Optima live™ and Optima predict™." See the organization website.

Optima Corporation. (2011). "Case Study Capital Region of Denmark Relies on Optima Predict to Develop Accurate, Real-World Simulation of Ambulance Services for Precision Planning." See the organization website.

Stout, J. (1989, April). "System Status Management." *JEMS Magazine.* See the organization website.

U.S. Department of Transportation, Federal Highway Administration. (2008). "Desktop Reference for Crash Reduction Factors" (Report No. FHWA-SA-08-011). See the organization website.

U.S. Department of Transportation, Federal Highway Administration. (2006, January). "Traffic Signal Preemption for Emergency Vehicles: A Cross-Cutting Study." See the organization website.

Key Terms

automatic vehicle location (AVL) System that makes use of the GPS to enable an ambulance service (or other agency) to remotely track the location of its vehicle fleet. AVL systems combine GPS technology, cellular or radio frequency communications, street mapping, and computer software to connect the pieces to a computer where vehicle location is displayed.

computer-aided dispatching (CAD) A suite of software used to initiate public safety calls for service, dispatch, and maintain the status of responding resources in the field. CAD systems consist of multiple modules including call input, dispatching, vehicle status maintenance, field unit status and tracking, and call disposition. CAD systems often include interfaces that permit the software to provide services to dispatchers, call takers, and field personnel.

deployment simulation software Integrates computer technology with operations research methods and techniques quickly and accurately.

global positioning system (GPS) Satellite-based navigation system that allows users to determine their exact location, velocity, and time 24 hours per day, in all weather conditions, anywhere in the world. GPS is used to support a broad range of military, commercial, and consumer applications.

in-vehicle navigation (IVN) Composed of a GPS receiver and specialized software that provides directions to a particular destination.

mobile data computers (MDC) Mounted in or used in vehicles, typically as the remote end of the CAD system data stream, as well as for storage, manipulation, and input of incident and response data.

syndromic surveillance (SS) systems Monitor ambulance (or other health) data sources in real time, and they alert users to sudden increases in specified levels of activity, with the intention of making authorities aware that there has been a sudden up-tick in a particular syndrome. For example, a sudden uptick in calls for service due to respiratory emergencies might be an indicator of the deployment of a chemical weapon.

traffic preemption system Allows the normal operation of traffic lights to be preempted or reordered to assist emergency vehicles, stopping conflicting traffic and allowing the emergency vehicle the right-of-way.

vehicle local area networking (V-LAN) Usually wireless, based in a vehicle, and allows computers and other devices on the vehicle to communicate with each other and remote sites (via the Internet or other media).

vehicle on-board monitoring and driver feedback systems (black boxes) Record vehicle operating parameters, communicate those parameters beyond the vehicle for later analysis, and provide feedback (usually audible) when a driver approaches or exceeds specified parameters.

CHAPTER 14

The Finance and Accounting Functions

SEAN CAFFREY, M.B.A., CEMSO, NRP, AND ASBEL MONTES, B.S.

Objectives

After reading this chapter, the student should be able to:

14.1 Describe the financial management and accounting roles and responsibilities in an organization.

14.2 Describe the standards and basic elements of accounting.

14.3 Compare and contrast cash versus accrual accounting.

14.4 Describe the basic financial statements and alternative names for those statements.

14.5 List common sources of ambulance revenue.

14.6 Describe the purpose of a budget.

14.7 Explain common ambulance productivity and financial measures.

14.8 List the steps in billing for ambulance service.

14.9 Describe the primary payment sources for ambulance services.

14.10 Explain common issues in ambulance billing and collections.

Overview

Ambulance services in the United States range in size from one ambulance operated by volunteers and managed by a community board of directors to large governmental agencies and even larger, private, for-profit corporations. This text presents information that the manager of an ambulance service, large or small, needs in order to keep the business solvent and provide clinically excellent service to the community.

Key Terms

accounting	cost per call	Generally Accepted	retained earnings/equity
accounts payable	days sales outstanding	Accounting	self-pay
accounts receivable	(DSO)	Principles (GAAP)	statement of cash
balance sheet	finance	income statement	flows
budget	financial	managerial	third party
chart of accounts	accounting	accounting	unit hour

WHAT WOULD YOU DO?

A large industrial facility in your community has recently indicated its intention to shut down within the next year. This facility is a major employer in the community and is responsible for a significant number of ambulance calls annually. The chief executive of your service has asked you to assist in analyzing the potential impact of this shutdown. In particular, your organization is concerned how this will affect ambulance revenues and what, if any, services might be able to be reduced or relocated. The chief executive has asked you to prepare projected or pro forma financial statements for the organization and develop a draft budget for next year. You will be conducting this analysis in partnership with the finance department of your service.

1. What information would need to be tracked regularly in order to estimate the impact of the facility closing described in this case?
2. Who would be responsible for tracking this information?
3. What information would be needed to understand the impact on revenue?
4. What information would be needed to understand the impact on expenses?
5. What methods could be used to estimate impacts if complete information were unavailable?

■ INTRODUCTION ——————————

Ambulance services, like most any type of organization, require financial resources to carry out their mission. Understanding where the money comes from and where it goes is an essential skill for the management of ambulance services. The services can be structured in a variety of ways, both in terms of how they are funded and how they operate. Despite these differences, all ambulance organizations have a **finance** function and all utilize standardized tools to understand their use of financial resources. This chapter reviews those common financial tools, explores financial measurements within ambulance services, and describes the basics of ambulance revenue stream management. Revenue stream management, although somewhat similar to other health care organizations, is among the most unique aspects of ambulance service administration.

■ WHY FINANCE AND ACCOUNTING ARE IMPORTANT

Although most managers understand the importance of funding, the details of finance and accounting, especially to managers with a response or clinical background, can be uninteresting. Mangers may feel that, much like operating a vehicle, an in-depth knowledge of how the engine works is not essential. This perspective can also be further magnified if specific individuals are responsible for the financial operations of the organization. What is important, however, is that senior leaders in an ambulance service have enough of a working knowledge of financial management and jargon to ensure that they understand where the money is coming from, how it is being expended, and especially how it is being tracked.

Although the financial community uses specialized terms such as **balance sheet**, **income statement**, *cash flow*, *time value of money*, *financial controls*, *audit*, and such, these concepts are not particularly difficult to learn. Learning about finance will not only allow a manager or executive to have a better understanding of how the money works but also will further serve to protect an organization from the potential for financial misconduct. Although misconduct is not common, a brief search using the terms *ambulance*, *fraud*, and *embezzlement* will show that the ambulance industry is not immune from the temptation to divert funds. This temptation can be especially strong in a small organization where very few people—or even only one person—handle the funds for the organization. Standardized accounting controls, however, are a great mechanism for preventing financial misconduct.

Revenue streams, such as Medicare, Medicaid, private insurance, tax funding, grants, and fund-raising, are also all subject to various rules, regulations, and policies that dictate how those funds must be requested and accounted for. Failure to understand or comply with those requirements jeopardizes an organization's ability to receive those funds, may require those funds to be returned in certain circumstances, and could even subject an ambulance service to criminal penalties.

Even the proper management of expenses and cash flow is a key to keeping an organization healthy. Understanding how to plan expenses, knowing how to effectively utilize vendor payment terms, and having a working knowledge of when it is appropriate or advantageous to borrow money are all skills that can allow an ambulance service to run most effectively. Unfortunately, none of these finance and accounting topics can be adequately covered in a single chapter, so this chapter is intended as an overview of major financial topics. College-level finance and accounting courses are an excellent way to build on these topics, and technical training on billing and collections methodologies would also serve to add to your knowledge of these topics.

■ GENERAL FINANCIAL MANAGEMENT

The finance function within any organization exists to monitor and effectively manage resources. In larger ambulance organizations, this function may be a separate department or may be housed outside of the ambulance organization if ambulance service is only part of a larger group of services, such as in a hospital or large municipal organization. In a smaller organization, all of the financial functions may be overseen by one person. Regardless of the size and scope of the financial organization, the responsibilities for finance activities often fall into two broad categories: the finance function that is responsible for management of funds and the accounting function that tracks funds throughout the organization.

Responsibilities and titles within a finance function may vary considerably. In many cases, the treasurer position is often an officer of the board of directors or an elected government official who is ultimately responsible for organizational funds. Treasurers also often take a lead role in establishing external audits of the organization's finances that may be required by law.

The chief financial officer (CFO), by contrast, is often a senior manager reporting to the chief executive. The CFO deals with financial issues related to both finance and accounting. The finance function is often also tasked with the preparation and monitoring of the organization's **budget**.

THE FINANCE FUNCTION

In general terms, the finance function manages money. Activities of the finance function may include some or all of the following:

- Establishing organizational bank accounts
- Developing procedures for disbursement of funds
- Securing and managing credit on behalf of the organization
- Establishing organizational budgets
- Determining organizational investments
- Ensuring the availability of cash when needed
- Planning for and financing capital purchases
- Managing or overseeing **accounts receivable** and collections activities
- Advising senior management on funding issues

As noted, titles for personnel in this area can vary considerably and may include such titles as chief financial officer, fiscal officer, financial manager, and so on. The finance function may also include additional areas of responsibilities, such as **accounts payable**, accounts receivable, credit management, petty cash, and such.

THE ACCOUNTING/CONTROLLER FUNCTION

The accounting function is often led by the controller, chief accounting officer (CAO), or comptroller. The controller's main responsibilities are tracking the organization's funds as well as preparing internal financial reports and standard financial statements for internal and external use. In addition, the accounting function is often involved with the filing and payment of taxes. The controller frequently develops and monitors financial controls within the organization. Accounting departments also often track major capital assets of the organization and, in conjunction with the finance function, may participate in their acquisition and sale.

RELATIONSHIP WITH OPERATING AND SUPPORT DEPARTMENTS

Although the finance function is responsible for the management and tracking of funds, its role is not to make key financial decisions for an organization. To the contrary, one of the responsibilities of finance and accounting staff is to ensure that managers responsible for all aspects of the organization have appropriate knowledge of available financial resources and the tools needed to monitor their specific financial activities. Although the CFO is often a participant in major organizational decisions, he or she is also responsible for allocating or obtaining the funding necessary to carry out major organizational activities or strategic initiatives.

Side Bar
How is financial management structured in your organization?
Who manages the money in your organization? Do you have a treasurer on the board of directors, a full-time chief financial officer, an independent accountant, or some combination of both? What is the role of the organization's

chief executive in establishing, reviewing, and approving financial transactions? How much do front-line managers in your organization know about revenues, expenses, and budgets?

■ OVERVIEW OF ACCOUNTING SYSTEMS

Accounting is the systematic recording, reporting, and analysis of financial transactions of a business according to a set of rules. Individuals who perform this function are often referred to as accountants. Accounting is accomplished through the use of a number of accounts that are used to follow the flow of funds through an organization. Unlike a bank account, accounts in the accounting context are not discrete amounts of money located at a financial institution but, instead, serve as a collection of categories that are used to track funds within an organization.

GENERALLY ACCEPTED ACCOUNTING PRINCIPLES

Generally Accepted Accounting Principles (GAAP) are rules that accountants are required to follow when tracking and reporting financial transactions. In the United States, most businesses, both for-profit and nonprofit, follow the procedures outlined by the Financial Accounting Standards Board (FASB). FASB is a nongovernmental organization. FASB rules must be followed by publicly held corporations and are often required for tax reporting purposes, giving them the force of law in many instances. FASB standards, however, do not define how to record specific transactions, but they often address the broader aspects of how the use of funds should be recorded. Standards are also changed over time to reflect the evolution of accounting practice and new situations that may be encountered. Governmental organizations in the United

States follow the generally accepted accounting principles outlined by the Governmental Accounting Standards Board (GASB), which is also a nongovernmental standard-setting organization. GASB standards are used by state governments, and state laws often require that local governments also follow GASB standards.

TYPES OF ACCOUNTING

Fundamental tools are used in all funds-tracking activities, whether the manufacturing of widgets or the operations of an ambulance service. These tools, once understood, become essential to understanding how organizations acquire and utilize funds at the organizational, departmental, and functional levels. Accounting concerned with users external to the organization is called **financial accounting**, and activities concerned with the internal use of funds is **managerial accounting**. Both forms of accounting are important to the ongoing financial health of an organization.

CHART OF ACCOUNTS

The **chart of accounts** is a collection of categories tied to the elements of the basic financial statements: general ledger, balance sheet, income statement, cash flow statement, and budget. In some organizations, hundreds of accounts can be used to categorize and subcategorize transactions. All transactions are coded to an account, and often a transaction in one account leads to a corresponding transaction in one or more different accounts. These corresponding transactions are described by the terms *debit* and *credit*, and they do not necessarily reflect a decrease or increase in funds, but instead reflect the impact of one activity on another. For example, the purchase of an item would increase an asset account and decrease a cash account. Although it is not important for a nonaccounting professional to understand the details of debit and credit transactions, it is important to know that these transactions serve as the basis of double-entry bookkeeping, which is a fundamental tenet of GAAP and essential to the preparation of financial reports.

GENERAL LEDGER

General ledger is an historic term for where all double-entry accounting transactions were recorded. Prior to computerized accounting systems, these transactions were often recorded in a large book and were collectively referred to as "the books" of a company or organization. Today, the general ledger is computerized and serves as a collection point for all of the transactions conducted by a business or government organization.

Accrual versus Cash Accounting

With a few limited exceptions, GAAP requires that most organizations utilize accrual accounting. Accrual accounting recognizes a transaction at the time it is made, as opposed to when cash changes hands. For an ambulance service this means that revenue is recorded when an ambulance call is billed. In keeping with the principles of double-entry booking, an increase in revenue is combined with an increase in accounts receivable. Correspondingly, when payment is received, cash is increased and accounts receivable is decreased. Similar principles play out on the expense side where loans are recorded at the time they are received for the full amount, despite the fact that cash may not be used to repay those loans for years. The primary purpose of accrual accounting is to be able to effectively record and easily understand the financial position of an organization within discrete time periods. Since cash often changes hands long after a bill is generated, or a loan is repaid, accrual accounting is much more useful than cash accounting. Considering just the example of an ambulance bill, imagine how

difficult it would be to determine annual revenue performance by only recording payments that may have occurred on ambulance bills this year, last year, or potentially years in the past.

BALANCE SHEET

The balance sheet, statement of financial position, or statement of net assets is a summary of an organization's assets, liabilities, and equity. The balance sheet, unlike other financial statements, is a snapshot of a particular moment in time. Other financial statements show activity over a period of time. The balance sheet is so named because it must balance using the formula of assets = liabilities + equity. Assets are the cash, investments, accounts receivable, inventory, and physical assets of an organization. Liabilities represent amounts owed by the organization. Equity is a combination of the paid-in capital and **retained earnings/equity** of an organization and may go by the terms *owner's equity, stockholder's equity, surplus,* or *retained earnings.* A balance sheet of a government-owned paramedic service is shown in Figure 14.1.

Balance sheets usually list assets from the most liquid (cash and cash equivalents) to the least liquid (property, plant, and equipment). Some assets, such as accounts receivable and equipment, are adjusted to reflect their likely actual value. Accounts receivable is offset by an allowance for doubtful accounts, which can be significant for health care organizations. Physical assets are often shown at their depreciated value. It is important to note, however, that these adjustments are an estimate of value and may not reflect the actual value of these assets if the organization were liquidated. Liabilities are also listed on the balance sheet from the most current to the least current financial obligations. Equity is usually listed with paid-in capital first, followed by

COUNTY OF WELD
STATE OF COLORADO

Statement of Net Assets
Proprietary Funds

December 31, 2009

	Business-type Activity	Governmental Activities
	Paramedic Enterprise Fund	Internal Service Funds
ASSETS		
Cash and short-term investments	$ 960,701	$ 9,170,486
Property taxes receivable	-	1,506,012
Receivables (net of allowance for uncollectibles):		
Accounts	1,488,136	585,852
Due from other County funds	-	16,200
Inventory	-	71,813
Other assets	-	36,556
Total Current Assets	2,448,837	11,386,919
Capital Assets:		
Land	48,496	-
Improvements other than buildings	55,728	580,500
Buildings	710,305	1,800,977
Machinery and equipment	1,286,367	32,750,701
Accumulated depreciation	(1,089,672)	(19,942,939)
Total Capital Assets	1,011,224	15,189,239
Total Assets	3,460,061	26,576,158
LIABILITIES AND FUND EQUITY		
Current Liabilities:		
Accounts payable	67,822	684,727
Accrued liabilities	299,328	1,743,643
Due to other County funds	823	2,958
Deferred revenue	-	2,476,293
Total Current Liabilities	367,973	4,907,621
Net Assets		
Invested in capital assets	1,011,224	15,189,239
Restricted for:		
Workers' compensation	-	879,753
Unrestricted	2,080,864	5,599,545
Total net assets	$ 3,092,088	$ 21,668,537

Some amounts reported for business-type activities in the statement of net assets are different because certain internal service fund assets and liabilities are included with business-type activities. — (397,544)

Net assets of business-type activities — $ 3,489,632

See accompanying notes to the basic financial statements

FIGURE 14.1 ■ Example of a balance sheet of a public paramedic service. *Source: Public Paramedic Service.*

retained earnings. In companies that pay dividends to the owners, equity is reduced when dividend payments are made. Nonprofit organizations often consider retained earnings to be a surplus. Based on the financial position of the organization, equity can be a negative or deficit number.

INCOME STATEMENT

The income statement is the most commonly known accounting statement and may be referred to using a variety of terms. An income statement may be referred to as a profit and loss (P&L), statement of financial performance, statement of operations, earnings statement, operations statement, or statement of changes in net assets. Unlike the balance sheet that reports financial condition at a specific point, the income statement captures performance over a period of time. Income statements usually measure performance over a month, quarter, or year. The statement is often divided into the two main areas of revenue and expense and may be further subdivided into operating and nonoperating categories (Figure 14.2).

The difference between income and expense is referred to as net income and is the figure most often referred to as the bottom line. Although net income is often the final calculation on the income statement, a number of the preceding calculations are used for other analytic purposes. Those fields that may appear could include gross profit or gross income, earnings before depreciation (EBD), earning before taxes (EBT), or earnings before interest, depreciation, taxes, and amortization (EBIDTA). Depreciation represents a noncash operating expense to reflect the use of assets in the operation of the business. The rate of depreciation may be dictated by useful life of the equipment and/or specific tax code requirements. In a similar vein, interest reflects the financing cost for an organization

to conduct business pretax income (EBT), which is a useful measure for private sector organizations to gauge profitability. Amortization is a collection of accounts that need to increase or decrease over time, which often represents the principle balance being paid on a loan. All of these calculations cumulatively are captured in EBIDTA and then are adjusted to net income in order for the organization to more fully understand its revenues and expenses.

In most ambulance organizations, income categories include patient billing fees, contractual revenue, training fees, public support (taxes, subsidies, etc.), and various subcategories. Nonoperating revenue may include interest income, grant income, and sale of assets. Based on the primary activities of the organization, categorization may vary between operating and nonoperating accounts.

Operating expenses include payroll costs, supplies, fuel, maintenance, rent, utilities, and any other areas or subcategories of expenses important to the organization. Most ambulance services also record a category of significant bad debt, uncollectible accounts, or contractual write-offs to reflect portions of ambulance bills that are expected to be unpaid. This amount often varies between 20 percent and 70 percent of revenue for most ambulance services and reflects a key financial consideration when providing emergency health care services. Most such write-offs are recorded after an account has been in collections for a period of time. As such, the income statement will usually reflect the amount billed in a period offset by the amounts written off during that same period. By this method, all accounts written off, regardless of their actual age, would be subtracted from the current year's revenue. This represents the collection rate on an accrual basis. A cash collection rate would be determined by calculating actual cash payments on accounts during a given period.

COUNTY OF WELD
STATE OF COLORADO

**Statement of Revenue, Expenses and
Changes in Net Assets
Proprietary Funds**

For the fiscal year ended December 31, 2009

	Business-type Activity	Governmental Activities
	Paramedic Enterprise Fund	Internal Service Funds
Operating revenues:		
Contributions	$ -	$ 11,056,492
Charges for services	7,426,884	8,796,968
Total operating revenues	7,426,884	19,853,460
Operating expenses:		
Bad debt expense	3,521,859	-
Personnel services	4,293,947	167,766
Supplies	299,732	1,835,244
Purchased services	903,899	3,932,245
Insurance and bonds	-	948,696
Depreciation	253,894	2,976,118
Other	28,077	107,690
Claims	-	12,341,260
Total operating expenses	9,301,408	22,309,019
Operating income (loss)	(1,874,524)	(2,455,559)
Nonoperating revenues (expenses):		
Taxes	-	1,497,239
Miscellaneous	30,820	100
Interest income	-	60,236
Fees	12,083	-
Federal grant	-	500,000
State Grant	84,750	-
Gain (loss) on disposition of assets	5,225	269,695
Judgements and damages	-	40,436
Total nonoperating revenues (expenses)	132,878	2,367,706
Income (loss) before contributions or transfers	(1,741,646)	(87,853)
Capital contributions	3,556	-
Transfers–in	1,385,000	1,000,000
Changes in net assets	(353,090)	912,147
Total net assets beginning of year	3,445,178	20,756,390
Total net assets at end of year	$ 3,092,088	$ 21,668,537
Some amounts reported for business-type activities in the statement of activities are different because the net revenue (expense) of certain internal service funds is reported with business-type activities.	(9,583)	
Change in net assets of business-type activities	$ (362,673)	

See accompanying notes to the basic financial statements

FIGURE 14.2 ■ Example of an income statement of a public paramedic service. *Source: Public Paramedic Service.*

In some cases, particularly in nonprofit and governmental organizations, separate income statements are kept for funds that may be managed or tracked independently. In private sector organizations, this accounting activity may be categorized by profit centers or service lines. Reasons for accounting for certain activities independently can occur for a variety of reasons, especially in large, complex organizations. The most common reasons in an ambulance service may be to account for specific grant funding, separate geographic locations, or for ambulance activity that is run as an independent business unit within a fire department or hospital.

CASH FLOW STATEMENT

The cash flow statement, or **statement of cash flows**, is specifically intended to track increases or decreases in cash over a period of time within an organization. As mentioned, some transactions are noncash in nature, such as depreciation. Other cash transactions are related to events recorded on an accrual basis that may have occurred in other accounting periods. In addition, some items, such as payments, are not recorded on the income statement using the accrual accounting method and must be reconciled to the balance sheet cash amounts. Although it is likely the least well-known financial statement, the cash flow statement addresses all of these issues and is often critical to running the organization. Cash flow statements are usually divided into operating, investing, and financing categories. They can be prepared using a direct or an indirect method; however, GAAP frequently requires use of the indirect method. Using the indirect method, the cash flow statement begins with the net income number from the income statement and reconciles to the change in cash and cash equivalents on the balance sheet (Figure 14.3).

Side Bar
Obtain financial statements from a local ambulance service. Review the elements of those statements and compare how they relate to the principles described in this section. If unable to obtain local examples, use a public filing such as can be found at www.airmethods.com/airmethods/investors.

Ambulance Service Revenue Sources

Ambulance services in the United States are primarily funded through the two sources of fees for service and public (tax) support. Although additional revenue sources exist, such as user subscriptions, membership drives, contract services or grant funding, in most cases these sources do not account for the majority of funding a service receives. Fee-for-service revenue is discussed in additional detail in "Revenue Stream Management: Life of a Chart," later in this chapter. It is common to fund an ambulance service exclusively through fees or exclusively through public funding. Some services are supported exclusively through donations. In many cases, however, ambulance organizations access a variety of revenue sources, and it is important for a manager of a service to fully understand all of the revenue sources applicable to the organization.

It is worth noting that public funding, regardless of its structure or source, is associated with substantial accountability and scrutiny by the governing body providing the funds. Although public funding is often more stable than fee-for-service revenue, it is subject to fluctuation and could be substantially modified or eliminated by the governing body that provides it. Public funding is also not exclusive to governmental agencies. In some cases, public funding is provided to privately owned providers through a contractual relationship. Funding of private organizations is often referred to as an operating grant or subsidy.

COUNTY OF WELD
STATE OF COLORADO

Combining Statement of Cash Flows
Proprietary Funds

For the fiscal year ended December 31, 2009

	Business-type Activity Enterprise Fund Paramedic Services	Governmental Activities Internal Service Funds
CASH FLOWS FROM OPERATING ACTIVITIES		
Cash flows from external customers	$ 5,242,769	$ 510,869
Cash flows from internal customers	-	19,417,273
Cash payments to external suppliers for goods and services	(987,897)	(17,960,872)
Cash payments to internal suppliers for goods and services	(556,297)	(191,520)
Cash payments to employees for services	(4,192,315)	(366,247)
Judgements/damages/losses	-	40,436
Miscellaneous revenues	-	100
Net cash provided (used) by operating activities	(494,341)	1,450,039
CASH FLOWS FROM NONCAPITAL FINANCING ACTIVITIES		
Taxes	-	1,495,839
Transfers/Advances	800,000	1,000,000
Grants	84,750	-
Other	42,903	-
Net cash provided by noncapital financing activities	927,653	2,495,839
CASH FLOWS FROM CAPITAL AND RELATED FINANCING ACTIVITIES		
Acquisition of capital assets	(185,436)	(3,207,920)
Proceeds from sale of capital assets	5,225	373,362
Net cash provided (used) for capital and related Financing activities	(180,211)	(2,834,558)
CASH FLOWS FROM INVESTING ACTIVITIES		
Interest on investments	-	60,236
Net Increase (decrease) in Cash and Cash Equivalents	253,101	1,171,556
Cash and Cash Equivalents at Beginning of Year	707,600	7,998,930
Cash and Cash Equivalents at End of Year	$ 960,701	$ 9,170,486
Reconciliation of operating income to net cash provided (used) by operating activities:		
Operating income (loss)	$ (1,874,524)	$ (2,455,559)
Adjustments to reconcile operating income to net cash provided (used) by operating activities:		
Depreciation expense	253,894	2,976,118
Judgements/damages/losses	-	40,436
Miscellaneous revenue	-	100
Change in assets and liabilities		
(Increase) decrease in accounts receivable	1,197,841	(44,102)
(Increase) decrease in due from other funds	-	280,479
(Increase) decrease in inventories	-	(28,106)
(Increase) decrease in other assets	197	-
Increase (decrease) in accounts payable	(48,929)	223,955
Increase (decrease) in accrued liabilities	(23,558)	375,368
Increase (decrease) in other liabilities	738	(16,502)
Increase (decrease) in deferred revenue	-	97,852
Total adjustments	1,380,183	3,905,598
Net cash provided by operating activities	$ (494,341)	$ 1,450,039
Noncash investing, capital, and financing activities:		
Contributions of capital assets from (to) government	$ -	$ (3,556)
Loss on Disposal of Asset	-	$ 15,667
See Accompanying notes to the basic financial statements		

FIGURE 14.3 ■ Example of a cash flow statement of a public paramedic service. *Source: Public Paramedic Service.*

BUDGETS

Budgets are the primary financial planning tool used by all organizations. They often exist at the organizational, departmental, work unit, and project levels. Budgets project revenue and set targets for expenditures over a given period of time and are usually tracked at the monthly, quarterly, and annual intervals. A budget can be viewed as an organizational plan expressed in monetary terms. Organizational budgets are often structured to reflect and measure the strategic goals of an organization. Performance against budget is also a standard analysis used by the management of an organization to measure financial health, validate forecasts, and monitor spending activity. In many cases, budgets are reflective of accounts used in the income statement; however, budgets used specifically for planning cash flow may be developed and followed. It is also common to develop specialized budgets for specific projects or capital purchases. Budgets developed for planning purposes to evaluate a future project or activity that may or may not occur are referred to as pro forma budgets and may be developed in conjunction with other pro forma financial statements.

In governmental ambulance services, budgets may be developed through a process specified in state or local regulations. Such budgets usually require the opportunity for public comment and adoption by elected officials. Although overspending a private budget likely only has consequences internal to an organization, overspending a public budget may have legal and regulatory implications.

In most cases, budgets rely on assumptions that must be evaluated and adjusted over time. Revenue targets, in particular, are projected for ambulance services based on anticipated call volume, collection rates, or tax receipts. Expenses are usually estimated based on historic experience. Major deviations from these assumptions may cause an organization

to rework its budget. In the event of a major change in assumptions or financial conditions, budgets may need to be adjusted or completely redone mid-cycle.

> ### Side Bar
>
> Review the HRSA rural ambulance service budget model at ftp://ftp.hrsa.gov/ruralhealth/AmbulanceBudgetModel.pdf. Would this budget model work in your ambulance service?

■ PRODUCTION MEASURES———

Measurement of productivity is an important activity for any organization. Productivity measurement provides an organization's leadership insight into how effectively the organization's resources are being used. Productivity is important regardless of the public or private nature of the organization. Ambulance service, as a personnel intensive activity, requires substantial investment in people in order to provide service. The productivity of the organization is based on the effective deployment of personnel and efficient management of the vehicles, equipment, and technology used to support ambulance response activity. Although organizations may chose to evaluate different factors in the measurement of productivity, measurements using unit hours and per call calculations are the most frequently used basis for this measurement.

UNIT HOUR COST

An ambulance **unit hour** represents the deployment of one ambulance for 1 hour of time. An ambulance that is deployed around the clock represents 24 unit hours per day or 8,760 (365×24) unit hours per year. In most ambulance services, a deployed unit represents a staffed unit ready for immediate response for a call. Large ambulance systems often measure their daily unit hours. A volunteer service can measure unit hours by determining the amount of time volunteers were available to respond to ambulance calls. It is also possible to calculate the amount of unit hours staffed with on-call or reserve personnel. This determination, however, becomes more difficult when an organization utilizes a variety of staffing methods as no standard adjustment is available to compare staffed units to on-call units or volunteer units. In some cases, it may not be possible to even measure the availability of volunteer units if no predetermined schedule of available response personnel is used.

Regardless of these complexities, a unit hour is the most common unit of production within the ambulance industry. Based on this measurement, unit hour cost is determined by dividing the annual expenses of the organization by the annual number of unit hours. Once calculated, cost per unit hour can be compared across periods, or even between organizations to get a relative sense of economic efficiency. A number of other calculations can also be made utilizing unit hours as a basis.

COST PER CALL

As an alternative to the unit hour method, overall costs can be divided by call volume to determine the **cost per call**. This method, however, is highly influenced by the call volume denominator and will cause smaller call volume services to appear more costly. Regardless of this issue, however, understanding cost per call, and secondarily cost per transport, gives a manager an estimate of how much revenue must be generated on a per call basis for the ambulance service to break even.

Side Bar

Review the most recent Ambulance Service Victoria annual report and financial report online (www.ambulance.vic.gov.au/Media/docs/AV%20Annual%20Report%202011-2012%20Web-d8ebb0d0-2bd2-402d-9dd2-4af241ab5506-0.pdf). Review the budget categories and calculate the cost per call for this Australian ambulance service. For added practice, calculate the changes in cost per call over multiple years.

■ FINANCIAL MANAGEMENT

Ambulance services can employ several modes of financial management tools to successfully evaluate and improve their financial stability and solvency.

DAYS SALES OUTSTANDING

Days sales outstanding (DSO) allows health care companies to determine the amount of time it takes from a patient encounter to account resolution. Since ambulance services cannot estimate or collect revenue for emergency transports prior to transport, there will always be an accounts receivable balance. Measuring DSO allows ambulance services to gauge the effectiveness of their collection practices and compare these efforts against other companies within the industry.

Calculating Days Sales Outstanding
The calculation is as follows:

$$DSO = \frac{Accounts\,Receivable}{Patient\,Encounters\,in\,Period} \times Days\,in\,Period$$

For example, ABC Ambulance Service transported 100 patients in the month of October, generating sales of $100,000. It began the month of October with $50,000 in receivables.

* The company collected $1,000 for a transport that occurred on October 5 prior to transport.
* The company generated invoices to various **third-party** payment sources for the balance of the transports, net 30 days payment terms. The total credit/invoice sales for October are $99,000. (The $1,000 the company received prior to transport and never invoiced to the customer cannot be factored into the credit/invoice sales. The DSO on that cash payment is 0.)
* During the month of October, the company received $45,000 in payments. So $50,000 + $99,000 − $45,000 = $104,000 in accounts receivable.
* $104,000 in accounts receivable is the result of $50,000 in accounts receivable prior to October *plus* the credit/sales of $90,000 invoiced in October *minus* the $45,000 in payments received in October. (It does not matter to what invoices the payments were applied. DSO only looks at what the accounts receivable is as of the end of October.)
* The accounts receivable at the end of October is $104,000. The DSO for the month of October would be $104,000/$99,000 × 31 (# of days in October) = 33.

The average DSO for ABC Ambulance Service to obtain payment is 33 days. This means that it takes an average of 33 days from the date of transport for payment to be received.

It is important to note that DSO is an efficiency measurement, not an effectiveness measurement, regarding collection efforts. We will continue to discuss other measurements that can be used, in conjunction with DSO, to evaluate collection efforts.

DAYS TO BILL

Days to bill is beneficial for determining how long it takes from the patient encounter to bill the invoice to the respective payer source. This calculation allows management to determine where process improvements need to be made. Lengthy days to bill are usually attributed to

inappropriate or incomplete documentation from field staff, delay in charge entry from billing staff, or a need for workflow changes.

Calculating Days to Bill
The calculation is as follows:

$$\text{Days to Bill} = \frac{\text{Date of Transport}}{\text{Date Claim Filed}}$$

For example, ABC Ambulance Service transports a patient on October 1. The paramedic completes the medical record and turns in the medical record. The business office inputs the medical record into its billing program on October 3. After review, the business office discovers that no insurance information is listed for the patient; however, the patient is over the age of 65. On October 4, the billing office calls the hospital that treated the patient to verify if the patient had insurance coverage. Insurance information is obtained on October 5 and filed to the insurance company.

* Transport occurred on October 1.
* Claim was filed to the insurance company on October 5.

The claim took 4 days to bill from the date of transport.

Delays in entering charges and submitting claims equate to free financing. It is important to file the claim as quickly as possible. Electronic medical records can reduce the amount of time it takes to bill a transport from the date of service.

REVENUE AND CASH PER TRANSPORT BENCHMARKS

Another metric that ambulance services use to determine if their collection programs are effective is revenue and cash per transport benchmarks. It is important for ambulance services to establish these benchmarks not only for budgetary reasons, but also to effectively evaluate insurance, facility, or government contracts.

Revenue per transport (RPT) is defined as the number of transports in a given period divided by gross revenue in the same given period. Cash per transport (CPT) is defined as the number of transports in a given period divided by the cash received in the same given period.

Cash Collections to Revenue Billed

By dividing cash collections into revenue billed, an ambulance company can determine the percentage of uncollectible income. Uncollectible income can be attributed to three main factors: (1) contractual relationships with Medicare, Medicaid, or other contracted insurance companies; (2) bad debt; and (3) poor collection practices.

How companies can set and implement appropriate key performance indicators (KPIs), benchmarks, and lean management techniques to improve cash collections is discussed later in this chapter. It is important to note here that contractual relationships with Medicare and Medicaid typically have mandated fee schedules that are set by federal and state governments. These fee schedules can be changed through legislative directives only.

REVENUE STREAM MANAGEMENT: LIFE OF A CHART

When viewed in the context of revenue stream management, the life of a chart refers to the length of time it takes from the date of transport to the payment or resolution of the transport.

Process improvements are recognized when management continually explores the life of a chart. Management can pose many questions, such as the following:

1. How can I improve my days to bill?
2. Is crew documentation sufficient to satisfy billing, federal, and state requirements?
3. Was the ticket coded appropriately for payment purposes?

4. If a denial was received from the insurance company, could it have been avoided if documentation had been sufficient or coding more accurate and specific?
5. Did the insurance company process the claim correctly the first time?
6. Are internal processes and procedures working effectively?
7. Are benchmarks appropriate?

Numerous other questions and processes can be explored for continuous process improvement by exploring the life of a chart.

■ HEALTH CARE PAYERS

Ambulance services are funded through two sources: fee for service and public (tax) funds. Fee-for-service ambulance providers, private and public, will typically bill the following revenue sources: Medicare, Medicaid, private health insurance, or some other contracted source.

MEDICARE

Medicare is a government-sponsored program that provides health insurance coverage to individuals over age 65 or who meet other specific criteria. This program is administered by the Centers for Medicare & Medicaid Services (CMS).

All individuals who have been legal residents of the United States for at least 5 years and are at least age 65 are eligible for Medicare. It is important to note that if the individual or the individual's spouse has not paid Medicare taxes for at least 10 years, a monthly premium will be required to enroll in Medicare.

Individuals under age 65 may also be eligible for enrollment if they meet the following requirements:

1. Disabled and have been receiving Social Security benefits for at least 24 months from the date of the disability; or
2. They have end-stage renal disease (ESRD) and require continuous dialysis treatment; or

3. They are eligible for Social Security Disability Insurance and have Lou Gehrig disease.

An individual who has qualified for insurance through both Medicare and Medicaid is known as a dual-eligible member. Medicaid will pay for the beneficiaries' Medicare Part B and D premium. We discuss Medicaid in the next section.

There are four types of Medicare:

- Part A is hospital insurance coverage.
- Part B is medical insurance coverage.
- Part C is coverage under a Medicare Advantage Plan.
- Part D is prescription drug coverage.

Ambulance services, unless hospital based, will bill all fee for services for Medicare recipients under Part B or to a Medicare Advantage Plan. Hospital-based services typically bill under Part A coverage.

Part B providers are paid at 80 percent of the current Medicare fee schedule, which is posted annually at the CMS website: www.cms.gov. If a Medicare recipient has not met his annual deductible, the payment will be reduced by the deductible amount.

Payments for Medicare services are administered through fiscal intermediaries who are contracted with CMS. These fiscal intermediaries are responsible for provider contracting and claims payment. Billing Medicare requires registration with the CMS. Individuals or organizations contemplating entry into the ambulance business must be aware that a National Provider Identifier (NPI) number is necessary before the organization can bill Medicare. This can be a lengthy process. Detailed information can be obtained from the Centers for Medicare & Medicaid Services (2012).

MEDICAID

Medicaid is a federally and state-funded program for individuals and families with low incomes and limited resources. Each state is responsible for administering this program with oversight from CMS since federal funds are distributed to the states to provide this care.

Title XIX of the Social Security Act of 1965 established or created the Medicaid system as we know it today; however, it is a voluntary program and states are not required to participate. All states do participate in Medicaid, and each state has employed a myriad of tactics to provide care to this specific population while working within budget constraints and the requirements of the program. Some states have created managed care organizations where private insurance companies contract directly with the state to manage these recipients for a fixed price per enrollee, while other states pay providers directly and manage the Medicaid dollars exclusively. Some states have privatized certain portions of the Medicaid program and manage the other portions directly. However the states decide to manage their Medicaid program, one common theme always prevails: *Yearly Medicaid Budget Crisis!*

Medicaid eligibility is determined by each state, so we will not go into too much detail regarding this. Medicaid is designed to provide insurance to individuals and their families who are at 133 percent of the Federal Poverty Level (FPL); however, there are exceptions to this rule.

PRIVATE HEALTH INSURANCE

Private health insurance is best defined as any insurance plan that is not funded by the government. There are two types of insurance policies that patients can have: (1) employer sponsored and (2) individual. The majority of individuals with private health insurance coverage are covered under an employer-sponsored program.

Most private health insurance covers emergency ambulance transportation. Each plan may subject the patient to a deductible and/or out-of-pocket expense, commonly referred to as co-payment or co-insurance.

Nonemergency transportation, such as hospital discharges to residence or nursing facilities, may or may not be covered under the patient's plan. It is important that ambulance services verify the patient's insurance benefit prior to transport. Insurance companies may also require that nonemergency transportation be preauthorized prior to transport.

Preauthorization requires the ambulance service to obtain an approval number from the patient's insurance company in order to receive payment for services. In the absence of an approval number, the ambulance service may not be paid for the transport.

CONTRACTED SERVICES

Contracted services are typically referred to as contractual agreements between the ambulance service and a contracted entity, typically a health care provider or government entity. Ambulance services can contract with government entities, such as the Veterans Administration or the U.S. Military, to provide ambulance services for a fixed price. These contracts are issued through a request for proposal (RFP) process.

Another type of contracted service would be an agreement between the ambulance service and a health care facility to provide services for that facility. Payment terms are usually outlined as part of the agreement. These agreements are subject to the Omnibus Budget Reconciliation Act, commonly referred to as the "Stark Law," which governs physician self-referral for Medicare and Medicaid patients. These contractual agreements should consider anti-kickback provisions as well.

It is important to always consult with legal counsel when entering into contractual relationships with federal, state, local, and private entities to ensure that there are no legal implications which may cause financial penalties and sanctions by the federal government.

■ PUBLIC FINANCING OF AMBULANCE SERVICES ——————

Public financing of ambulance services, achieved through tax subsidies, is a common method of financing ambulance services. In certain areas of the United States, ambulance services are fully subsidized by tax dollars, while other counties receive partial subsidies and bill Medicare, Medicaid, and private health insurance companies to balance their budgets.

It is becoming more and more popular for local governments to respond to a request for proposals (RFPs) in a bid to have their emergency and nonemergency transport services provided by private ambulance companies. Some local governments will subsidize these services with a monthly subsidy, while others will not. Typically these RFPs are written with specific deliverables, including response criteria, coverage requirements, and sometimes rate caps. Public financing of ambulance services requires a vote from residents, and any increase in the subsidy through tax dollars must be voted on by local government.

■ BILLING OPERATIONS——————

Ambulance services, as well as most health care entities, will perform billing functions in house or contract with an agency to perform all billing functions and pay a per-transport fee or a percentage of cash collected. For a myriad of reasons, ambulance services decide to outsource their revenue cycle to an external agency.

These reasons include, but are not limited to, the following:

1. Availability of personnel with revenue cycle knowledge, specific to ambulance reimbursements

2. Cost analysis that shows it would be cheaper to outsource
3. Prioritization of resource allocation

Typically, it is cheaper for an ambulance service with a high volume of transports to perform its billing functions in house. An ambulance service should always conduct a cost analysis prior to contracting with a billing agency. This cost analysis can be performed by an internal accounting department or an external consultant who is not tied to obtaining the business of the ambulance service.

■ SELF-PAY MANAGEMENT

Self-pay management is an area that continually plagues the ambulance industry. Since ambulance services are not allowed to screen emergency transports or refuse to treat patients who present with an emergency medical condition, patients without insurance continue to be transported and innovative solutions must be explored to obtain payment from this group of patients after the fact.

Ambulance services should implement a self-pay management process, geared to the organization's revenue cycle, in order to determine if these patients qualify for supplemental financial resources or Medicaid. These services may be available by contracting with an outside vendor or creating an internal workflow or process to analyze the data to identify the patient's ability and capacity to pay for medical services.

EARLY OUT

One way for ambulance services to manage self-pay accounts is to institute an early-out program. This program utilizes a third-party agency to collect, for a nominal percentage fee, from patients who are self-pay within 90 days from the transport. This requires the ambulance service to send this agency the customer account within 28 days from the date of service. An early-out agency will develop a program to collect on these accounts for 90 days for a percentage of what it collects. Early-out programs should not be confused with hard collections. Early-out agencies are an extension of the ambulance service, and the patient is not aware that the account has been referred to this agency.

COLLECTION AGENCIES

Another avenue to self-pay management is to utilize a collection agency to collect on those accounts where the ambulance service has been unable to obtain payment. A collection agency is typically used when an ambulance service has exhausted all efforts to collect payment. Due to the Fair Debt Collection and Practices Act and the many requirements associated, ambulance services typically contract with an agency or agencies to handle external collections and credit reporting.

Larger companies with extensive self-pay receivables may use several agencies in order to have comparative analysis among the agencies they use. It is important to provide the collection agencies with benchmarks to hold them accountable to results. These agencies will typically charge a percentage of collections that is negotiated based on revenue volumes.

Second placement agencies are typically used after the first collection agency has had the account for at least a year. Some ambulance services will retract the accounts from the first agency if no payment has been received by the patient and will send it to the second placement. Due to the age of these accounts, second placement agencies will typically charge a recovery fee of 40 percent to 50 percent.

CHAPTER REVIEW

Summary

Ambulance service financial management methods are similar to those used by many other private and public sector organizations and are heavily influenced by the same health care payment mechanisms as the rest of health care. Ambulance service managers should have a fundamental understanding of basic accounting and financial management practices and should be familiar with the major financial issues related to the provision of ambulance service. The analysis of financial performance and the projection of future performance are key to the budgeting process that establishes how ambulance service will be provided. As most ambulance services charge for service, it is also imperative that ambulance managers understand the billing and collection cycle.

WHAT WOULD YOU DO? Reflection

With the help of the finance team, you have completed the analysis of the revenue generated by ambulance runs to the closing industrial facility and found that it accounts for only 1 percent of the annual revenue generated by your service. You have further determined that the loss of this call volume will decrease the unit hour utilization of your night-shift units, yet will only decrease the revenues of your service by 1 percent. You have also estimated a small increase in the amount of Medicaid and self-pay calls once the facility closes. Overall, you anticipate this will allow for a reduction in the amount of night-shift coverage and an increase in uncollectible accounts. You have prepared pro forma financial statements reflective of these changes that will be shared by the CEO with the board of directors.

Review Questions

1. Describe the difference between the finance and accounting functions.
2. Explain the role of accounting standards.
3. What are the key elements of the balance sheet and what must "balance"?
4. What are the differences between the balance sheet, income statement, and cash flow statement?
5. Describe what managerial accounting measures are important for ambulance services.
6. What is the role of the budget?
7. Describe the major sources payment for ambulance service.
8. List the steps in the ambulance billing and collections cycle.

References

American Institute of Certified Public Accountants. (2012). "Statements on Quality Control Standards." See the organization website.

Centers for Medicare & Medicaid Services. (2012a). "National Provider Identifier

Standard (NPI)." See the organization website.

Centers for Medicare & Medicaid Services. (2012b). "Medicare Claims Processing Manual. Chapter 15 – Ambulance." See the organization website.

Financial Accounting Standards Board. (2010). *FASB Codification (2010 Edition).* Norwalk, CT.

Office of Inspector General. (2006). "Medicare Payments for Ambulance Transports." See the organization website.

Siciliano, G.(2003). *Finance for Non-Financial Managers.* Madison, WI: McGraw-Hill.

State of Colorado, County of Weld. (2009). "2009 Comprehensive Annual Financial Report." See the organization website.

Key Terms

accounting The systematic recording, reporting, and analysis of financial transactions of a business according to a set of rules.

accounts payable Any amount owed to another business as the result of a purchase of goods or services on a credit basis.

accounts receivable Any amount owed from another business as the result of a purchase of goods or services on a credit basis.

balance sheet A statement of the financial position of a business on a specified date.

budget Inclusive list of proposed expenditures and expected receipts of any person, enterprise, or government for a specified period, usually 1 year. Budget estimates are based on the expenditures and receipts of a similar previous period, modified by any expected changes.

chart of accounts A list of numbered accounts containing account names and numbers showing classifications and subclassifications that are affected by the financial transactions of a business.

cost per call The annual cost of providing service divided by the number of ambulance calls.

days sales outstanding (DSO) An analysis that provides general information about the number of days on average that customers take to pay invoices.

financial accounting Used primarily by those outside of a company or organization. Financial reports are usually created for a set

period of time, such as a fiscal year or period. Financial reports are historically factual and have predictive value to those who wish to make financial decisions or investments in a company.

finance The management of revenues; the conduct or transaction of money matters generally, especially those affecting the public, as in the fields of banking and investment.

Generally Accepted Accounting Principles (GAAP) Rules that accountants are required to follow when tracking and reporting financial transactions.

income statement An accounting of income and expenses that indicates a firm's net profit or loss over a certain period of time, usually 1 year.

managerial accounting Used primarily by those within a company or organization. Reports can be generated for any period of time, such as daily, weekly, or monthly. Reports are considered to be future looking and have forecasting value to those within the company.

retained earnings/equity The portion of net income that is retained by the corporation rather than distributed to its owners as dividends.

self-pay A person who pays out of pocket for a health-related service in absence of insurance to cover the costs of that service.

statement of cash flows A financial statement that shows how changes in balance sheet accounts and income affect cash and cash equivalents, and breaks the analysis down to operating, investing, and financing activities.

third party An organization other than the patient (first party) or health care provider (second party) involved in the financing of personal health services.

unit hour Measurement based on an hour when an ambulance is staffed and on duty.

The Regulatory Environment of Ambulance Services

SEAN M. CAFFREY, M.B.A., CEMSO, NRP, AND D. RANDY
KUYKENDALL, M.L.S., NREMT-P

Objectives

After reading this chapter, the student should be able to:

15.1 Describe the need for regulation of emergency medical services.
15.2 Describe the objectives of regulation.
15.3 Compare and contrast statutes, regulations, and policy.
15.4 List the areas of ambulance service that are regulated.
15.5 Describe the role of local, state, and federal regulation.
15.6 Explain the role of nongovernmental organizations in EMS regulations.
15.7 List the major national EMS organizations.
15.8 Describe advocacy and lobbying.
15.9 Explain regulatory conflict.

Overview

Ambulance services in the United States range in size from one ambulance operated by volunteers and managed by a community board of directors to large governmental agencies and even larger, private, for-profit corporations. This text presents information that the manager of an ambulance service, large or small, needs in order to keep the business solvent and provide clinically excellent service to the community.

Key Terms

advocacy	**licensure**	**regulation**
certification	**policies**	**statute**

WHAT WOULD YOU DO?

You have recently heard of an ambulance manager in your state that is being charged with Medicare fraud by the U.S. attorney. You have also heard from another local service that it owes hundreds of thousands of dollars in back overtime pay. And you have just been notified by the state EMS office that one of your employees has falsified the educational records required for her to renew her EMT card. As the chief executive of an ambulance service, you must be aware of the EMS regulatory environment and of changes in regulations that affect your organization. You must be aware of state and local regulations pertaining to EMS as well as a variety of federal and state regulations that affect how your service operates. Virtually every area of EMS is subject to regulation, and keeping up on existing and changing requirements is key to the success of your service. To be best prepared to succeed, you must also engage in the development of policies that affect you and be prepared to lobby elected and appointed officials. Are you prepared?

1. What governmental agencies are responsible for enforcement of the issues described in this case?
2. What does an EMS manager need to know about the issues in this case?
3. What should an EMS organization do to avoid running afoul of regulatory agencies?
4. What is the best way to avoid being the respondent in a regulatory action?

■ A NOTE ON TERMS

Throughout this chapter, the term *licensing* or **licensure** is used frequently and refers to the official permission granted by a governmental entity that is legally required before a service can be performed. Although some governmental entities may refer to licensing by other names, such as **certification**, *authorization*, or *accreditation*, the generic term *license* is used where applicable.

Certification, when used, refers to an endorsement and attestation that is given by a nongovernmental organization (NGO) when minimum criteria have been met. It is common within EMS for the terms *license* and *certification* to be used interchangeably.

In most cases, however, certification by the government is effectively the granting of a license regardless of the actual term used, provided that certification is legally required to perform a service or function.* The National Registry of Emergency Medical Technicians (NREMT, 2013) has provided a detailed opinion by a legal subject matter expert that clarifies this often-misunderstood topic.

Accreditation refers to a process used by an NGO to verify that an organization has met a set of standards that have been established by one or more private organizations. In some cases, certification and/or accreditation are prerequisite requirements of licensure by a governmental organization.

INTRODUCTION

Health care in the United States and most of the world is a highly regulated activity. This regulatory history stretches back well over a century and has become quite complex in recent decades. Efforts to reform health care in the United States will also increase this complexity. Heath care **regulation** has a number of purposes, including protecting public health and safety, ensuring quality, maintaining access to services, and controlling costs. Regulation is also exercised to varying degrees by local, state, and federal governmental agencies. As a public safety function, ambulance service is also subject to significant public oversight at the local and state levels. As such, ambulance managers must understand a wide variety of regulations, be able to ensure their organizations operate in compliance with rules and regulations, and be prepared to be accountable to officials at all levels of government on an ongoing basis.

OBJECTIVES OF REGULATION

The primary purpose of the regulation of health care in general, and ambulance services in particular, is the protection of public health and safety. Since emergency medical care is a specialized field and is provided in a wide variety of circumstances, it is difficult for most users of these services to evaluate the qualifications of providers or evaluate the utility, quality, and value of care they receive. To address this imbalance, and to prevent unqualified services or providers from taking advantage of patients, a multilayered regulatory scheme has been put in place by states. Layers of this regulation include the following:

- Establishing educational standards
- EMS instructor qualifications
- Educational program certification/accreditation
- Provider criminal background check requirements
- Provider testing/performance requirements
- Scope of practice regulation
- Physician oversight
- Continuing education requirements
- Service inspection and licensing requirements
- Emergency and trauma center designation programs

QUALITY OF CARE

A secondary, and closely related, area of regulation relates to quality of care. This activity is tied to protection of the public but may also relate to access-to-care issues. In many cases, quality-of-care regulation also involves NGOs that may serve as mandatory or voluntary agents of the regulatory system. The most widely known organization of this type is the Joint Commission on the Accreditation of Healthcare Organizations (JCAHO). Other major organizations in the EMS arena include the Commission on Accreditation of Allied Health Educational Programs (CAAHEP), the National Registry of EMTs, the Commission on Accreditation of Ambulance Services (CAAS), the Commission on Medical Transportation Systems (CAMTS), and the American College of Surgeons Committee on Trauma. These organizations do not exercise direct regulatory authority, but they do develop and enforce standards that are often used as a basis for governmental regulation or as a voluntary standard within an industry. Use of these NGO programs may also serve to restrict the number of providers in a market.

In addition to NGOs, it is increasingly common for governmental regulators to directly require that active oversight and ongoing quality monitoring programs exist for ambulance services. This trend follows a longer history during which physicians and hospitals have been granted some legal protection from liability if they engage in peer review or quality assurance activities. The most common form of quality monitoring, however, is the requirement that ambulance service clinical activities be overseen and evaluated by a physician medical director.

Side Bar
The primary purpose of regulation is protection of public health and safety.

ACCESS TO CARE

Access to care is another fundamental element of health care regulation. In the predominantly free market health care system in the United States, it should be noted that emergency care must be delivered by certain hospital providers under the requirements of the Emergency Medical Treatment and Active Labor Act (EMTALA) regardless of a patient's ability to pay. In addition, most ambulance services are required to respond to emergencies through contractual arrangements or regulations imposed by local governments. Such mandatory requirements are almost exclusive to EMS and hospitals.

Another mechanism for ensuring access to care is the state-controlled certificate of need (CON), which regulates exclusive provider arrangements that allow for only a single or limited number of providers to operate within a certain area or market. Although states take various views of the use of CONs, governmental creation of limited monopolies and their obligation to regulate these monopolies are important concepts. Ostensibly, these programs are designed to ensure that a provider can obtain a sufficient economy of scale to successfully operate and remain in an area. An argument should also be noted, however, that the limiting of providers in a market could potentially decrease efficiency and

quality while driving up costs. However, the geography, population density, and payer mix of some jurisdictions require that appropriately regulated monopolies exist in order to ensure adequate emergency services coverage and actually serve to contain costs and efficiencies in such environments.

COST CONTROL

The final purpose of health care regulation is to control costs. Most health care in the United States is paid for by governmental programs (i.e., Medicare and Medicaid) or by third-party insurers. In addition, most health care fees are not readily available to the public and are based on a fee-for-service model. This combination of factors has made the overall costs of U.S. health care very expensive and a matter of significant concern to the governmental agencies and private insurers that pay for care. A number of regulations imposed by governmental health care programs have a major impact on ambulance services, and these efforts to control costs are expected to increase as large numbers of baby boomers begin to be enrolled in the Medicare programs and recent health reform legislation begins to expand the state-federal Medicaid program for the poor.

■ HISTORY OF EMS REGULATION

Modern health care regulation began in the late nineteenth century with the adoption of physician licensing requirements. In an effort begun by the American Medical Association to prevent the practice of medicine by unqualified practitioners, most states had physician licensing requirements in place by the early twentieth century. In addition to the public protection benefits of physician licensing, the supply of doctors was also limited and physician incomes rose substantially.

Throughout the twentieth century, a number of allied health professions also developed licensing programs. Professions including nursing, athletic trainers, ultrasound technicians, physical therapists, and many others have developed formal educational programs, scopes of practice, and testing requirements and exercise self-regulation through state boards, commissions, or other regulatory bodies. The NREMT was formed in 1970 based on a recommendation to form a national certification organization for ambulance technicians, following the 1966 white paper "Accidental Death and Disability: The Neglected Disease of Modern Society" (National Academy of Sciences, 1966). Throughout the 1970s, most states developed emergency medical technician credentialing programs as the basis for improving out-of-hospital care to medical and accident victims.

Hospitals are highly regulated in the health care system. Modern hospitals emerged in the late nineteenth century as medical science advanced to the point where a dedicated location was required to perform increasingly complex medical tests and procedures. The American College of Surgeons (ACS) issued its first standards for hospitals in 1917 on a one-page document. In 1951, the Joint Commission on Accreditation of Hospitals (JCAH) was formed by a number of stakeholder groups. Beginning in 1965, JCAH-accredited hospitals were deemed "substantially compliant" for Medicare payment purposes. A hospital accredited by JCAH did not have to be separately inspected by Medicare or the state to receive Medicare payments. Now known as The Joint Commission on Accreditation of Healthcare Organizations (JCAHO), this independent, not-for-profit authority accredits more than 20,000 health care organizations and programs, including hospitals, laboratories, other health care facilities, and managed care organizations. JCAHO accreditation continues to be a standard for Medicare and

many state-licensing programs. JCAHO has also recently taken an aggressive stance on patient safety, quality improvement, and unannounced inspections (Joint Commission on Accreditation of Hospitals, 2013).

Commercial insurance programs began in the 1930s, primarily as a result of hospitals that developed prepaid "blue cross" programs for hospital care. The programs later expanded to "blue shield" programs that paid for outpatient services. These programs expanded dramatically during World War II, when government wage controls created an opportunity by freezing wages, while allowing employers to increase employee benefits programs. As a result of this situation, employer-sponsored health insurance became the primary method by which employers competed for employees, and these benefits continued as a standard in the postwar years. A significant milestone in health insurance occurred in the late 1960s when the Medicare Act was passed to provide health care to the elderly. The state-federal Medicaid insurance program developed shortly thereafter. Another major change occurred in the late 1970s when health maintenance organizations began to develop in earnest.

The Emergency Medical Treatment and Active Labor Act (EMTALA) was passed in 1986, making the provision of emergency care a requirement for all hospitals accepting Medicare funds (Legal Information Institute, n.d.). The American College of Surgeons Committee on Trauma began verification of trauma centers shortly thereafter in 1987. The Commission on Accreditation of Ambulance Services (CAAS) was founded in 1990, primarily due to the efforts of the American Ambulance Association (Commission on Accreditation of Ambulance Services, 2013). The Committee on Accreditation of Medical Transportation Systems was formed the same year by a number of organizations to accredit air ambulance programs. The Committee on

Accreditation of Educational Programs for the EMS Professions (CoAEMSP) was founded in 1983, when the American Medical Association identified emergency medical services as a distinct allied health care profession, enabling training programs to become voluntarily accredited (Committee on Accreditation of Educational Programs for the EMS Professions, 2010).

Although the regulations in each state evolved over time, most were the direct result of the EMS Act of 1973 (National Institutes of Health, 1973). This far-reaching **statute** was implemented by the U.S. Department of Health, Education and Welfare (currently the Department of Health and Human Services). Most state EMS offices, as well as most state-level EMS regulations, were implemented throughout the 1970s and 1980s. Today, state EMS offices exist in all U.S. states, all territories, and the District of Columbia. Most state offices manage EMT credentialing programs and regulate the provision of ambulance services. Most state EMS offices also manage a number of other programs, including EMS data collection, trauma center designation, EMS scope of practice, and disaster preparedness programs (National Association of State EMS Officials, 2013a).

Local governments have an inconsistent history of involvement with the regulation of EMS. In a few states, such as California and North Carolina, county governments take an active role in EMS regulation. In California, EMS was historically regulated at the county level, although in recent years there has been a move toward statewide regulation. According to the California Emergency Medical Service Authority's website:

> Since the inception of EMS in California, local agencies have played a pivotal role in EMS system development. While county-by-county regulation of EMS evolved, there was frequently no inter-county or statewide coordination. Currently, the Local EMS Agency (LEMSA) serves as the lead agency for the EMS system at the local level and is responsible for coordinating system participants within its jurisdiction. This decentralized approach has historically enabled the development of local EMS systems that have addressed local needs and spawned many of California's innovative EMS programs. (California Emergency Medical Services Authority, 2007)

In North Carolina, EMS is a "mandatory service" that, pursuant to state law, must be ensured by every county government. North Carolina counties are required to establish EMS systems, and to comply with state regulations governing EMS systems (North Carolina Department of Health and Human Services, 2009). Florida counties regulate ambulance service within the county through the "certificate of public convenience and necessity" (COPCN) process (Florida Department of Health, 2009).

Considering that states vary widely in the level and type of local control exercised, the regulation of local EMS is inconsistent or in many states nonexistent at the local level. In some states (so-called "Dillon's Rule" states), municipalities (cities) or counties may only regulate a particular subject if the state has expressly granted authority to do so (Lang, 1991). In others ("home rule" states), municipalities may regulate in a wider arena.[1] Lack

---

[1]In the United States, the authority granted to local governments varies by state. In some states, known as "home rule" states, cities, municipalities, and counties have the authority to pass laws to govern themselves as they see fit, as long as they obey the state and federal constitutions and perhaps some overarching state laws. In other states, only limited authority has been granted to local governments by the state legislature. In these states, a municipality must obtain permission from the state legislature if it wishes to pass a law or ordinance that is not specifically permitted under existing state law. Most nonhome rule states apply the principle known as "Dillon's Rule" to determine the extent of a municipal government's authority. See also http://nmml.org/wp-content/uploads/dillon.pdf for an in-depth look at Dillon's Rule.

of local involvement may or may not be balanced by additional state involvement. Some localities have highly developed regulatory and oversight programs, up to and including the actual provision of services. However, local EMS system regulation cannot be generalized.

Clearly, the regulatory history of U.S. health care, and that of EMS, is a shared effort between private NGOs, state regulators, and the federal government. In many cases, regulatory lines are blurred and governmental interests overlap with the interests of **advocacy** groups and organizations that finance the delivery of health care. This complex regulatory web is likely to continue and may likely become more complex over time.

> **Side Bar**
>
> Regulatory agencies and nongovernmental accrediting both have roles in encouraging a consistent and high quality of care.

■ REGULATORY HIERARCHY————

The origin of all regulation is specific legal authority. In the United States, the basis of all law is the Constitution of the United States, which provides the framework for and grants specific powers to the federal government. Powers not granted to the federal government are reserved for the states or the people as described in the Tenth Amendment.[2] Every state also has a state constitution, which serves as the basis of state government and state law. State constitutions also frequently describe the division of authority among local, county, and state governments. This division of authority varies substantially among states with some having a strong centralized state government and others delegating significant powers to local and county governments.

In almost all cases, EMS in particular and health care, public health, and public safety in general receive little mention in constitutional documents. Therefore, laws or statutes enacted by federal and state governments serve as the basis for the regulation of EMS. The original federal law in this area was the National Highway Safety Act of 1966 (Public Law 89-564, 23 U.S.C. 401), which began the federal government's involvement in EMS following the National Academy of Science white paper "Accidental Death and Disability: The Neglected Disease of Modern Society" (National Academy of Sciences, 1966). A number of other federal laws have been passed regarding EMS, including Public Law 94-573, the Emergency Medical Services Amendments, which required states to develop EMS regulatory structures in order to receive federal EMS funding.[3] This law was the origin of most state EMS offices. At the state level, almost every state and territory has an EMS Act that defines the regulatory framework for EMS within that state. At the state and federal levels, these laws are referred to as the statutory basis of EMS regulation. Subsequent EMS regulations and **policies** are derived from this statutory authority.

Statutes are laws created by the legislative branch and implemented or enforced by the executive branch of the state or federal government. Rules or regulations, by contrast, are promulgated by departments or other

---

[2]While many in the United States seek stronger federal leadership in the emergency medical services arena, the concept of EMS is not mentioned anywhere in the U.S. Constitution. Therefore, a strong case can be made that EMS is a state, not a federal, matter.

[3]Use of federal spending power to encourage states to comply with federal wishes in areas where the federal government does not have specific legislative authority has a long history in the United States. See *New York v. United States* 505 US 144 (1992) for a discussion of this subject by the U.S. Supreme Court. See also www.famguardian.org/Publications/PropertyRights/spndpwr.html.

agencies of the executive branch of government. Rules cannot be created without statutory authority, and often deal with issues in greater detail. Rules are often also easier to change and update, although statutory changes require the action of a legislature. In some cases, a single administrator adopts rules; in other instances, adoption is through a board or commission. Nearly every state has an EMS act or EMS statute and a comprehensive set of EMS regulations (also known as administrative rules, administrative code, or similar title). Although promulgated by executive branch agencies, these laws may carry criminal or civil penalties or other enforcement sanctions.

Policies represent the final form of regulation that usually represent an official interpretation of a statute or rule by a regulatory agency. Policies, however, are the easiest form or regulation to change or challenge.

Of note is that statutes, rules, and policies are all potentially subject to challenge in the courts and subsequent judicial review. Review by the courts, when it occurs, usually leads to a finding or judgment that creates precedent that must be taken into consideration in the future when implementing regulations.

■ CONTROLLED SUBSTANCES——

The most notable, and perhaps the most confusing, area of federal involvement in EMS is the regulation of the procurement, storage, and distribution of controlled substances, typically used by paramedics for pain control, sedation, and the control of seizures. The U.S. Drug Enforcement Administration (DEA), an arm of the Department of Justice, is responsible for federal drug enforcement and regulatory actions. The Office of Diversion Control within the DEA investigates and enforces drug security and accurate record keeping. Diversion investigators work closely with dispensers of controlled substances and may issue citations for violations. Depending on the severity of the offense, the consequences of a DEA violation can include fines, revocation of practitioner licenses and certifications, and/or imprisonment.

This is a very challenging area for ambulance service managers. The language in the DEA regulations that applies to ambulance services was not written with ambulance services in mind—it contemplates a physician's office or midlevel practitioner workplace (U.S. Department of Justice, 2013). The EMS medical director must be the purchaser of record and is completely responsible for everything involving controlled drugs. This requires a DEA registration for the ambulance service and, depending on the ambulance service's operating practices, may require a license for every EMS station. There are specific requirements for documenting the purchase, receipt, storage, distribution, and administration of controlled substances, violation of which can result in significant monetary penalties. The medical director must also be individually registered with the DEA, as the person licensed to dispense (and to order, via standing orders or online medical control) the administration of controlled substances.

As of this writing, numerous professional associations, both medical and administrative, are working through the federal legislative and executive branches to modify and clarify these regulations to address ambulance service concerns. As a result, a complete exploration of the issue is not possible. To further complicate this area, some state pharmacy regulations also apply to the ambulance service environment. A number of high-dollar enforcement actions recently have garnered great publicity, so ambulance service managers and medical directors need to constantly monitor changes to these regulations.

■ FEDERAL REGULATION

The federal government does not directly regulate the provision of EMS or ambulance service, but it does indirectly regulate a number of areas important to EMS. The federal government also provides support for various EMS activities.

The U.S. Department of Transportation, National Highway Traffic Safety Administration (NHTSA), is the current home of the federal EMS office. The NHTSA Office of EMS provides support for planning and coordination of EMS activities and has played an active role in developing and maintaining EMS educational standards. NHTSA's Office of EMS works closely with the National Association of State EMS Officials (NASEMSO) on a variety of projects that affect EMS on a national level. NHTSA also manages the Federal Interagency Committee on EMS (FICEMS), which coordinates the EMS efforts of a number of federal agencies. More recently, NHTSA also manages the National EMS Advisory Council (NEMSAC), which is comprised of EMS stakeholders who advise on federal EMS policy. The NHTSA Office of EMS website is an excellent starting point for information about federal involvement in EMS (NHTSA Emergency Medical Services, n.d.).

In addition to NHTSA, the U.S. Department of Health and Human Services (HHS), primarily the Health Resources and Services Administration (HRSA), the Assistant Secretary for Preparedness and Response (ASPR), and the Centers for Disease Control and Prevention (CDC) also provide federal support to EMS. These agencies are involved in EMS planning activities and provide financial support to a number of EMS programs, such as the national EMS for Children program (Emergency Medical Services for Children, n.d.).

The United States Fire Administration (USFA) resides in the Federal Emergency Management Agency (FEMA) of the U.S. Department of Homeland Security (DHS) and provides advanced level EMS educational programs through the National Fire Academy. The DHS Office of Health Affairs also participates in FICEMS and assists with the coordination of national EMS policy. The DHS is believed to be the largest federal employer of EMS personnel, through such agencies as Customs and Border Protection, the Secret Service, and the U.S. Coast Guard.

Other federal agencies that provide or support EMS and participate in FICEMS include the Indian Health Service, Federal Communications Commission, Department of Defense, and General Services Administration.

In addition to the support of EMS, a number of federal agencies influence or regulate various facets of EMS. The most influential agency concerning EMS finance is the Centers for Medicare & Medicaid Services (CMS), located in HHS. In 2010 CMS administered 21 percent of the federal budget or $743 billion for the Medicare, Medicaid, and children's health insurance programs. It is estimated that the Medicare program alone funded more than $3 billion in ambulance service payments in 2002. State-directed Medicaid programs and many private insurers also adopt Medicare payment policies. As such, the Medicare program likely has more influence on ambulance service than any other federal organization.

CMS also administers the Clinical Laboratory Improvement Amendments (CLIA), which sets standards for medical laboratories and establishes a waiver process for certain simple tests, such as EMS blood glucose monitoring.

Payment of EMS professionals, usually the largest single expense for an ambulance service, is regulated to a large degree by the U.S. Department of Labor, Wage and Hour Division, which administers the Fair Labor Standards Act (FLSA). The FLSA establishes federal minimum wage requirements and overtime payment rules. Section 207(k) of the act establishes overtime rules for firefighters and police officers. The eligibility of EMS providers to qualify under this section has been hotly debated and litigated in the recent past. Most recently, the Third U.S. Circuit Court of Appeals found that City of Philadelphia "fire service medics" who were trained in firefighting as well as emergency medicine, but who did not engage in fire suppression activities and who were in fact prohibited from doing so, did not qualify for the 207(k) exemption and thus must be paid overtime. The U.S. Supreme Court has denied review of this case (*Lawrence v. City of Philadelphia*, 2008). The FLSA also establishes requirements for on-call pay and withholding of sleep time for shifts greater than 24 hours. Many states also apply additional wage and hour payment regulations.

The Occupational Safety and Health Administration (OSHA) is also part of the Department of Labor that maintains and enforces occupational health regulations applicable to a number of employers. OSHA regulations such as 29 CFR 1910.120 regulate hazardous materials emergency response and such as 29 CFR 1910.1030 regulate management of blood-borne pathogen hazards (U.S. Department of Labor, n.d.). These and other regulations, even if they do not apply to certain employers, often serve as the standard for occupational health practices.

Unlike OSHA, the National Institutes for Occupational Health and Safety (NIOSH) is a nonregulatory research arm of the CDC that occasionally conducts research on EMS-related matters.

In recent years, the HHS Office of Civil Rights has also been tasked to enforce the privacy rule of the Health Insurance Portability and Accountability Act (HIPAA) of 1996, which ensures the protection of patient medical records (U.S. Department of Health and Human Services, n.d.). Many states may have medical record privacy requirements in addition to HIPAA requirements.

In addition to the support and regulation of ambulance service, a number of federal agencies are also involved in the direct provision of EMS. Federal organizations such as the Indian Health Service, Department of Defense, and National Park Service directly operate ambulance services. Other agencies, such as the U.S. Coast Guard, also provide EMS services and may interact closely with local ambulance services. Many other federal organizations, such as National Laboratories, U.S. Mints, U.S. Forest Service, Bureau of Land Management, U.S. Secret Service, and Federal Bureau of Investigation, have EMS providers among their ranks.

■ STATE REGULATION———————

Most regulation of EMS and ambulance services occurs at the state level. State governments for the most part have jurisdiction over public safety issues, health care systems, and the occupational licensing of health care providers, including EMS providers. States also regulate health insurance through their insurance commissioners and directly manage state Medicaid programs. In addition, states have public health powers that may be used in a pandemic or other large-scale crisis involving health or health care.

Occupational licensing of EMTs (all levels), as well as most other health care providers, is performed by the states. This licensing function represents the vast majority of influence that states exercise over the health care system and in most cases involves the direct regulation of thousands of EMTs and other health care providers in each state. Although standards of EMS provider licensure vary from state to state, all require successful completion of an educational program and an exam that may include written and practical components to measure technical competency. In addition, the majority of states utilize certification by NREMT as the technical basis to issue a state license. It should be noted, however, that certification by NREMT is not official permission to act as an EMS provider in any state. States may also have additional requirements for EMS provider licensure, with the most common being a criminal or driving record check. Other requirements may include certification by a local medical control authority, affiliation with a licensed EMS service, or proof of legal residence in the state or the United States. States may or may not charge a licensure fee to the individual. Although fees are commonplace in most professions, they may be waived for EMS providers, particularly in states with large numbers of volunteer EMS providers, when fees may cause a hardship or exacerbate an existing shortage of EMS providers.

In addition to initial licensure requirements, renewal requirements are also regulated by the states. In most cases, states also have the authority to investigate complaints against EMS providers and mete out discipline for misconduct. Unlike many regulated professions, however, it is rare for the disciplinary process to include or be managed by members of the EMS profession. In most cases, this authority is vested in administrators at the state or local level.

It should also be noted that in some instances states do not exercise jurisdiction over EMS providers. Examples may include federal or tribal enclaves such as military bases, Department of Veterans Affairs hospitals and clinics, and Native American reservations. State licensing jurisdiction may also be suspended during certain types of disaster declaration or for assistance requests between states under the authority of an Emergency Management Assistance Compact (EMAC). It should be noted that federal exceptions to licensing requirements only apply to limited locations and circumstances, and it is quite common for federal or tribal EMS providers

to hold state certifications in order to effectively perform services. Performing EMS on land owned by the federal government, however, does not guarantee that state occupational licensing laws do not apply.

Ambulance service managers have a distinct responsibility to ensure that personnel providing services are appropriately licensed and/or certified to do so. In order for the ambulance service to receive payment, regulations governing Medicare and Medicaid programs in all states require that personnel providing services be currently credentialed to do so. Utilizing inappropriately credentialed personnel to provide service to Medicare or Medicaid beneficiaries exposes the service to potential penalties in terms of reimbursement as well as to civil liability for torts such as "negligent hiring" or "negligent retention." Maintaining an effective continuing education program and local oversight of credentialing is an important component of providing ambulance services.

Although most states do not directly require that ambulance service be provided to communities, the qualifications, inspection, and licensing of ambulance services is a function performed by most states. In those states that do not directly regulate ambulance service, this authority is most often found at the county level. Most state regulations require that an organization meet a variety of minimum standards in order to be licensed as an ambulance service. Standards also exist for the vehicles and equipment that must be used to provide ambulance service. Fees are also common for this type of licensing, but they may also be waived for public policy reasons. Despite the fact that the provision of ambulance service is almost universally regulated, the provision of rescue or nontransport EMS services is often not regulated, or is regulated to a far lesser extent.

Based on the regulatory structure, either individual EMS providers or EMS organizations are required to obtain and maintain physician oversight services. This oversight may also be directly or indirectly tied to the scope of practice for EMS providers. Some states may also delegate these functions to local or regional authorities.

Some states also exercise more extensive regulatory authority over ambulance service, including the granting of certificates of need, granting of exclusive operating areas, or regulation of ambulance rates. Certificates of need or exclusive operating areas are usually used as a mechanism to ensure that a provider can obtain an adequate-size market area in order to be economically feasible (National Conference of State Legislatures, 2012). In some cases, this market can include emergency and/or interfacility ambulance service. Absent this state-level authority, individual local jurisdictions often also have the authority to designate an exclusive ambulance provider, particularly for emergency response. Direct regulation of ambulance rates is not particularly common at the state level; however, it does occur in some jurisdictions.[4]

An evolving area of EMS regulation at the state level is data collection. With the advent of the National EMS Information System (NEMSIS) in recent years, it has become increasingly common for states to require ambulance services, in particular, to submit patient care reports to the state EMS agency. This trend continues as electronic medical records become the standard of care. Although there is a desire to aggregate these records to better understand overall EMS care at the state and national levels, most of this analysis work is in its infancy. Most data collection regulations do, however, protect the privacy of individual records. North Carolina has required all EMS agencies to submit data to the Prehospital Medical Information System (PreMIS) since 2004 (National EMSC Data Analysis Resource Center, 2003).

In terms of health care payments that affect ambulance services, states operate the federal/state Medicaid health insurance program for the poor within each state. Medicaid in many states pays for emergency and nonemergency medical transportation services. Since most direct control of Medicaid rests with the states, and states usually have limited financial resources in comparison to the federal Medicare program, regulations usually restrict eligibility and limit payment rates. In addition to Medicaid, state insurance regulators, often through an insurance commissioner, also regulate acceptable practices regarding health insurance and health insurance payments. Although direct regulation of rates is rare, acceptable coverage requirements and prompt payment regulations are common and may apply to ambulance services.

State agencies may also regulate other areas related to EMS, including occupational health and safety, emergency vehicle operations in traffic, patient privacy, storage and distribution of pharmaceuticals, and labor issues. In some cases, this regulation is in addition to federal regulations that may also apply.

Since the beginning of the twenty-first century, states also have been provided far-reaching public health powers that may be used during a health crisis or other public health emergency. In many cases, these emergency regulations consider an expanded role for EMS providers in a public health emergency. States also operate emergency management programs that contemplate certain roles for ambulance services in the event of a large-scale disaster. State emergency management procedures may also specify how an ambulance service can obtain assistance in a disaster affecting its jurisdiction.

Some states have also created regional EMS organizations or structures that may

---

[4]Arizona is perhaps the best known exception to the general rule. See Arizona Department of Health Services (2013).

perform or coordinate some regulatory func-tions. The coordination of medical protocols and medical direction is a common function among these organizations. Other coordina-tion activities such as mutual aid, distribution of grant funding, educational services, and ambulance destination policies may also be performed by these groups. Pennsylvania's EMS system is a highly visible example of state delegation of regulatory processes to regional EMS organizations.[5]

Side Bar
Most regulation of ambulance services occurs at the state level.

LOCAL REGULATION

Based on the division of authority in state constitutions, local or county involvement in EMS may be almost as extensive as the state functions or very limited. In most cases, how-ever, local governments have the authority to determine how EMS is provided in their jurisdiction and/or to provide it as a govern-mental function.

In most states, county or local govern-ments are not required by law to provide EMS, or to even ensure that it is provided. Despite the fact that ambulance service or EMS is often not mandated as an essential service, most communities desire to have ambulance service available to their commu-nities. In addition to this desire, many local governments have the authority to set the

standards regarding how ambulance service is provided in their jurisdiction or to provide it directly. In some cases, various units of local government may also join together to form authorities or create independent districts that can provide or contract for ambulance service. In some cases, this function is adminis-tered through a department of the govern-ment such as public health, emergency management, or the fire department. Regard-less of the local structure, the ambulance serv-ice manager should understand how this process works locally, and actively engage with local governments where ambulance service is provided.

Local jurisdictions may also have special event regulations in place that pertain to large venues such as sports stadiums, concert events, or outdoor sporting events that require EMS coverage. A special events ordinance will serve to protect the local EMS system against extraordinary, unanticipated demands for service brought on by an unusual influx of visitors, or the unusual sales of alcohol at a particular venue. An excellent example is the approach taken by the Boston Public Health Commission, parent agency to Boston EMS (Boston Public Health Commission, 2009). These coverage requirements can potentially benefit local ambulance services through the generation of standby or coverage fees. The opposite also can be true if local regulations, or the absence thereof, allow for any ambu-lance provider to serve a large event.

NONGOVERNMENTAL ORGANIZATIONS

As noted previously, a number of NGOs play a prominent role in EMS. The most well-known of these organizations is the NREMT, which plays an active role in EMS provider education and credentialing nationwide. Although NREMT works closely with state

---

[5]Pennsylvania's EMS system is defined by Act 45 of 1985, Pa C.S. §6921–6938, new regulations published October 14, 2000, and the Statewide EMS Development Plan. The state's EMS system includes sixteen regional EMS coun-cils, the Statewide Advisory Council, and the Pennsylvania Trauma Systems Foundation.

regulators, it has no direct regulatory authority over EMS providers or ambulance services. It does, of course, drive how many organizations deliver continuing education through recertification requirements. Although the use of the NREMT credential is voluntary in some states, it is directly tied to state licensure in others.

Another well-known credentialing body is the Board for Critical Care Transport Paramedic Certification (BCCTCP) that administers the certified flight paramedic (FP-C) program, which has evolved as a popular voluntary standard among air medical programs. Unlike NREMT, BCCTCP certification is not currently used as the basis for state licensure.

Some NGOs have been created to develop standards. The National Fire Protection Association (NFPA) is one such organization that has developed a variety of standards for building codes, electrical codes, fire protection, and fire and EMS equipment and operations. Like other standard-setting organizations, such as ASTM International, NFPA uses an extensive development process to create and issue standards. Although NFPA or ASTM standards have no force of law on their own, it is not uncommon for jurisdictions to adopt these standards in governmental regulations. It is also not uncommon for standards to be cited in civil litigation as the industry standard or standard of care for emergency operations.

Another common EMS standard is the General Services Administration (GSA) Standard KKK-A-1822 for automotive ambulances used by the federal government to purchase ambulances. It represents a government purchasing standard that has been adopted by the industry for the construction of ambulances.

Voluntary accreditation programs also exist for ambulance services. The Commission on Accreditation of Ambulance Services (CAAS) and the Commission on Accreditation of Medical Transport Systems (CAMTS)

are NGOs that accredit both ground and air ambulance programs, respectively.

Paramedic educational programs are also accredited by the Commission on Accreditation of Allied Health Educational Programs (CAAHEP). As of 2013, NREMT will require paramedic candidates to have successfully completed a CAAHEP accredited paramedic program to be eligible for NREMT certification. Considering the large number of states that use the NREMT certification as a basis for state licensure, this is an excellent example of how an NGO can initiate requirements that directly impact governmental programs: in this case, through the use of requirements promulgated by yet another NGO.

Labor groups also play a role in EMS organizations and politics. Although labor groups do impose requirements on ambulance services through labor contracts, they do not have any regulatory authority. How a labor organization or potential labor organization is dealt with, however, is subject to regulation of the National Labor Relations Board (NLRB) and applicable state labor regulations. Labor groups, such as the International Association of Fire Firefighters (IAFF) are often very active in local and national politics.

Many nongovernmental advocacy organizations also exist within the EMS community. Examples of these organizations include:

- National Association of EMTs (NAEMT)
- National EMS Management Association (NAEMSMA)
- Advocates for EMS
- National Association of State EMS Officials (NASEMSO)
- National Association of EMS Physicians (NAEMSP)
- National Association of EMS Educators (NAEMSE)
- American Ambulance Association (AAA)
- National EMS Labor Alliance (NEMSLA)

- International Association of EMS Chiefs (IAEMSC)
- International Association of Fire Chiefs—EMS Section (IAFC)
- International Association of Flight Paramedics (IAFP)
- Association of Air Medical Services (AAMS)

In addition to these organizations, a number of state and local EMS organizations may also exist. The primary purpose of these organizations is usually to communicate, coordinate, educate, and lobby on behalf of the organization's membership. As such, once of its primary roles is lobbying regulatory organizations and legislative bodies on behalf of EMS and ambulance services.

INTERACTION WITH REGULATORS AND LEGISLATURES

The First Amendment of the U.S. Constitution guarantees the right to petition the government for redress of grievances. This right allows citizens to lobby or advocate for their positions elected officials and administrative departments in all levels of government. To this end, it is common for ambulance services to interact regularly with local governments and elected officials, particularly if they are private ambulance services. This relationship with the local government customer is often essential to maintaining the ability to provide emergency ambulance service to a community. It is also common for ambulance organizations to form state-level associations or to work directly with state government. As ambulance services are subject to a variety of state regulations, it is often helpful to have an ongoing relationship with the state EMS office. In many cases, state executive departments that regulate EMS also have an appointed board that advises on the development of state-level policy.

In addition to working with executive departments, lobbying of state legislatures to pass laws favorable to EMS is also common. As noted earlier, state legislatures pass laws (statutes) that serve as the basis for EMS systems and EMS regulations statewide. Ambulance managers would be well advised to understand that regulatory structure and participate either directly or through state associations in state legislative lobbying activities. Some large EMS organizations and state associations may also employ professional lobbyists to advocate on a regular or full-time basis for EMS needs.

Lobbying for EMS at the federal level is conducted to a large extent by national EMS organizations such as Advocates for EMS, the American Ambulance Association, or the International Association of Fire Chiefs. Advocacy at the federal level often involves working with representatives and senators on legislative matters. Members of Congress also play a key role in advocating for constituents to other parts of the federal government. EMS organizations may also deal directly with federal agencies involved in policy or regulation that affects EMS and ambulance service. Ambulance managers would also do well to support these organizations and keep abreast of federal activities related to EMS.

REGULATORY CONFLICT

Ambulance services are highly regulated by many levels of government and by a large number of regulatory agencies. This complexity requires an ongoing commitment on behalf of ambulance service administrators to understand, comply with, and work to improve these regulations. It is also clear that various regulators have conflicting interests. For example, the Medicare and Medicaid programs are attempting to contain costs, whereas local EMS regulations often specify system minimum capacity and universal access to EMS. These competing interests create a situation in which government payments to EMS decrease as local requirements become more expensive.

One of the better-known regulatory conflicts involves the regulation of air medical services. State EMS agencies claim the authority to regulate air ambulance services, particularly rotary-wing air ambulances, under the state's authority to regulate medical and health care services in general (Figure 15.1). Some air medical service vendors, seeking to avoid detailed state medical regulations, have argued that state regulation of air medical services is preempted by federal regulation of aircraft and flight crews. This conflict has sometimes led to protracted and intense litigation. A number of resources on this topic have been assembled for easy access by the National Association of State EMS Officials (2013b).

Ambulance managers should be aware of these conflicts and work to provide the highest-

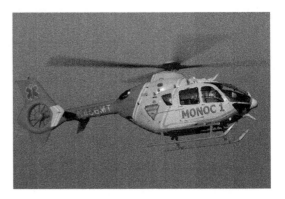

FIGURE 15.1 ■ Air medical services exist in both the federal and state regulatory domains. Thus, confusion and conflict occasionally result. *Source: MONOC, by permission.*

quality service that is compliant with regulations while lobbying to reduce negative regulatory impacts and support regulatory changes that may enhance efficiencies and opportunities.

CHAPTER REVIEW

Summary

As a health care and public safety service, ambulance service is a highly regulated activity. Although most EMS regulation is conducted at the state level, local and federal regulations also impact ambulance services. Regulations run the spectrum from licensing, system design, and personnel requirements to data collection, payment systems, pharmaceutical management, and clinical oversight.

Many ambulance services also voluntarily submit to outside accreditation programs or industry standards that add additional organizational burdens. Although this environment requires ongoing efforts on behalf of ambulance service leaders, compliance with these various regulations demonstrates a commitment to responsible and accountable service to the patients and communities they serve.

WHAT WOULD YOU DO? Reflection

Your state EMS office has recently formed a committee to take input on the update of ambulance licensing regulations for your state. Being well informed on the issues in the state, local, and federal regulations that affect ambulance service, you join the committee and are able influence the new regulations, which improves them to better meet the needs of ambulance services throughout the state and the state government.

Review Questions

1. Which levels of government regulate most aspects of the delivery of ambulance service?
2. What governmental office issues legal authorization to practice as an EMS provider in most states?
3. List examples of nongovernmental accreditation organizations involved in EMS.
4. What are the elements of EMT licensing?
5. What role does local government play in ambulance service regulation?
6. What federal agency regulates controlled medications?
7. What is regulatory conflict?
8. Give examples of organizations involved in EMS advocacy.

References

Arizona Department of Health Services. (2013). "Programs & Services." See the organization website.

Boston Public Health Commission. (2009). "Emergency Medical Services Regulation." See the organization website.

California Emergency Medical Services Authority. (2007). "EMS Systems Division—NHTSA EMS Assessment of California." See the organization website.

Commission on Accreditation of Ambulance Services. (2013). "Brief History." See the organization website.

Committee on Accreditation of Educational Programs for the EMS Professions. (2010). "EMS Accreditation Fact Sheet." See the organization website.

Department of Health and Human Services, Office of Inspector General. (2006). "Medicare Payments for Ambulance Transports." See the organization website.

Emergency Medical Services for Children. (n.d.). "EMSC National Resource Center." See the organization website.

Florida Department of Health. (2009). Florida Administrative Code (F.A.C.). Section 401.25, Florida Statutes & Chapter 64J-1.002, & 64J-1.003. See the organization website.

Joint Commission on Accreditation of Hospitals. (2013). "About The Joint Commission." See the organization website.

Lang, D. (1991). "Dillon's Rule and the Birth of Home Rule." *The Municipal Reporter.* See the New Mexico Municipal League website.

Lawrence v. City of Philadelphia. (2008). See the United States Court of Appeals for the Third Circuit website.

Legal Information Institute. (n.d.). "42 USC Sec. 1395dd: Examination and treatment for emergency medical conditions and women in labor." See the organization website.

National Academy of Sciences. (1966). "Accidental Death and Disability: The Neglected Disease of Modern Society." See the organization website.

National Association of State EMS Officials. (2013a). "State EMS Agencies." See the organization website.

National Association of State EMS Officials. (2013b). "Air Medical." See the organization website.

National Conference of State Legislatures. (2012). "Certificate of Need: State Health Laws and Programs." See the organization website.

National EMSC Data Analysis Resource Center. (2003). "State-of-the-Art EMS Data Collection Systems: The North Carolina PreMIS System." See the organization website.

National Institutes of Health, Office of NIH History. (1973). P.L. 93-154. See the organization website.

National Registry of Emergency Medical Technicians. (2013). "Certification v. Licensure." See the organization website.

NHTSA Emergency Medical Services. (n.d.). "About NHTSA EMS." See the organization website.

North Carolina Department of Health and Human Services. (2009). 10A NCAC 13P .0201(a); Authority G.S. 131E-155(a)(8), (a)(9), (a)(15); 143-508(b); (d)(1), (d)(5), (d)(9); 143-509(1); 143-517. See the organization website.

U.S. Department of Health and Human Services. (n.d.). "Health Information Privacy: The Privacy Rule." See the organization website.

U.S. Department of Justice, Drug Enforcement Division. (2013). Title 21 CFR, Part 1300–1399. See the organization website.

U.S. Department of Labor, Occupational Safety & Health Administration. (n.d.). Regulations (Standards – 29 CFR). See the organization website.

Key Terms

advocacy Working to influence a legislative body, public officials, or public policy individually or on behalf of a group.

certification Attesting to a truth; in the EMS context, it represents that a minimum standard has been met by a person or organization.

licensure Formal permission from a governmental or other official body to conduct business or perform a profession.

policies Courses of action established by an organization in order to carry out its objectives.

regulation Establishing conformity with rules, principles, or common practice

statute An enactment of a legislative body expressed through a formal document or law.

CHAPTER 16

Legal and Compliance Issues for Ambulance Services

DAVID M. SHOTWELL JR., J.D., NREMT-P

Objectives

After reading this chapter, the student will be able to:

16.1 Create a compliance program meeting the current criteria specified by the Department of Health and Human Services, Office of the Inspector General.

16.2 Evaluate an existing compliance program to determine adequacy.

16.3 Recognize the value of having a compliance program in place.

Overview

Ambulance services in the United States range in size from one ambulance operated by volunteers and managed by a community board of directors to large governmental agencies and even larger, private, for-profit corporations. This text presents information that the manager of an ambulance service, large or small, needs in order to keep the business solvent and provide clinically excellent service to the community.

Key Terms

audit

corporate integrity
   agreement (CIA)

code of conduct

compliance committee

compliance officer

compliance program

Federal Register

federal sentencing
  guidelines

fraud

Medicare

WHAT WOULD YOU DO?

A letter is received from a recovery audit contractor (RAC), indicating its authority to audit Medicare claims and recover fraudulent payments. The letter lists claims submitted by your agency and requests you produce all the documentation to support 212 claims. The auditors will arrive at your facility in one month, on July 2.

After the audit, you receive a letter from the RAC, indicating that the review identified 94 claims that are being disallowed, and for which they will recoup the payments. Further, they are considering extrapolating the error rate (44 percent) to recover on all claims during the past 2 years. Of the 94 claims disallowed, the RAC claims 47 were "upcoded" to the "ALS Emergency" billing rate when they should have been billed as "BLS Emergency"; 7 were billed as "specialty care transport" (SCT) when they should have been billed as "BLS nonemergency" transport, and 40 ambulance trans-

ports were entirely disallowed as the patient's condition, documented in the patient care report (PCR), did not warrant ambulance transportation.

1. It's the beginning of the summer. A substantial portion of your office staff is on vacation, and the parking lot is being resurfaced while the staff is off. What steps can you take to get ready for the impending audit?

2. In speaking with the billing staff, you are informed that they "bill 'em the way they look." Your dispatch staff relies on the caller to tell dispatch whether an emergency response or a nonemergent response is needed, and whether the patient requires ALS, SCT, or BLS care. Could the billing department be the source of the alleged billing errors?

3. Review with the field staff indicates a mix of crew reactions to obtaining signatures and supporting documents. Could the field staff be contributing the number of errors in billing?

■ INTRODUCTION ————————

A compliance program provides a focal point for finding and determining the rules that regulate provision of health care services in the ambulance industry — and living within them regardless of the source. Although this section will have primary focus

on the federal reimbursement scheme (**Medicare**), the precepts should be applied to any regulatory scheme, including state payment programs (Medicaid), grant administration, privacy, financial practices, safety, and almost any framework requiring accountability.

The recently enacted Patient Protection and Affordable Care Act (PPACA) allows the

2

Secretary of Health and Human Services to designate certain types of providers that will be required to have compliance programs in place.[1] At this writing, the types of providers have not been designated.

A logical starting place for developing or evaluating an EMS compliance program is the Compliance Program Guidelines (CPG) for Ambulance Suppliers promulgated by the Office of the Inspector General (Office of Inspector General, 2003). Prior to the CPG, programs were developed by referring to **corporate integrity agreements (CIAs)** imposed on health care institutions that have previously been subject to federal enforcement actions. Continued monitoring of developments regarding CIAs may be useful in keeping a compliance program current.

The CPG for ambulance suppliers published in the *Federal Register* does not contain any novel elements when compared with existing CIAs. Essentially, there are seven components to a comprehensive compliance program:

1. *Written standards.* The development and distribution of written standards of conduct and policies and procedures that promote the agency's commitment to compliance. This must also address specific areas for potential **fraud** (upcoding) and financial relationships.
2. **Compliance officer** and **compliance committee.** Designating a compliance officer and other appropriate entities, such as a compliance committee, along a direct reporting relationship to the governing body and CEO.
3. *Training and education.* Regular and effective education and training programs for employees.
4. *Detection, monitoring, and reporting process.* Processes for finding and correcting problems and to receive information.

5. *Response process.* A process for responding to allegations or improper or illegal activities and the enforcement of disciplinary actions against employees who have violated internal compliance policies, applicable laws, regulations, or requirements.
6. *Open lines of communication.* Establishing and maintaining means by which employees, customers, vendors, and patients can communicate easily with the compliance officer.
7. *Enforcing standards.* Implementation of appropriate corrective actions, including discipline, termination, removal, and remediation for violation of policies. The corrective actions should be established and well publicized within the written policies.

■ WRITTEN STANDARDS

A written, published, and distributed **code of conduct**, along with consistent written policies and procedures, demonstrates the ambulance service's commitment to compliance.

It is tempting, convenient, and sometimes efficient to use prepackaged documents and policies to meet this requirement. Off-the-shelf programs can be used as templates but will probably require modification to accurately describe the policy or process used by each agency.

The standards should reflect the actual flow of work, reporting, and accountability as it exists in the organization. In some cases, the agency may need to change the way the work flows to ensure compliance. The CPG in the *Federal Register* specifically offers an example of a policy indicating 100 percent review of PCRs. The CPG suggests against indicating 100 percent review if the agency is capable of neither performing nor enforcing such.

Some agencies will choose to publish the code of conduct on their public website as well as distributing it throughout the

---

[1]Public Law 111-148, 124 Stat. 119, to be codified as amended at scattered sections of the Internal Revenue Code and in 42 U.S.C.

organization via the employee handbook, newsletter, wall poster, or promotional handouts. A code of conduct should include a statement from the CEO that the agency is committed to conducting business with integrity, to meeting the highest ethical standards, and being in compliance with all applicable regulations and laws. It should include recognition of the agency's obligation to its employees, stakeholders, customers, and patients. A well-developed code of conduct will address the roles of the policies and procedures, risk management, internal controls, conflicts of interest—and perhaps use of assets, employee expense reimbursement, proprietary interests, intellectual property, and compensation schemes—and how these interests relate to the agency's stated ethical standards.

Compliance policies and procedures must go through the same approval process as the agency's other policies and procedures. This is true whether the policy requires approval from the CEO, action by a public governing body, board of directors' approval, membership consensus, or some other process.

Compliance policies and procedures must be as accessible to employees as any other policy, and perhaps more so in certain areas of the agency. Failure to meet the requirements for accurately billing Medicare can have disastrous implications for the entire agency. By way of example, reimbursement claims must be supported by several types of documents, including physician certification statements of medical necessity, PCRs, patient consent forms, assignments of billing rights, and advance beneficiary notices. Policies that ensure this documentation has been obtained, reviewed, stored, and protected must be in place. Of course, the steps required if a deviation from the procedure occurs must also be part of the policy. Accessibility and familiarity can enhance and ensure compliance.

COMPLIANCE OFFICER AND COMPLIANCE COMMITTEE

Some organizations by virtue of size, tradition, or economy will combine compliance officer functions with another position. In many cases, the organization's legal counsel may simultaneously serve as the chief compliance officer. This may be efficient from an organizational standpoint, but there are drawbacks. From a best-practice standpoint, dividing the roles of general legal counsel and compliance is strongly preferred. The division of roles is supported by ethical standards that apply to general counsel, Office of the Inspector General comments, and review of **federal sentencing guidelines** and corporate integrity agreements. Smaller EMS agencies may lack the personnel and resources to divide the roles, despite the increased risk of conflict between the two roles.

The CPG indicates that a compliance officer should be a "high-level individual" who reports directly to the CEO, upper management, or board of directors. A review of corporate integrity agreements makes it clear that the compliance officer must not be subordinate to the general counsel or to the chief financial officer. Following this guidance should ensure the compliance officer of a degree of autonomy and prevent any actual or perceived influence from other areas in the agency.

The Office of Inspector General (OIG) explicitly recognizes that the compliance officer function may be combined with additional functions or tailored to meet agency-specific needs. An agency may choose to have additional compliance areas—such as Occupational Safety and Health Administration (OSHA), Federal Communications Commission (FCC), intellectual property, environmental regulations, or traditional risk management—handled by a compliance officer who is also handling the reimbursement-related areas.

The compliance officer should also chair the compliance committee. Although the CPG does not specify members for a committee, it will be useful to include responsible parties from billing, **audit**, coding, operations, clinical, education, and legal sections. It may also be helpful to include technical support staff, security, finance, and perhaps representatives from other health care agencies serviced by the agency.

Best Practice

Avoiding the Notice of Audit

As is his habit, toward the end of his workday John scanned the performance dashboard on the company's internal website. The dashboard is a display that only company managers can access. It shows up-to-the-minute information regarding call volume, in-service and out-of-service units, and response time averages overall and for individual units on the current shift. It also has links for weather, traffic diversions, hospital bypass, and recent shifts.

As the compliance officer, John had little use for the dashboard, but it gave him some insight as to how things were going for his co-workers in the field. It had been snowing heavily for two days, and the average response time was the highest number John had ever seen. When he glanced at the individual unit times to see who was on the various units, he noticed that only one nonemergent unit had arrived on time all day, and curiously, the trip was canceled a few minutes after the crew called on location. Sympathetic about the crew's frustration, John noted the assignment number and pulled the job up on his screen to see who was on the crew that undoubtedly had planned their arrival prudently in order to be on time under the adverse conditions. What John immediately noticed while scanning the trip was that the assignment was the first leg of a dialysis trip, that the trip was canceled due to "Patient Not Ready," and that no other unit had been assigned for a later pickup. With concern that a patient was stranded without the means to get to dialysis, John reached out to the EMS supervisor, Jennifer, to check on the matter.

Jennifer indicated she was aware of the situation and that the patient's family had informed the crew that the patient was shopping at the mall. The patient would be delayed from getting home in time for the ambulance pickup because plowed snow had been piled in the handicapped parking spots and she'd had to drive around the mall for a long time to find an open handicapped parking spot. With a backlog of storm-related calls, Jennifer had immediately made the crew available for reassignment, rather than wait for the patient to arrive home. Both the crew members, and Jennifer, having participated in regular Medicare compliance training, were aware that ambulance transport is only appropriate when a patient cannot be transported by other means safely. Clearly, the patient who can drive herself in near blizzard conditions falls into the category of patients who can be transported by other means safely. At John's suggestion, Jennifer informed the family of the patient that the ambulance would not return for the pickup, and she suggested that they have the dialysis center staff or the physician call the dispatch center if a return trip was needed later that day.

John accessed the patient records and located the Certificate of Medical Necessity. The certificate, issued the previous month, indicated that the patient was bed confined and could not be transported safely by other means. The certificate was signed by the patient's attending physician. Further, the patient had been transported to and from the dialysis center on 11 days, generating 22 PCRs, all by ambulance. John began reviewing the PCRs. He noted that the crews sometimes found the patient in a reclining chair watching television on the first floor of her home, other times found the patient sitting on the front porch. Various crews recorded "transferred to stretcher via sheet lift" or "ambulated to stretcher" on multiple occasions, but no crew recorded findings suggestive of weakness, fatigue, or distress in any form. Prior to the next scheduled shift, John requested an EMS clinical supervisor visit to the patient at home in order to evaluate the patient and follow up with the patient's physician if necessary. After meeting with the patient, the clinical supervisor reported that all pending trips for the patient should be canceled. The patient and her husband, when informed of the requirements for ambulance reimbursement, claimed

surprise that she had ever been classified as bed confined and that, when the patient started dialysis treatment, she was simply told that the ambulance would transport her and never inquired as to the reason.

John then advised the billing department to rescind the Medicare reimbursement requests and refund any Medicare payments received, indicating that the Certificate of Medical Necessity was in error. To prevent future incidents, all repetitive-trip patients are screened by an EMS clinical supervisor prior to the first trip, and at least monthly field supervisors are encouraged to drop in on routine and repetitive trips. The PCR assessments and findings for such trips are now getting the same scrutiny that the emergent PCRs receive.

TRAINING AND EDUCATION

3

Training and continuing education are essential elements of every compliance program. As with health care providers' licenses and certifications, compliance training and education must be documented and retained. Following the CPG, two types of training should be considered: general compliance training and job-specific education.

GENERAL COMPLIANCE TRAINING

General compliance training will probably be offered during the employee orientation phase for new hires. When establishing a new compliance program, general training must be offered to all employees to ensure that they have the baseline education offered to the new hires. This training should include an overview of where the program fits in the agency; the focus areas, including, but not limited to federal and state reimbursement and privacy regulations; the policies and procedures that apply; and how and when to access compliance program

resources. In addition, the initial training may include examples and solutions to common compliance problems and some that may be unique to the agency or specific response areas. When establishing a new program, consider providing general compliance training to vendors and customers as well.

It may be helpful to discuss reported violations and outcomes, including the effect the violations had on specific agencies, employees, and the industry. Real cases are fairly easily found by reviewing trade publications and Internet searches. Employees are usually more impressed with the facts and application of law from real events than they are with hypothetical events. High profile events, such as the Health Insurance Portability and Accountability Act (HIPAA) violations in the St. Vincent Infirmary Medical Center case in Little Rock, Arkansas, in July, 2009 (Health Imaging, 2003), or the Medicare fraud in the Americare Ambulance Service case stemming from indictments in June 2007 are of instructive value and will make a lasting impression (Federal Bureau of Investigation, 2009).

JOB-SPECIFIC EDUCATION

Job-specific training offers the benefit of tailoring the presentation to the task that the employee will be performing. Obvious areas for specific training are billing and patient care. In most agencies, the personnel involved in the billing process are not the same personnel who provide patient care. Consideration of cross-training the two groups may result in increased awareness of the challenges each endures to comply with regulations.

Compliance training should not be restricted to patient care and billing personnel. All employees, including those whose employment responsibilities are unrelated to billing and patient care, should be aware of the regulatory framework within which the company operates. It may not be necessary to educate engineering and fleet management personnel in signature and patient privacy requirements, but it is likely to foster a general agency awareness of regulatory requirements and ethical practices. Personnel not normally involved in billing or patient care may have a broader perspective and offer increased vigilance in areas that would otherwise go unnoticed.

Documentation of completed training must be maintained. Effectiveness of the training is usually established through post-training tests, reviewing employee performance, and audits.

Agencies may find it beneficial to include affiliate agencies, vendors, and customers in compliance training. An agency might routinely be dispatched with another agency, such as a fire department that relies on a separate ambulance service for transport; an EMS agency might be assigned with law enforcement first responders; or a specialized transport service or special response team might interface with a variety of hospitals, first responders, and EMS agencies.

Nonemergency trips and interfacility trips have different compliance considerations than 9-1-1 trips, and the supporting documentation for reimbursement will originate within another agency. An agency may rely on vendors for a variety of functions, such as information technology, archive services, or routine building maintenance. Regulatory requirements imposed on the agency will not be relaxed because of the interface, origination, or outsourcing scheme. It is incumbent on the agency to ensure and document that all compliance considerations are intact. Consideration should be given to obtaining such assurance by providing appropriate education and training to the involved entities. An example of this is providing awareness education to skilled nursing facilities regarding Medicare requirements for ambulance transports, such as the Certificate of Medical Necessity (CMN) or Physician Certification Statement (PCS).[2] Another example would be HIPAA training for contracted maintenance personnel.

---

[2]The Centers for Medicare & Medicaid Services (CMS) has long held that a PCS was not conclusive evidence of medical necessity of a nonemergency transport, and that an ambulance service's documentation must independently establish the medical necessity of the transport. As this manuscript was in development, a federal court has held to the contrary: *Moorecare Ambulance Serv., LLC v. Dep't of Health and Human Services,* Civ. No. 1:09-0078, 2011 WL 2682987 (M.D. Tenn. July 11, 2011), and *Moorecare Ambulance Serv., LLC v. Dep't of Health and Human Services,* Civ. No. 1:09-0078, 2011 WL 839502 (M.D. Tenn. March 4, 2011). There, the court held that a PCS is conclusive of medical necessity and rejected the arguments of Health and Human Services (HHS) that the *Medicare Benefit Policy Manual* provisions or other CMS guidance imposed additional requirements that ambulance providers must also meet. Since this decision, CMS has revised its rules to require that ambulance documentation support medical necessity, in addition to requiring the CMS, in a manner that avoids the reasoning of the decision in *Moorecare.* Ambulance services should carefully monitor information on this topic from the Office of Inspector General (OIG) and should be aware that a case in one federal circuit may not be controlling in other venues.

▓ MONITORING, DETECTION, AND REPORTING

Monitoring processes are another essential element of a functional compliance program and will typically be accomplished through a combination of automated and personnel functions.   4

The agency's computer billing system should include system edits to ensure that the information required to submit claims is included in each claim. Claims that do not meet the data requirements should be identified by the system to allow the claim to be completed properly or removed prior to submission to prevent incomplete or fraudulent claims. Computer systems should not automatically insert missing information.

A regular schedule of claims reviews should be conducted as well. Reviewers should analyze a sampling of claims for appropriateness and completeness. Reviewers should not analyze claims they have personally prepared. Reviewers may lack objectivity when assessing their own work. Whether claims are prepared in-house, or through outsourced operations, the agency should give consideration to engaging third-party reviewers as part of a comprehensive compliance plan.

Reviews may be limited to claims ready for submission or already submitted, along with the supporting documentation for each claim. These target-specific audits are the most common form of review and may be classified as billing reviews.

A better and more comprehensive review can be performed by including every aspect of the claim, from the initial request for service through to the payment and posting process. A deficiency anywhere in the system can expose the agency to liability for improper claims. These "patient" reviews will involve the billing process and the supporting docu-

mentation but will also expand to the call intake process, and perhaps dispatch protocols, which are areas not typically considered for billing compliance.

The most comprehensive review can be achieved by developing the list of events to analyze or audit from a list other than claims made. This comprehensive "event review" analysis may identify areas where revenue has been lost if all events (billed, unbilled, and unbillable) are all included in the analysis. Many agencies assign an incident number to every incoming request, whether or not it results in a dispatch, patient encounter, or a billable event. When performing a comprehensive internal "event" review or audit, including the nonbilled events in the review will expose additional aspects of the agency's operations to review. In addition to reimbursement schemes, such a review would also include HIPAA, OSHA, and state regulatory compliance. A review may extend beyond the documents and could involve crew interviews to assess compliance with issues that may not appear in routine documentation, such as vehicle documentation and equipment checks, payroll accuracy, use of vehicle warning equipment, personal safety equipment, product recall replacements, and medical waste disposal.

The comprehensive review of the event may be beyond the capabilities of the compliance officer, but it should be manageable by drawing on the expertise of the members of the compliance committee. Although certain aspects of such an event review exceed the areas normally included in the compliance program, before discarding those aspects an agency should consider if the excluded components are subject to internal review by any other responsible party. Agencies that use an after-action review process for large incidents will find the concept of the event review to be similar, albeit typically focused on a much smaller event, such as request for an ambulance for possible injury at a motor vehicle accident (MVA) or establishing a repetitive patient schedule for cancer therapy.

The wide variety of sizes, organizational structure, and population demographics will present an equally diverse array of risk areas. Regular review of industry newsletters and the U.S. Department of Health and Human Services' website (http://oig.hhs.gov) will help identify risk areas that merit special attention. Attention to areas identified by the OIG in the CPG must be included in the reviews. Areas of regular note include unallowable costs, medical necessity, upcoding, repetitive trip patients, and billing for co-pays and deductibles. Additional areas will be identified based on experience, and from print and online sources. Additional areas for review can be found in the Medicare Claims Processing Manual, OIG Fraud Alerts, and OIG Advisory Opinions as well as monitoring regular and industry news sources.

Analyzing denied claims may reveal a pattern and suggest areas in need of further employee education, or perhaps a change in the agency's practices. If the rationale for the denial cannot be determined, request clarification from the payor. If the denials are inappropriate, the agency should request reconsideration and appeal the denial.

Federal law prohibits using Medicare funds to pay for services provided by firms or individuals that have been placed on the Excluded Parties List. Agencies should check the list before hiring or contracting with individuals or firms. At this writing, the list, along with instructions on its proper use, can be accessed at http://oig.hhs.gov.

If the agency utilizes customer or patient satisfaction surveys, the compliance committee or the compliance officer should be kept aware of the information that may be returned to the agency, including the number and frequency of "No Such Address" or "Unknown at This Address" returns. Evaluate undeliverable mail carefully. It may indicate identity theft or other fraud. Completed surveys may contain questions or allegations that merit the attention of the compliance officer.

RESPONSE PROCESS

Of course, it's not enough to simply identify a problem. Conduct that is discovered but not corrected will likely continue and ultimately result in agency and personal liability. Every agency must have a plan for responding to areas in need of improvement and to correct mistakes. A written policy that includes time frames will demonstrate the agency's commitment to compliance.

Upon detecting or receiving a report of possible noncompliance, the compliance officer or other high-level manager should initiate action to investigate the conduct and determine if a violation of the compliance program, law, or regulation has occurred. Agency personnel directly involved, particularly in the billing and claim generation areas, should be permitted, and encouraged, to stop a process that may result in a violation. For example, a policy could explicitly state that "a claim for reimbursement that is missing supporting documentation shall be suspended by the employee processing the claim, pending receipt of the documentation."

The investigating manager or compliance officer must also initiate the steps to halt and correct the violation. If appropriate, referral to criminal and civil authorities, reporting to government entities and other affected parties, development of a corrective action plan, and refunding overpayments also must be initiated. Any disciplinary action taken should be in accordance with the agency's written disciplinary policy.

In the CPG, the OIG has identified specific risk areas that should be included when developing response policies and procedures: medical necessity, documentation, billing and reporting risks, Part A "under arrangement" services, compliance with Medicaid regulations for matters not covered by Medicare, and anti-kickback regulations. Additional areas include "no transport" calls, multiple patient transports, and multiple ambulance responses.

OPEN LINES OF COMMUNICATION

Employees, vendors, customers, and patients should all have unrestricted means of reporting to, and inquiring of, the compliance officer. The use of a hotline is recommended. This should be a publicized toll-free number offering anonymity to the caller. Anonymous e-mail reporting can also be offered. Publicizing the hotline number, as well as additional means of communication, should be part of every compliance education event and included on HIPAA notices, available at the agency's websites, and posted at all work sites, such as EMS stations.

Employee newsletters, blogs, and in-service education events also serve to foster communications with employees. If the agency publishes a customer or community newsletter, consideration should be given to compliance-related topics and inclusion of the hotline number. Customer satisfaction surveys may also include compliance-related topics.

ENFORCING STANDARDS

The CPG recommends policies and procedures that include disciplinary mechanisms when employees or contractors negligently or intentionally violate compliance policies, laws, or regulations. Of course, disciplinary activity taken pursuant to agency policy should be uniform and consistent. Guidance in developing and managing compliance programs, whether originating with federal authorities or nongovernmental entities, predominantly focuses on disciplinary measures for inspiring cooperation with standards. Initiatives for inspiring conformity with regulations using other incentives may be viable, but they have received substantially less attention.

Best Practice

Lines of Communication

1. Establish a written code of conduct. Publicize it inside and outside the agency.
2. Designate a compliance officer and establish a compliance committee with a direct reporting relationship to the CEO and governing board.
3. Provide training and education on regulatory compliance topics upon hire and regularly thereafter.
4. Establish and maintain provisions for detecting, monitoring, and reporting problems.
5. Establish and maintain response protocols for allegations and findings of illegal or unethical activity.
6. Establish and maintain open lines of communications between compliance personnel and employees, patients, customers, vendors, contractors, and the general public.
7. Enforce the established standards, and document actions taken to enforce the standards.
8. Regularly review these steps for areas that require improvement or change.

Consideration should be given to expedited resolution of compliance policy violations. Ongoing or repetitious events that become the subject of government enforcement actions may be subject to sanctions levied on a per-occurrence or per-diem basis.

CHAPTER REVIEW

Summary

Compliance programs have not been mandated by the federal government for agencies in good standing, although this may change under the Patient Protection and Affordable Care Act. Compliance programs are found in well-managed EMS agencies and can serve as a resource for all aspects of the agency's efforts to provide service and to ensure compliance with the regulatory framework necessary to sustain revenue.

WHAT WOULD YOU DO? Reflection

Given the depth and breadth of the regulatory problem existing in the agency, a compliance program is needed. A senior manager must be selected to be responsible for the program, and an initial compliance committee must be formed that includes key operations and billing department personnel.

The current risk to the company includes an offset of more than tens of thousands of dollars and the potential for criminal charges and civil action. A robust comprehensive compliance program would have provided written guidelines for the billing and dispatch departments to avoid assigning levels of service and coding that were inappropriate to the required and appropriate level of service. A regular routine of audits would have identified deficiencies in documentation to support claims, including missing or unsupportive Certificates of Medical Necessity and miscoded (downcoded or upcoded) trips. A response process would address the cause of the mistakes, including refunding payment on claims inappropriately submitted and paid, training and education for employees in the assignment of appropriate resources, collection of supporting documentation, and coding and submission of claims. When a compliance program is functioning well, denied claims can often be appealed with confidence and successfully resolved for the appellant, rather than absorbed as losses.

1. An audit is unlikely to occur at a convenient time. You might be tempted to scramble to collect the requested files in time for the audit, recall staff from vacation, pay overtime, and delay the parking lot work in order to appear organized and accommodating, A phone call and follow-up letter to the RAC will probably allow you to propose a date a few weeks or a month later, and allow your staff to pull and review files for completeness without compromising vacations, hiring temporary staff, or incurring overtime, thus allowing the parking lot maintenance to stay on schedule. Provide the auditors with a reasonable work space where they can work undisturbed. Designate an employee to interface with the auditors. The employee

should be a person who can be easily available to the audit team and will have access to key managers if the auditors have questions. Let the audit team know where they can park and where the restrooms, fire exits, and nearby convenience stores and restaurants are located.

2. In this case, the billing department's practices are exacerbating a problem that starts the moment the phone rings in the dispatch center. Written guidelines are often used in dispatch. If the agency has control of the dispatch center, proper billing practices can start when the call taker begins obtaining information from the caller and properly identifies the call type as emergent or non-emergent, wheelchair service, ambulance service, or specialty care. Likewise, the billing staff should be working from written

guidelines when coding the service for reimbursement by Medicare or other reimbursement programs. Undoubtedly, experienced staff will become proficient at typing and coding services, but convenient reference to written standards should always be at hand. Regular internal auditing can reinforce accurate dispatch and billing practices and remind experienced personnel of the guidelines.

3. Field staff complacency in obtaining signatures will undoubtedly result in financial loss from disallowed claims. The lack of compliance with signature requirements is likely to also be found with failure to adhere to other Medicare requirements, such as a legible name and title of the signatory. Signatures, printed names, and titles of signatories are a fairly easy target for auditors.

Review Questions

1. A local hospital frequently requests your service to handle emergency department (ED) discharges for patients returning to skilled nursing facilities (SNFs). An audit results in Medicare disallowing several claims previously paid, all originating at the local hospital and going to local SNFs. How might a compliance program have prevented this result? How might a compliance program affect the response to the disallowance?

2. A billing assistant in your agency notices that nearly half of the signatures on the physician certification statements (PCS) appear to be identical in many respects, although they are for different names. The letters are consistently the same height, appear in the same place on the page, and are on the signature and printed name lines. The assistant notes the trend for a few months before he mentions it to his supervisor. Her response is "Just do your job." How will a well-developed compliance program affect the billing assistant's choices in

addressing his concerns? What are the possible consequences to the agency of not having a compliance program in place? What avenues would be open to the compliance officer if she received the report from the billing assistant anonymously? Would the situation be handled any differently if the report were received after the billing assistant appealed progressive disciplinary measures by the supervisor for continuing to note the occurrence of similar signatures in the PCS forms?

3. When should training and education in the requirements of the compliance program be introduced to employees? Are the same education and training appropriate for all employees? What, if any, jobs in your agency require specialized training in regulatory requirements?

4. What lines of communication should be in place for patients who believe they are being billed improperly? For an employee who

believes a patient could be safely transported by wheelchair but is being transported by ambulance? For vendors, contractors, or subcontractors with concerns about the agency's adherence to regulations? How will patients, employees, vendors, and contractors know about these lines of communication?

5. A manager is alerted by an ambulance crew that it will be running behind schedule. The crew arrived at the home of a dialysis patient for a scheduled stretcher transport. On arrival, the patient's husband advised that the patient is on her way home from the local mall and should be home soon. The crew has been asked by the patient's husband to wait for her to return and then transport her to her dialysis appointment. How should the manager respond to this situation?

6. What are the advantages of having a written code of conduct? Are there any advantages or disadvantages to publicizing a code of conduct on an employee website? On a public website?

References

Federal Bureau of Investigation. (2009, May). "Last Two Defendants Convicted in Ambulance Fraud Case Sentenced." See the organization website.

Health Imaging. (2009, July). "Three Arkansas Health Workers Plead Guilty to HIPAA Violations." See the organization website.

Office of Inspector General. (2003, March 24). *Federal Register 68*(56). See the organization website.

Schoenmann, J. (2009, April). "It Pays EMTs to Dot i's and Cross t's: In Vegas They Get Bonus for Properly Completed Paperwork but City Touts Savings." *Las Vegas Sun*. See the organization website.

Key Terms

audit An examination of an organization's records conducted by the organization, a regulatory agency, or a third party to assess compliance with one or more sets of laws, regulations, or other standards.

corporate integrity agreement (CIA) An agreement between the Office of Inspector General and a health care provider as part of a settlement for alleged civil wrongdoing relating to federal health care laws.

code of conduct A written set of rules governing the behavior of an organization and its employees or members.

compliance committee An interdepartmental committee bringing together managers and resources from various areas of the organization to address risk areas and concerns specific to regulatory issues and to provide a route for disseminating information to and from the compliance officer on a regular basis.

compliance officer A senior manager responsible for operation of the compliance program.

compliance program An organized set of procedures and personnel tasked with ensuring that regulatory requirements are met.

Federal Register The daily publication in which federal agencies publish regulations.

federal sentencing guidelines A detailed set of instructions for judges to determine appropriate sentences for federal crimes.

fraud 1. A knowing misrepresentation of the truth or concealment of a material fact to induce another to act to his detriment. 2. A misrepresentation made recklessly without belief in its truth to induce another to act. 3. An unintentional deception or misrepresentation that causes injury to another. 4. Fraud that has been made illegal by statute and that subjects the offender to criminal penalties.

Medicare A federal system of health insurance for people over age sixty-five and for certain other people.

CHAPTER 17

Safety Considerations for Ambulance Services

PETER DWORSKY, M.P.H., EMT-P

Objectives

After reading this chapter, the student should be able to:

17.1 Identify the role of the incident safety officer.
17.2 Explain the limitations of technology for creating a safer work environment.
17.3 Compare the relationship between the EMS safety officer and the ISO.
17.4 Describe why the investigation of a near miss event is important.
17.5 Explain the difference between a regulation and a standard.

Overview

Ambulance services in the United States range in size from one ambulance operated by volunteers and managed by a community board of directors to large governmental agencies and even larger, private, for-profit corporations. This text presents information that the manager of an ambulance service, large or small, needs in order to keep the business solvent and provide clinically excellent service to the community.

Key Terms

DART rate	**incident safety officer**	**Occupational Safety**	**Ryan White**
EMS safety officer	**(ISO)**	**and Health**	**Comprehensive**
EMS Voluntary	**National Fire**	**Administration**	**AIDS Resources**
Event Notification	**Protection**	**(OSHA)**	**Emergency**
Tool	**Association**	**personal protection**	**(CARE) Act**
exposure control	**(NFPA)**	**equipment**	**sentinel event**
plan	**near miss**	**risk management**	

WHAT WOULD YOU DO?

You, the EMS safety officer, were notified that one of your agency's units was transporting a critical patient from one hospital to another for an intervention in the cardiac catheterization lab at another facility. While off-loading the patient from the ambulance, the stretcher collapsed and the crew dropped the patient. The crew moved the patient to the emergency department and, once cleared, continued to the catheterization lab. Upon returning to the station at the end of the shift, the crew notified the supervisor of the incident because one of the crew members claimed to have hurt his shoulder while attempting to prevent the stretcher from falling. A quick evaluation of the stretcher showed that it did not have the traditional locking mechanism because it was dedicated to the critical care fleet. Further investigation revealed that the EMT assigned to the unit for the day had never worked on a critical care unit before and was just filling in.

1. What are your agency's policies for reassigning staff from unit to unit?
2. What is your protocol for dealing with equipment failures?
3. What documentation do you maintain for proof of training and for retraining staff on the use of equipment?
4. What policies do you have in place for notification of sentinel events?

■ INTRODUCTION

This chapter will focus on the roles and responsibility of the EMS or ambulance service safety officer, which encompass the development of safety programs, **risk management** processes, and compliance with **Occupational Safety and Health Administration (OSHA)** regulations and the **National Fire Protection Association's (NFPA)** standards and wellness programs. When functioning in the area of administrative responsibilities, the **EMS safety officer** is often referred to as the health and EMS safety officer (HSO). However, when deployed to an incident or preplanned event, the EMS safety officer will assume the role of **incident safety officer (ISO)** and take on site-specific functions that will be discussed. In this dual role, an agency's EMS safety officer is typically responsible for the following:

- Responding to incidents of significance
- Assessing personnel at incident for signs of stress

- Identifying and correcting safety hazards
- Possessing knowledge of applicable laws and regulations and standards
- Investigating all on-the-job worker injuries
- Investigating injuries to patients
- Keeping accurate training records
- Maintaining inspection and service records
- Investigating collisions and other events
- Managing infection control issues including blood-borne pathogens and respiratory protection

■ SAFETY CONSIDERATIONS FOR AN EMS AGENCY ⎯⎯⎯⎯

Ambulance service employees respond to many calls that are anything other than routine. Today, incidents involving ambulance services are often complex in size and nature, and they frequently involve multiple agencies and resources. In many circumstances, responders are exposed to hazards that they may not have the experience or the training to manage appropriately, including mass casualties, biohazards, chemical hazards, explosives, acts of terrorism, and natural disasters.

EMS has existed in its current format for less than 50 years, while ambulance services have been around for several centuries. In recent years, dramatic advances have been achieved in communication systems, medical treatment, and transport support services. Largely ignored, though currently the subject of greater attention, has been the safety of our most precious resources: the EMTs, paramedics, and others who staff our ambulances and other emergency vehicles.

Recent visible efforts to enhance the safety of ambulance paramedics include the following (also see "Your Web Connection" at the end of this chapter):

- The creation of the National Association of EMTs' "Taking Safety to the Streets" course,

an effort to increase the awareness of safety across many potential areas of risk
- The work of Objective Safety and the EMS Safety Foundation to improve the safety of our ambulance design and construction
- The EMS Culture of Safety Project, funded by the National Highway Traffic Safety Administration and managed by the American College of Emergency Physicians

The discipline of safety in EMS systems is relatively new and predominantly draws experience from the fire service and hospitals. However, some agencies have been slow to join for numerous reasons, include budgeting issues, lack of staff, lack of resources, and lack of internal expertise.

Capturing data about occupational illnesses and injuries in EMS is limited as there is not a national repository or lead agency collecting information about these issues. Some states have begun to develop reporting systems to capture this data; however, the data remain fragmented or incomplete and are often abstracted from multiple sources, including OSHA injury logs, police reports, and workers' compensation loss-run reports. However, comprehensive injury data collection has been proven feasible if an industry effort is put forth and an entity is created to a lead agency, as is the case with the fire service. It is known that each year approximately a hundred firefighters die in the line of duty and that heart disease is responsible for nearly 45 percent of these deaths. Since 1977, the U.S. Fire Administration (USFA) has tracked firefighter line-of-duty deaths (Figure 17.1). In 1998, Congress established the Firefighter Fatality Investigation and Prevention Program within the National Institute for Occupational Safety and Health (NIOSH). Among the goals established by the NIOSH programs are the investigation of all firefighter line-of-duty deaths, determining contributory factors, and publishing reports on specific fatalities with

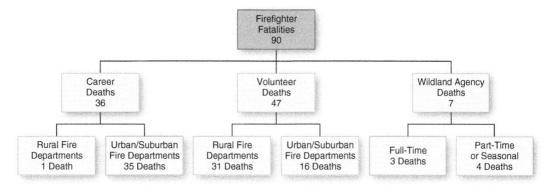

FIGURE 17.1 ■ A breakdown of the causes of firefighter fatalities in the United States in 2009. *Source: Courtesy of U.S. Fire Administration.*

the goal of implementing changes that will result in the reduction of fatalities. Every year, the USFA and the National Fire Data Center release a report detailing firefighter fatalities in the United States. Within the report is a breakdown of the findings surrounding the death, including the type of duty the firefighter was involved in, the cause of the fatality, and the nature of the injury (U.S. Fire Administration, 2010).

A national database of EMS provider injuries and fatalities does not exist, although some data are captured based on the provider type. For example, if the injury or fatality originates in a fire-based EMS service, injuries will be tracked by the USFA through the National Fire Incident Reporting System (NFIRS), and the International Association of Fire Fighters (IAFF) will track injuries from career departments if they are represented by the IAFF. Neither organization tracks injury data from unrepresented departments, volunteers, or seasonal or part-time firefighters. Thus, not all injuries are accounted for.

In 2010, the Center for Leadership, Innovation and Research in EMS (2013) released the **EMS Voluntary Event Notification Tool** (E.V.E.N.T.). E.V.E.N.T. is a collaborative effort between the EMS Chiefs of Canada, the National EMS Management Association and the North Central EMS Institute. The purpose of E.V.E.N.T. is to allow for the anonymous reporting of **sentinel events**, **near misses**, equipment and medical device failures, and lessons learned. The near miss is an event that has all of the dynamics of an actual incident—be it a collision, wrong medication administration, patient drop, and so on—but it does not actually occur. For example, a paramedic picks up the wrong medication but does not actually administer it.

However, even data collected by E.V.E.N.T. and other systems are incomplete and fragmented. Not every injury from every agency is going to be reported if there is not a mandate to do so. In addition, agencies and individual providers are often unwilling to report when, where, and the circumstances surrounding an injury due to fear of penalties and reprisals, especially if an investigation may reveal that the injury was caused by a policy violation (Rajasekran, Fairbanks, and Shah, 2008).

Even obtaining an accurate count of responders is difficult. Nationally, the American Ambulance Association estimates that there are nearly 840,000 EMS responders (American Ambulance Association, 2007). Based on statistics captured by the National Association of Emergency Medical Technicians (2013), the breakdown of providers is as follows:

First Responder: 11 percent

EMT-B: 53 percent

EMT-I: 9 percent

EMT-P: 41 percent

Registered Nurse: 8 percent

On an annual basis, these nearly 1 million EMS providers will respond to 31 million requests for emergency service, and possibly an equal number of nonemergency responses, and will ultimately treat more than 22 million patients (EMS Magazine, 2006).

The Institute of Medicine (IOM), in its "To Err Is Human" report, examined the impact of errors on patients in the hospital setting. The IOM estimates that there are between 44,000 and 98,000 annual deaths due to medication and procedural errors. Medical errors are the leading cause of death, followed by surgical complications and mistakes. More Americans will die from medical errors than breast cancer, AIDS, or motor vehicle accidents. In all, 7 percent of all hospitalized patients will experience a serious medical error. These errors will add upwards of 25 billion dollars annually to the costs of health care (Kohn, Corrigan, and Donaldson, 1999). The cost is not broken down to track EMS's responsibility due to the fragmented nature and the lack of standardization within EMS systems.

Relatively few safety standards apply specifically to EMS agencies. Most standards arise from other regulatory entities and are modified in order to be applicable to EMS as EMS operates outside the normal environment for which the standards were designed. In either case, many managers are not aware of all the standards that apply or even of the regulatory agencies that may govern their activities (Figure 17.2).

For example, the Centers for Medicare & Medicaid Services (CMS) issued a memo in 2007 clarifying its policy on medical gas storage (Centers for Medicare & Medicaid Services, 2007).

■ DRIVING

For several reasons, the area of greatest concern for EMS safety is transportation-related incidents. The National Highway Transportation

---

Best Practice

Free Consultation Services

Both the Public Employees Occupational Safety and Health (PEOSH) and the Occupational Safety and Health Administration (OSHA) offer free consultation services to employers to aid them in identifying potential hazards in the workplace and improving safety and health management systems. The safety and health consultation program is completely separate from the inspection effort, and no citations are issued or penalties proposed unless the employer fails to correct an imminent danger or serious hazards.

The employer's only obligation will be to commit to correcting serious job safety and health hazards—a commitment that is expected to be made prior to the actual visit and carried out in a timely manner.

In rare instances, during the walk-through the consultant may find a situation that presents imminent danger. If so, immediate actions must be taken to protect all employees. Other situations—those that would be judged a serious violation under OSHA criteria—require the employer and the consultant to develop a plan and schedule to eliminate or control the hazard.

NFPA
JCOHA
ASTM
CAMTS
CAAS
OSHA
PEOSHA
NIOSH
EPA
DEP

FIGURE 17.2 ■ Numerous federal, state, and local agencies promulgate regulations and standards that affect the safety of EMS operations.
Source: Reprinted by permission from MONOC Mobile Health Services.

Safety Administration (NHTSA) estimates that over 8,500 EMS-related collisions occur every year. In the 10-year period between 1991 and 2002, NIOSH reported that 300 fatal ambulance collisions occurred, resulting in 357 deaths of EMS providers, patients, and passengers (Centers for Disease Control and Prevention, 2003). The numbers are staggering: Nearly 75 percent of EMS line-of-duty deaths result from transportation-related incidents. Of these, 20 percent of the fatalities are from the EMS provider being struck by another vehicle at the scene. The remaining 80 percent of EMS deaths are as a result of the ambulance being involved in a collision (Maguire, Hunting, Smith, and Levick, 2002). The majority of collisions are preventable through the use of administrative tools, training, and technology. It should also be noted that the actual number of collisions are thought to be significantly underreported. The predominant reason is fear of management reprisal—that is, staff are afraid of getting in trouble for getting into an accident or getting hurt.

Additional research has shown that crashes were the leading causes of civil suits against EMS providers, with a 10-year study revealing that nearly 72 percent of the claims were for transportation-related incidents and accounted for over 50 percent of the insurance monies paid, compared to the 35 percent that was paid for medical negligence (Colwell, Pons, Blanchet, and Mangino, 1999; Wang, Fairbanks, Shah, Abo, and Yealy, 2008).

Due to the potential severity of motor vehicle collisions, the agency must be committed to reducing these negative events. One of the first steps is to change the attitude of all involved. Collisions should not be referred to as "MVAs" or "accidents," when analyzed; a causal factor can almost always be identified. The collision should be classified as preventable or unpreventable. In one urban system, nearly 45 percent of the collisions were deemed to be preventable, and a primary causal factor was a policy violation.

The process involved in reducing the total number of collisions is multifaceted and involves harnessing the entire management team, technology, and behavior modification, and it involves four types of action:

1. Prevention efforts include maintaining up-to-date policies and procedures regarding the use of emergency warning devices, keeping the staff educated about current trends, and regulations, and evaluating current technology.
2. Managing the incident includes collecting data for analysis and identifying causal factors.
3. Implementation of corrective processes includes, as warranted, re-education, retraining, review of existing policies, and discipline.
4. Legal issues associated with collisions should be reviewed.

Everyone must be involved in prevention. This includes implementation and enforcement of policies, which at a minimum should address speed, the use of lights and sirens, seat belts, cell phone use, and the use of backers or spotters.

In general, any motor vehicle collision prevention program must be clearly communicated to the staff and management team. Specifically, prevention programs should address policies and procedures that govern the use of lights and sirens. Often agencies leave the decision to use lights and sirens up to the vehicle operator, within certain parameters. Other agencies allow their communication center to determine the level or type of emergency response; this is most common for interfacility transports. In either situation, certain guidelines or policies must be in place as research has shown that the use of emergency devices does not speed the transport time or positively affect patient outcome. In one study, O'Brien, Price, and Adams (1999) had an observer vehicle travel the same route to the hospital as the ambulance, which was using lights and sirens. Upon arrival at the hospital, the observer proceeded to the patient location and noted the medical interventions accomplished at the hospital prior to the observer's arrival. This study found that the ambulance arrived 3 minutes and 50 seconds sooner than the observer vehicle. However, of the 75 patients involved in the study, only 4 were felt to have benefited clinically by the time saved. The authors concluded that lights and sirens shorten the transport time, but the time saved is not usually associated with immediate clinical significance.

Another published study (Brown, Whitney, Hunt, Addario, and Hogue, 2000) concluded that lights and sirens in an urban EMS system reduced ambulance response times by an average of 1 minute and 45 seconds. Although statistically significant, this time saving is likely to be clinically relevant in only a very few cases, thus exposing the crew and patient to a high-risk activity that has limited benefit.

VISIBILITY

All agencies should also establish policies governing the use of seat belts and cell phones, and those need to be clearly communicated to all staff. In addition, agencies should mine their data on collision history for patterns or trends. For example, collisions resulting from the vehicle operator backing into an object are 100 percent preventable events and can often be controlled with a policy mandating a spotter or the implementation of backup cameras.

A system review should be in place to address the visibility of ambulances. All too often the agency paint scheme is what it is and never changes over the years, and, if it does change, it is often due to a marketing agenda and not safety concerns.

A number of interrelated factors affect the visibility of an emergency vehicle to other drivers, both during a response and while parked at the scene. These variables include the vehicle's size, color scheme (*aka* livery), passive conspicuity features such as marker lights and retroreflective striping, and the presence/operation of active warning devices including emergency lighting systems or audible sirens and horns. Environmental conditions also influence visibility; chief among these are time of day, ambient lighting, weather, and the presence of driver distractions or visual clutter in the surroundings.

Conspicuity refers to the ability of a vehicle to draw attention to its presence, even when other road users are not actively looking for it. Although a high degree of visibility is usually a desirable characteristic for emergency vehicles, at times public safety personnel do not want their vehicles to be readily visible. While parked off the roadway at an incident, emergency vehicles should reduce their conspicuity both to avoid being hit by drivers who are potentially attracted to activated warning devices and during law enforcement support operations.

Historically, emergency vehicle operators primarily relied on active signaling, using various mechanical devices to enhance their vehicles' visibility and conspicuity while responding to, and on the scene of, emergency incidents. These technologies include emergency warning lights and audible systems designed to attract surrounding drivers' attention. Although active devices will likely always be needed to promote emergency vehicle visibility/conspicuity, passive treatments using retroreflective sheeting and other materials are increasingly being used to complement lights and sirens (U.S. Fire Administration, 2009).

During the past 10 years, the British government researched and deployed a set of visibility/conspicuity standards now used on law enforcement vehicles throughout the country (Harrison, 2004). Efforts to develop conspicuity specifications in the United Kingdom were undertaken with several objectives in mind:

* Be recognizable at a distance of 200 to 500+ meters (650 to 1,650+ feet)

* Assist with high-visibility policing
* Be readily identifiable nationally as a police vehicle, with room for local markings
* Be acceptable to at least 75 percent of the staff using it

In 2004, the United Kingdom Home Office, Scientific Development Branch, published a subsequent specification detailing a "high conspicuity" livery for police vehicles used in cities and towns. In addition to the "full Battenburg" scheme used on patrol cars primarily assigned to high-speed roadways, the 2004 document specifies a "half Battenburg" pattern for patrol vehicles deployed in the urban environment (Figures 17.3 and 17.4). Public safety agencies across the United States have begun exploring the concepts from the United Kingdom high-conspicuity liveries, including the Battenburg pattern, to their vehicles.

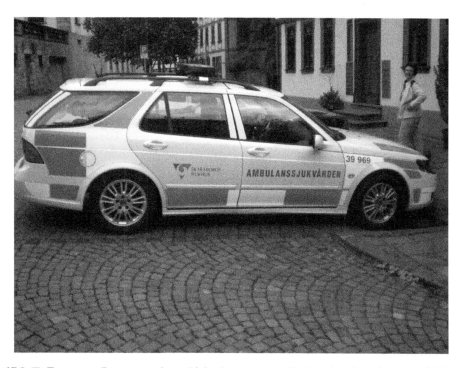

FIGURE 17.3 ■ European first responder vehicles have standardized their color scheme, which includes the Battenburg pattern. *Source: Used by permission from MONOC Mobile Health Services.*

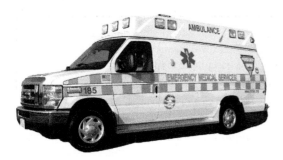

FIGURE 17.4 ■ MONOC Mobile Health Services displaying a modified Battenburg pattern. *Source: Photo courtesy of MONOC Mobile Health Systems.*

In contrast to the United Kingdom, there is currently no evidence of a U.S. industry standard for the visibility/conspicuity of law enforcement vehicles. As a best practice, however, many U.S. agencies apply retroreflective treatments to patrol cars, motorcycles, and other vehicles.

Recent editions of national standards for U.S. fire apparatus and ambulances (NFPA 1901 and the draft version of NFPA 1917) require the increased application of retroreflective striping and markings to enhance visibility and conspicuity, including corner markings, chevrons, and striping (National Fire Protection Association, 2009b; National Fire Protection Association, 2011).

Visibility and identity are influenced by the color schemes and patterns in which emergency vehicles are painted. Case in point: Many people think that fire trucks are always red, although we know that not to be the case, and it is possible to mask the vehicle so as to confuse the motorist.

Different marking patterns can also change driver responses. The association of the down-and-away chevron pattern with a message of "Danger" or "Slow down" is related to its widespread use on traffic barriers, as specified in the *Manual on Uniform Traffic Control Devices* (MUTCD), and which may account for the recent trend toward the application of this marking on fire engines and ambulances (U.S. Department of Transportation, 2009). There

also exists the notion that drivers steer toward bright lights, such as those used to increase the visibility of emergency vehicles. This is often referred to as "moth effect," or phototaxis. Several recent studies, however, suggest that while bright lights may not be the cause, drivers' fixation on roadside objects can cause their steering to drift in the direction of their gaze.

In 2008, the NFPA formed a committee to draft a new standard, NFPA 1917: Standard for Automotive Ambulances, which is scheduled to be released in 2013. The committee was tasked with developing a new baseline standard to replace the Government Services Administration's KKK–version F specifications. The committee is made up of a weighted cross-section of stakeholders representing insurance companies, manufacturers, special experts, end users, research agencies for testing, and others. The Department of Homeland Security's Science and Technology Directorate Human Factors and Behavioral Sciences Division project in conjunction with NIOSH has begun to look at the human factors design of ambulances to improve the safety of the provider and occupant (Figure 17.5).

Perhaps the best methodology for reducing collision is the simplest and least expensive—changing driver attitudes. Staff needs to be educated in the local vehicle and traffic codes and the agency's policies requiring compliance. In many post-collision interviews, drivers often express the belief that they had the right-of-way. It is incumbent upon management to ensure that vehicle operators know exactly what they are allowed to do and to expect that other drivers may not understand their personal responsibility as evidenced by poor compliance with move-over regulations.

Staff also needs to understand the capability and limitations of the vehicles they are driving (Figure 17.6). Often new employees may never have driven an ambulance before and do not understand that their vehicle is much larger, has many blind spots, and may weigh several times that of the car they drove

Ambulance Type	Car
I – 10,500 lbs	Nissan Versa – 2,751 lbs
II – 9,000 lbs	Jeep Grand Cherokee – 3,968 lbs
III – 10,500-11,000 lbs	Chevy Silverado – 4.709 lbs

FIGURE 17.5 ▨ A comparison of the GVW vehicle weights of ambulances and commercial vehicles, emphasizing the need for better driving training. *Source: Courtesy of the Institute for Highway Safety.*

to work and that it and maneuvers differently. The most important variation is the braking distance. Basically, the heavier the vehicle, the longer it will take to stop.

As an adjunct to changing vehicle operator behavior, the agency should look to investing in a commercially available driver training program. Simply having all employees take an emergency vehicle operations course or defensive driving course provides the opportunity and forum to discuss company policy and legal obligations. For example, many emergency vehicle operators believe they have the legal ability to run red lights. Each state has its own laws governing the use of lights and sirens and the ability to disregard them. The agency's policies should address this.

In New Jersey, the statute is as follows:

Title 39:4-91. Right of way of emergency vehicles; liability of drivers

a. The driver of a vehicle on a highway shall yield the right of way to any authorized emergency vehicle when it is operated on official business, or in the exercise of the driver's profession or calling, in response to an emergency call or in the pursuit of an actual or suspected violator of the law and when an audible signal by bell, siren, exhaust whistle or other means is sounded

Number of Violations (Last Five Years)	Number of Accidents (Last Five Years)			
	0	**1**	**2**	**3 (or more)**
No Minor Violations	Clear	Ok to Drive	Borderline	Can Not Drive
1 Minor Violation	Ok to Drive	Ok to Drive	Borderline	Can Not Drive
2 Minor Violations	Ok to Drive	Borderline	Can Not Drive	Can Not Drive
3 Minor Violations	Borderline	Can Not Drive	Can Not Drive	Can Not Drive
4 or More Minor Violations	Can Not Drive	Can Not Drive	Can Not Drive	Can Not Drive
Any Major Violation	Can Not Drive	Can Not Drive	Can Not Drive	Can Not Drive

FIGURE 17.6 ▨ Agencies should work with their insurance carriers to develop a Drive/No Drive decision table. *Source: Reprinted by permission from MONOC Mobile Health Services.*

from the authorized emergency vehicle and when the authorized emergency vehicle, except a police vehicle, is equipped with at least one lighted lamp displaying a red light visible under normal atmospheric conditions from a distance of at least five hundred feet to the front of the vehicle.

b. This section shall not relieve the driver of any authorized emergency vehicle from the duty to drive with due regard for the safety of all persons, nor shall it protect the driver from the consequences of his reckless disregard for the safety of others. Nothing in this section shall be construed to limit any immunity or defense otherwise provided by law.

In addition to a classroom training session, such as the Coaching the Emergency Vehicle Operator (CEVO) course, adding the opportunity for the student to have some actual driving time with an instructor will give the driver an opportunity to see how a larger ambulance functions in a controlled setting. This training, whenever possible, should be conducted annually. In addition, there should be a review of all drivers' driving history through the state's Division of Motor Vehicles annually and after any unpreventable collision. A retrospective study examining 11 years of fatal ambulance crash data concluded that 41 percent of the ambulance drivers involved in crashes had poor driving records and were classified as high-risk drivers (Kahn, Pirrallo, and Kuhn, 2001).

Working with the agency's insurance carrier, managers will find that they have established baselines for chargeable occurrences that when exceeded will not provide coverage for the driver. Therefore, an ambulance service needs a policy governing what happens when a staff member loses the ability to drive. The staff member may have a specified time period during which to reduce the number of points through a defensive driving program while taking a leave of absence; it may involve a suspension or termination or reassignment of job functions, assuming driving is not part of the job description, or another option.

Another area related to driving is general operations on roadways. Traditional EMS uniforms are dark blue pants and jackets, thus making EMTs and paramedics almost invisible during nighttime and low-light operations. In 2007, the Federal Highway Authority Act, 23 CFR 634, went into effect. This act mandated that all persons working within the right of way on any federal highway wear personal protective clothing that meets the ANSI standard for Class II or III safety vests. This requirement has been adopted by the MUTCD. Therefore, if an agency does not provide high-visibility uniforms to staff, it must have a high-visibility safety vest for each crew member. This is extremely important as nearly 20 percent of EMS provider transport fatalities occur from being struck and killed while at the scene of an incident. Other options include a complete change to a high-visibility uniform. Turnout gear does not have enough reflective material to meet the MUTCD standard for high-visibility clothing so the vests must be worn in addition.

The ambulance service should conduct frequent, detailed training about highway operations for its personnel. Good-quality highway operations safety training programs are available from a variety of sources. Specific training should include, as a minimum, the following:

- Proper positioning of vehicles, and the use of heavy vehicles such as fire apparatus as scene barricades
- Proper lighting of accident scenes, including use of mobile signboards for long-term incidents and the reduction of emergency lights while stationary at the scene to aid traffic flow
- Proper use of personal protective equipment at highway incident scenes (Figure 17.7)

TECHNOLOGY

The implementation of technology is a must. This includes choosing lighting colors and patterns, siren types and placement, and vehicle

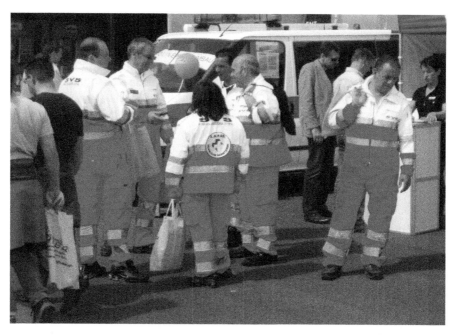

FIGURE 17.7 ■ Many European EMS agencies have adopted high-visibility uniforms for everyday use, as opposed to the minimal standards set forth by the U.S. Federal Highway Act of 2007. *Source: Photo courtesy of MONOC Mobile Health Systems.*

markings. For example, red and blue lights take advantage of the Purkinje shift effect, during which the human eye sees red best during daylight and blue best at night. After white, yellow is the color most easily seen. Many agencies will only use red and, in some states, other colors are prohibited.

Several "black box" types of devices are commercially available to provide real-time feedback to the vehicle operator by providing an audible warning when preset parameters are being reached or exceeded. The Road Safety System uses an onboard computer that detects and records vehicle speed, RPM, ignition, and other user-defined digital inputs that can monitor braking force, turn signal usage, and activation of emergency lights and siren. The driver logs onto the system by use of an electronic key fob, so the system can create a history of driver performance regardless of

what vehicle is being used. Additional sensors can be added to track seat belt usage, vehicle abuse, and other functions. An onboard computer provides automated downloading of vehicle metrics. The system can also be tied into a GPS receiver. One study showed that the implementation of black box technology in an urban system led to a decrease in "penalty counts, increase in seatbelt use, and decrease in maintenance savings with no change in response times" (Levick and Swanson, 2005).

Another option is the installation of a windshield or dash-mounted video recording system such as Drive Cam (Figure 17.8). Such systems will typically have a dual-lens camera system with one lens facing outward at what the driver is seeing and another facing inward. When choosing a camera, make sure it has the ability to record audio. These systems are typically triggered by a change in G-force that is

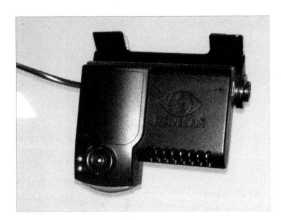

FIGURE 17.8 ■ A windshield-mounted video recording device can be a useful tool for reviewing driver behavior and allegations of aggressive driving. *Source: Photo courtesy of MONOC Mobile Health Systems.*

caused by hard braking, rough use, or a collision. Many cameras can be set with pre- and post-recording times that will allow a manager to review the event leading up to the collision. Newer technology allows for the cameras to be uploaded to a server via a built-in cellular capability, so vehicles stationed at outlying posts will still have data transferred without the need to bring the vehicle to a main facility or send a manager to download the footage.

Installing a simple backup camera will clearly reduce the number of backing accidents, but it should not alleviate the driver of the need to have a spotter. Some systems employ a device that requires the spotter to depress a button on the rear of the ambulance to allow it go in reverse. The addition of a backup camera, supported by appropriate training and policy, may be the best possible investment of safety dollars, having the potential to avoid both property damage and personal injury events.

DATA COLLECTION

The safety officer should also be involved in the development of post-collision standard operating procedures (SOPs) as some post-collision activities can be time sensitive. Once a collision occurs, a process must be in place to manage the functions that need to be accomplished in a timely manner. This may involve delegating tasks to other managers. All injuries must be attended to, vehicles may need to be towed, the driver may need to be drug tested (Figure 17.9), and photographs and evidence must be collected. It is often a good idea to develop a task list to ensure that all details are covered.

The majority of the data collected should be analyzed for patterns and trends, and then feedback (which may or may not include discipline, if a policy violation is found) should be given to the staff member.

To an agency, it may be acceptable as a measure of success to reduce the overall number of collisions, and to another it may be equally acceptable to reduce the severity of each collision, although the obvious goal should be to reduce both as this will have an impact on auto insurance premiums. Although counting the number of actual collisions is simple, one must have a standardized scale for severity. One agency developed the criteria listed in Figures 17.10 and 17.11.

Federal Motor Carrier Safety Admin, DOT SS 382.303 post accident drug testing criteria

Collision involving loss of life or Bodily injury with immediate medical treatment away from the scene or Disabling damage to any motor vehicle requiring tow

FIGURE 17.9 ■ The U.S. Federal Motor Carrier Safety Administration has developed post-accident drug-testing criteria. *Source: Reprinted by permission from the US FMCA.*

Green category are the following criteria:
- No damage to either vehicle
- An injury occurred, but resulted in an RMA
- Damage to both vehicles/objects combined < 1000.00

Yellow category are the following criteria:
- An minor injury occurred, but resulted in transport to an ED
- Damage to both vehicles/objects combined > 1000.00
- Either vehicle needs to be towed
- An animal was hit

Red category are the following criteria:
- An injury occurred, but resulted in an admission to a hospital or lost work time
- Damage to both vehicles/objects combined > 10,000.00
- A fatality occurred

If any of the following are identified as a compounding factor, severity is raised to the next level:
- Violation of law or policy
- Patient onboard
- Use of Lights and Sirens
- Deliberate act or negligence

FIGURE 17.10 ■ An objective scale should be used for categorizing the severity of collisions to develop trends and aid in focused education programs. *Source: Reprinted by permission from MONOC Mobile Health Services.*

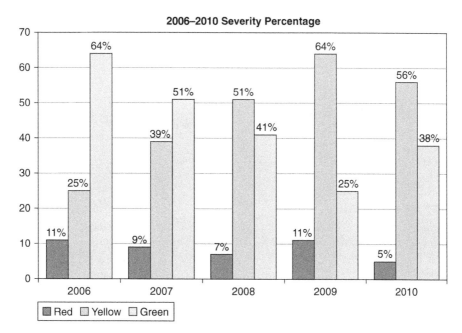

FIGURE 17.11 ■ A graphical representation of collisions based on the Severity Scale will give a quick view of trends being developed. *Source: Reprinted by permission from MONOC Mobile Health Services.*

Collisions must be analyzed for other factors to account for a true cost to the agency. These include the obvious: loss of life or injury, the impact of negative publicity, loss of the vehicle, and any revenue associated with that vehicle. Hidden costs may include litigation expenses, increased insurance premiums, loss of the employee and costs of hiring a replacement, medical disability costs, and increased workers' compensation claims. Once the historical costs of collisions are known, it may be justifiable to invest money in a collision reduction program. For example, a steel step bumper may cost $1,000 and a retrofitted backup camera $350. Analysis may show that it is cheaper to invest in the cameras than to replace the bumpers, although if there is strong compliance with policies and a spotter is used, there may not be a history of backing collisions.

Only through data collection will you be able to know where to invest your financial resources (Figure 17.12). One agency utilizes an

---

Motor Vehicle Collision Incident Report

Date of Collision: Time of Collision: Call #:
Incident Location: Town: State:
Unit ID #:   Vehicle #:
Unit Type: □ MAV □ BLS □ ALS □ SCT
Vehicle Type: □ Van □ Box □ Car □ Other

Driver: Age: Seat belt □ Yes   □ No
Certification Level: □ EMT □ EMT-P □ RN □ RN/EMT or RN/EMT-P
Time shift started:
Injured: □ Yes □ No

Other personnel:
Name: Where in vehicle were they seated?
Seat belt □ Yes □ No
Certification Level: □ EMT □ EMT-P □ RN □ RN/EMT or RN/EMT-P
Injured: □ Yes □ No

Name: Where in vehicle were they seated?
Seat belt □ Yes □ No
Certification Level: □ EMT □ EMT-P □ RN □ RN/EMT or RN/EMT-P
Injured: □ Yes □ No

Patient onboard: □ Yes □ No   Where in vehicle were they?
Seat belt □ Yes □ No
Patient injured: □ Yes □ No

Status at time of accident:
□ Responding to a 911 call   □ En route to medical facility with a patient
□ Responding to a non-emergency assignment   □ Non-emergency transport
□ En route to medical facility without a patient   □ On scene
□ Not on an assignment
□ Entering/exiting station
□ Other

FIGURE 17.12 ■ Some EMS agencies develop internal motor vehicle collision reports for capturing data not typically contained in standard incident reports. *Source: Reprinted by permission from MONOC Mobile Health Services.*

Accident Location:
☐ Roadway ☐ Parked ☐ Intersection ☐ Other:

Road Characteristics:
☐ Straight & Level ☐ Uphill ☐ Downhill ☐ Curve

Road System:
☐ Interstate ☐ State Highway ☐ County Highway
☐ Municipal ☐ Private Property

Road Surface Type:
☐ Concrete ☐ Blacktop ☐ Gravel ☐ Steel Grid ☐ Dirt ☐ Other:

Road Surface Condition:
☐ Dry ☐ Wet ☐ Snow ☐ Ice ☐ Slush ☐ Water ☐ Sand/Mud/Dirt ☐ Other:

Road Divided by:
☐ Guide Rail   ☐ Concrete Barrier   ☐ Concrete Island
☐ Grass Median   ☐ Painted median   ☐ None   ☐ Other:

Road Construction:
☐ Yes   ☐ No   ☐ Workers Present

Number of lanes in your travel direction:

Weather: ☐ Clear ☐ Rain ☐ Snow ☐ Fog ☐ Sleet ☐ High Wind ☐ Overcast

Light Condition: ☐ Daylight ☐ Dawn ☐ Dusk ☐ Dark ☐ Other

What were you doing just before the collision?
☐ Going Straight Ahead ☐ Making Right Turn ☐ Making Left Turn
☐ Making U-Turn ☐ Starting from Parking ☐ Starting in Traffic
☐ Slowing or Stopping ☐ Parking ☐ Parked ☐ Changing Lanes ☐ Merging
☐ Backing ☐ Driverless ☐ Other:

Collision Type:
☐ Head-on ☐ Rear-end ☐ Broadside ☐ Roll-over ☐ Pedestrian struck
☐ Vehicle vs. Object ☐ Other:

Emergency Warning Devices used
☐ Lights ☐ Lights & Siren ☐ None

Police Report Generated:
☐ Yes   ☐ No

Vehicle towed
☐ Yes   ☐ No

Supervisor notified
☐ Yes   Who_____   ☐ No   Why not_____

Description of Collision:

FIGURE 17.12 ▧ (*Continued*)

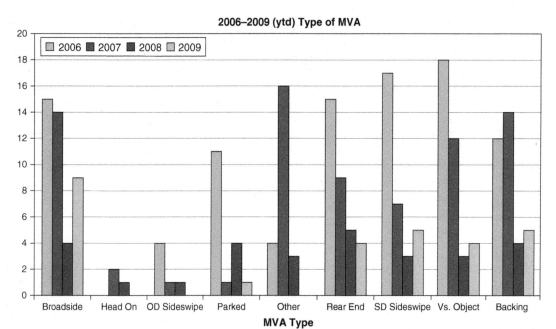

FIGURE 17.13 ■ A graphical representation of MVA by type will give a quick view of trends and can assist with the development of training programs. *Source: Reprinted by permission from MONOC Mobile Health Services.*

electronic data collection tool that has nearly fifty forced-answer questions that the driver must answer after every collision. The information obtained provides feedback to the management team and staff about potential issues, which for some services have included policy violations, driver fatigue issues, poor awareness at intersections, and lack of seat belt usage.

Once data are collected, targeted education of staff can be used. In the chart below, broadside accidents (either striking or being struck) had the highest rate of occurrence (Figure 17.13). This led to a retraining campaign highlighting the dangers involved in intersection collisions.

■ VIOLENCE AGAINST EMS PERSONNEL———————

Assaults against ambulance paramedics appear to be a growing problem in the United States (National Association of State EMS Officials,

2009), the United Kingdom (Calkin, 2011), Canada (Kollek, Welsford, and Wanger, 2010), and Australia (Mayhew and Chappell, 2009). According to an article in *EMS World*, the National Association of EMTs, in a study released in 2005, revealed that 52 percent of American EMTs have been assaulted on the job. It also reports that on January 17, 2009, EMT Melissa Greenhagen was shot to death in Glasgow, Montana. A few days later, EMT Mark Davis was shot to death while responding on an ambulance call in Cape Vincent, New York. Yet there is a paucity of attention given to this subject in either preservice or in-service education of ambulance paramedics (EMS World, 2009).

At a recent "Escaping Violent Encounters" class for fire and EMS personnel, the instructor asked the group, "How many of you have been assaulted in the line of duty?" A small number raised their hands. Then the instructor asked, "How many have been punched?" "Kicked?" "Spat upon?" "Scratched?" By the end of that series, every hand in the room had been raised, some multiple times. It was clear to those present that the definition of *assault* is not well understood (personal conversation with K. Tietsort, May 22, 2012).

EMT and paramedic training is generally devoid of information about violence directed at ambulance paramedics. The common wisdom is that paramedics should avoid entering dangerous or potentially violent scenes, waiting instead for the law enforcement officers to secure and stabilize the scene. Although it is generally believed that ambulance paramedics comply with this guidance, it fails to take into account the concept of the changing or deteriorating scene, and the not-uncommon lack of prompt availability of law enforcement officers.

Given the lack of training, two scenarios are likely when paramedics are confronted with violence. First, the provider may freeze, panicked into immobility and subject to further assault. Second, the provider may overreact, as is believed to have happened when a Denver paramedic responded to violence with violence and was subsequently sentenced to 12 years of imprisonment for assault (Larson, 2009).

Why is this issue not better addressed in EMS preservice and in-service education programs? There is precious little data about why. However, experts in the subject area suggest several reasons:

1. Paramedics are rescuers who regularly place the interests of themselves over the interests of others.
2. We have evolved a culture of acceptance of violence against us, unlike any other workplace culture. Even law enforcement officers, who have extensive training in the area, usually have a zero-tolerance policy for assaults on police officers.
3. Often, senior members will regard being assaulted as a rite of passage or will mock younger members who report incidences of violence against them.

4. Sometimes, organizational processes—lengthy reports, investigations or interviews by untrained supervisors, mandatory visits to occupational medicine providers, and lack of organizational support for the prosecution of those who attack ambulance paramedics—serve as reporting barriers.
5. Ambulance service managers, unfamiliar with the subject matter, develop misplaced "legal" concerns about "teaching medics to fight."

Ambulance services, as employers, have a legal duty to provide their employees with a workplace that is as safe as possible, with known hazards reduced or eliminated. This statute is known as the OSHA General Duty Clause[1] and deals with areas of occupational risk that are not addressed by a specific OSHA standard. Given the growing body of evidence about the issues of violence in EMS, the hazard is more clearly known—placing this burden more clearly on employers to be addressed as part of a workplace hazard mitigation program.

Violence against ambulance paramedics is believed to be similar in nature to violence in hospital emergency departments, which has attained a much higher profile. The Emergency Nurses Association has developed a strong program to address the concerns of its members (Emergency Nurses Association, 2010).

Every ambulance service should strive to develop a workplace culture that effectively addresses violence against staff. The following elements are recommended:

1. Organizational leaders should strive to develop a culture that encourages reporting of assaults against ambulance paramedics.
2. An organizational policy should declare violence against ambulance paramedics unacceptable, and establish mandatory reporting and prosecution of all incidents.

---

[1] 29 U.S.C. § 654, 5(a)1.

3. Barriers to employee reporting should be removed, and onerous or burdensome processes should be minimized as much as possible.

4. All paramedics should be trained to avoid, de-escalate, and escape from violent encounters. Senior staff should be aware that police-style defensive-tactics training is not recommended for paramedics. Police *defensive tactics* is defensive in name only—the goal of all police hands-on encounters is custody and control of the violent person, while the goal of paramedics is to escape uninjured. Moreover, law enforcement techniques rely on pain compliance, which is known to be ineffective when used against drunk, drugged, or demented persons. Similarly, self-defense training offered by local martial arts studios should also be avoided. Personal self-defense is different from safely escaping from a violent situation, and self-defense courses based in the martial arts often are focused on fighting techniques that may not be appropriate for use in the health care environment.

Violence directed toward paramedics is an important issue that should be addressed by every organization's leadership. Effectively doing so is important to the well-being of the provider and the ambulance service, both in the immediate (violent) environment and later in the media and in the courts. A properly constructed and instructed program can help to ensure a successful outcome in each of these important arenas.

■ OSHA

OSHA estimates that 5.6 million workers in the health care industry and related occupations are at risk of occupational exposure to blood-borne pathogens. As a subset of this group, 1.5 million EMS providers have an exposure risk to needlestick- and other sharps-related injuries for being exposed to a blood-borne patho-gen (U.S. Department of Labor, n.d.). This risk is substantial based on these professions' work environments: motor vehicle collisions and trauma, unlit areas, and unstable environments with limited personnel.

HISTORY

In 1966, President Lyndon Johnson directed then Secretary of Labor Willard Wirtz to develop a comprehensive national program to protect workers. On December 29, 1970, President Richard Nixon signed into law the Williams-Steiger Occupational Safety and Health Act (P.L. 91-596), which gave the federal government the authority to set and enforce safety and health standards for most U.S. workers. Currently twenty-two states have plans administered by OSHA that cover both governmental and private sector employees. The remaining states have plans that are administered under the Public Employees Occupational Safety and Health (PEOSH) Act, which covers government workers. PEOSH requires these other states' plans to be as stringent as the OSHA plan.

On paper, it is quite simple to comply with OSHA standards; in reality, an employer must overcome many barriers. The majority of violations involve employee compliance. For example, it is not enough to supply **personal protective equipment (PPE)** and training to staff; the employer also must ensure that the staff is using the equipment properly. However, this is not always practical, given the environment in which EMS operates. Constant education and reminders are imperative.

HUMAN RESOURCES

Typically, the human resources (HR) department is responsible for maintaining the documentation of injuries and illness. However, the EMS safety officer should be involved in the review of the OSHA Form 300 log of work-related injuries and illnesses (Figure 17.14).

OSHA's Form 300 (Rev. 01/2004)

Log of Work-Related Injuries and Illnesses

Attention: This form contains information relating to employee health and must be used in a manner that protects the confidentiality of employees to the extent possible while the information is being used for occupational safety and health purposes.

Year 20___

U.S. Department of Labor
Occupational Safety and Health Administration

Form approved OMB no. 1218-0176

You must record information about every work-related death and about every work-related injury or illness that involves loss of consciousness, restricted work activity or job transfer, days away from work, or medical treatment beyond first aid. You must also record significant work-related injuries and illnesses that are diagnosed by a physician or licensed health care professional. You must also record work-related injuries and illnesses that meet any of the specific recording criteria listed in 29 CFR Part 1904.8 through 1904.12. Feel free to use two lines for a single case if you need to. You must complete an Injury and Illness Incident Report (OSHA Form 301) or equivalent form for each injury or illness recorded on this form. If you're not sure whether a case is recordable, call your local OSHA office for help.

Establishment name _____

City _____ State _____

Identify the person

(A) Case no.	(B) Employee's name	(C) Job title (e.g., Welder)	(D) Date of injury or onset of illness

Describe the case

(E) Where the event occurred (e.g., Loading dock north end)	(F) Describe injury or illness, parts of body affected, and object/substance that directly injured or made person ill (e.g., Second degree burns on right forearm from acetylene torch)

Classify the case

CHECK ONLY ONE box for each case based on the most serious outcome for that case:

Death (G)	Days away from work (H)	Remained at Work — Job transfer or restriction (I)	Remained at Work — Other recordable cases (J)

Enter the number of days the injured or ill worker was:

Away from work (K)	On job transfer or restriction (L)
days	days

Check the "Injury" column or choose one type of illness:
(M)

Injury (1)	Skin disorder (2)	Respiratory condition (3)	Poisoning (4)	Hearing loss (5)	All other illnesses (6)

Page totals ▶

Be sure to transfer these totals to the Summary page (Form 300A) before you post it.

Public reporting burden for this collection of information is estimated to average 14 minutes per response, including time to review the instructions, search and gather the data needed, and complete and review the collection of information. Persons are not required to respond to the collection of information unless it displays a currently valid OMB control number. If you have any comments about these estimates or any other aspects of this data collection, contact: US Department of Labor, OSHA Office of Statistical Analysis, Room N-3644, 200 Constitution Avenue, NW, Washington, DC 20210. Do not send the completed forms to this office.

Page ___ of ___

FIGURE 17.14 All private companies are required to fill out the OSHA Form 300 log, which tracks on-the-job injuries and illnesses. *Source: Courtesy of OSHA.*

This log is used to classify work-related injuries and illnesses and to note the extent and severity of each case. When an incident occurs, specific information giving the details about what happened and how it happened must be recorded on the log. A summary form, OSHA Form 300A, shows the totals for the year in each category. OSHA requires that the Form 300A be posted each year by February 1 in a visible location so that staff members are aware of the injuries and illnesses that have been occurring in the workplace. The form must remain posted until April 30.

Let's start with a question. Last year an EMS agency had ten recordable injuries. Did it do a good job or a poor job protecting its staff? The answer depends on three factors:

- How many employees worked for the EMS agency
- How many hours were worked by those employees
- The industry of the employer

For example, if an EMS agency employed ten EMTs who worked 40 hours per week, then ten injuries (10 injuries per 400 hours =1 injury every 40 hours) would be a very bad record. However, if a similar EMS agency employed 80 EMTs who worked an average of 40 hours per week, ten injuries would not be as significant (10 injuries per 3,200 hours = 1 injury every 320 hours). Furthermore, the ten injuries may be considered high in a low-hazard industry such as a dispatch center. Those same ten injuries may be considered very low in a high-hazard segment of the EMS industry.

Your record is dependent on these factors. Each company employees a different number of employees, and we rarely speak in terms of how many injuries we had. In fact, OSHA doesn't typically ask "How many injuries did you have?" Instead, it will ask "What is your injury and illness incident rate?" or "What is your **DART rate**"? (DART stands for <u>D</u>ays <u>A</u>way from work, job <u>R</u>estrictions and/or job <u>T</u>ransfers).

The DART rate is the gold standard for benchmarking any organization's safety record. DART rate calculations provide individual businesses with the data necessary to effectively and accurately benchmark their safety records as well as track their progress toward enhancing workplace safety over time. The DART rate is calculated by adding up the total number of injuries and illnesses that had one or more lost days, that had one or more restricted days, or that resulted in an employee transferring to a different job within the agency, and multiplying that number by 200,000 (a constant), and then dividing that number by the number of labor hours at the agency. The incidence rate is a trending number based on your injury and illness rates if you had worked 200,000 hours.[2]

The following is the empirical formula:

$$\text{DART rate} = \frac{\text{Total Number of DART incidents} \times 200{,}000}{\text{Number of Employee Labor Hours Worked}}$$

This statistical measurement of an employer's safety record is highly revered by OSHA. It is a standard calculation used to identify workplaces with the highest occupational injury and illness rates. OSHA is beginning to target agencies with high DART rates. Using a DART rate will also enable an agency to benchmark itself against other public safety agencies. As a general rule of thumb, you want your DART rate to be lower than your incidence rate.

Every year, OSHA publishes a list of the top ten violations for the preceding year (Figure 17.15). Although the majority of the violations are not applicable to EMS, two almost always

---

[2]OSHA use the 200,000-hour benchmark to set a baseline based on the fact that 200,000 hours are the number of hours worked by 100 employees, averaging 40 hours per week, over a 50-week span (2 weeks taken away for holidays).

OSHA Top 10 workplace violations - 2010	
Scaffolding	Electrical Wiring
Fall Protection	Ladders
Hazard Communication	Powered Industrial Trucks (Fork Lifts)
Respiratory Protection	Electrical
Lock out/Tag out	Machine Guarding

FIGURE 17.15 ■ Each year, OSHA publishes the top ten violations based on the number of citations issued. *Source: Courtesy of OSHA.*

are cited: Hazard Communications and Respiratory Protection.

OSHA may conduct inspections for a variety of reasons, often related to complaints by the members of services, injury rates, mandatory reporting requirements, or notification of accidents. The specific reporting process is outlined in 29 CFR 1904.39. Within 8 hours after the death of any employee from a work-related incident or the inpatient hospitalization of three or more employees as a result of a work-related incident, the fatality/multiple hospitalization must be reported by telephone or in person to the OSHA area office that is nearest to the site of the incident. The report also may be phoned in via the OSHA toll-free central telephone number: 1-800-321-OSHA (1-800-321-6742).[3]

When OSHA initiates the investigation, it will cite a specific reason for the investigation. If a citation is issued, it will be for a specific reason, such as not having an **exposure control plan** or failure to provide annual fit testing. If a specific standard does not apply to a work function, OSHA will apply the General Duty Clause, which states in section 5:

a. Each employer–
   1. Shall furnish to each of his employees employment and a place of employment which are free from recognized hazards that are causing or are likely to cause death or serious physical harm to his employees;
   2. Shall comply with occupational safety and health standards promulgated under this Act.
b. Each employee shall comply with occupational safety and health standards and all rules, regulations, and orders issued pursuant to this Act which are applicable to his own actions and conduct

When OSHA initiates an investigation, it may conduct a site visit, interview staff, conduct surveillance testing for environment issues, and review records, such as OSHA Form 300 logs and injury sharps logs, for the previous 5 years. If a violation if discovered, OSHA will define a specific time period within which to abate the issues. This may include retraining of staff, purchasing new or additional safety equipment, and updating policies. OSHA may also issue a monetary penalty up to $7,000 if the violation is deemed to be serious. Repeated violations are deemed to be willful and can carry a penalty up to $70,000 for each violation. An appeals process is detailed in the written citation that can substantially reduce the monetary penalties.

BLOOD-BORNE PATHOGENS

Infection control issues constitute another area that the EMS safety officer must manage.

---

[3]29 CFR 1904.39: Standard for Reporting Fatalities and Multiple Hospitalization Incidents.

One of the major activities will include developing and maintaining an exposure control plan as required by OSHA's 29 CFR 1910.1030 blood-borne pathogen standard. The exposure control plan is designed to eliminate or minimize the employee's risk of exposure to dangerous pathogens in the workplace. The plan must be customized to the workplace. Various components of the plan include selection of personal protection equipment, enforcement of policies pertaining to the use of cleaning and disinfecting equipment, and training and education of staff on the contents of the plan.[4]

NIOSH conducted a study in California and found that nearly 22 percent of the paramedics had an occupation exposure to blood in the course of a year (National Institute of Occupational Safety and Health, 2010). One section of the plan will deal with engineer and work practice controls. Through the use of policies and procedures and, in certain cases, changes in equipment design or use, the purpose is to prevent exposure from occurring. This will include SOPs on hand washing and waste management (e.g., biohazard red bags). Another section should specify how the ambulances and work spaces are to be maintained in a sanitary condition. Within this section one should find the details on how uniforms, once contaminated, are handled; the main purpose of this standard is to prevent staff members from bringing contaminated uniforms home to be laundered.

When a provider functions at the advanced life support level, another level of complexity is added to the operations plan: sharps management. The plan must address all engineering control and use of safety devices, a review process for all needlestick injuries, and methods for following up on all exposures (Figure 17.16). You also must document that all staff

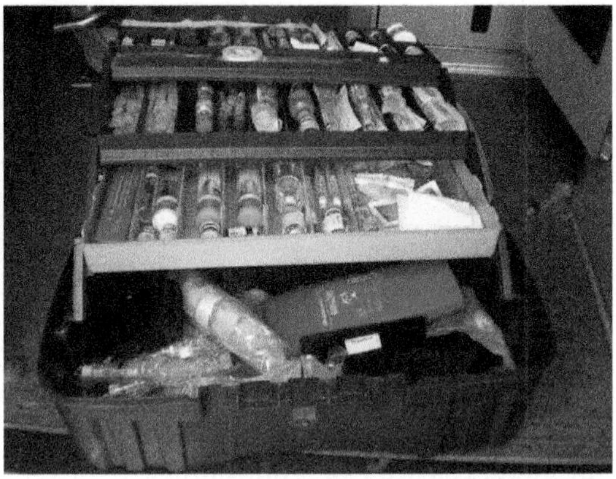

FIGURE 17.16 ■ Although they vary in size, OSHA mandates that sharps containers be brought to wherever a sharp is being used. *Source: Photo courtesy of MONOC Mobile Health Services.*

have been in-serviced in the use of these devices.

Perhaps the most difficult task addressed in the plan deals with the follow-up for all documented exposures and needlestick injuries. In many instances, hospitals own or operate the local EMS agency, and it is incumbent upon the infection control department to ensure that the hospital's exposure control plan covers the EMS department. For unaffiliated EMS agencies, this becomes the responsibility of the safety officer. EMS agencies not closely affiliated with hospitals may not have sufficient internal expertise to manage a comprehensive exposure control program. The EMS safety officer should establish a relationship with infection control departments to assist them with compliance, training, and follow-up information.

For EMS agencies that are not hospital based, it is particularly important that procedures be in place that would allow for accurate and timely notification should paramedics be exposed to a potentially infectious pathogen. A law that helps address this, but is not known by many in health care other than hospital infection control departments and EMS, is the

---

[4]29 CFR 1910.1030: Standard for Blood Borne Pathogens.

Ryan White Comprehensive AIDS Resources Emergency (CARE) Act. The law was named after a thirteen-year-old hemophiliac from Indiana who inadvertently became infected with HIV during a blood transfusion in the 1980s. Shortly after his death in 1990, Congress passed the Ryan White CARE Act, intended to improve the quality and availability of care for low-income, uninsured, and underinsured individuals and families affected by HIV and AIDS. The Ryan White program also funds and provides technical assistance to local and state primary medical care providers, support services, health care providers, and training programs.

In Part G of the act, "Notification of Possible Exposure to Infectious Diseases," the law outlines several situations that allow for the sharing of protected health information between hospitals and EMS in order to protect emergency response employees. Two of the main situations addressed in the law include these:

1. *When a patient is transferred to a health care facility and is found to have an airborne infectious disease.* In this case, the medical facility must notify the designated officer of the emergency response employee who transported the patient as soon as possible, but no later than 48 hours after the determination has been made.

2. *When emergency response employees believe that they have possibly been exposed to an infectious disease by a patient who they have transported to a medical facility.* In this case, after collecting the appropriate information about the incident and making a decision that his emergency response employee may have been exposed, the designated officer for the agency will contact the receiving medical facility and request a determination of whether or not the employee was exposed to an infectious disease. Upon investigation of the request, the medical facility will notify the designated officer in

writing of its determination. *Source: Centers for Disease Control and Prevention [cdc.gov]*

One of the most frightening experiences for an emergency services provider is occupational blood-borne exposure. Despite two decades of safety engineering advancements, such as the introduction of self-capping needles and the adoption of standard precautions, occupational exposures still occur. Fortunately, significant advancements in available antiviral post-exposure prophylaxis (PEP) medications and the laboratory's ability to rapidly assess whether the source patient is actually infected with HIV or hepatitis C help those exposed receive treatment more accurately and quickly.

As the art and science of occupational exposure have developed, another important concept has emerged: *nonexposure*. A nonexposure occurs when emergency workers come in contact with potentially infectious materials (i.e., blood and body fluids) from a patient, but they're deemed without risk of disease transmission on the basis of the circumstances of the exposure. Often, nonexposures occur because of the proper use of standard precautions. The simplest example of a nonexposure would be getting blood on gloves.

Another way to define a nonexposure is to define an exposure. Any situation that doesn't meet the criteria of an exposure constitutes a nonexposure, which doesn't warrant medical evaluation. The Centers for Disease Control and Prevention (CDC) uses the following definition (Centers for Disease Control and Prevention, 2001):

> An exposure that might place HCP [Health Care Personnel] at risk for HBV, HCV, or HIV infection is defined as a *percutaneous injury* (e.g., a needlestick or cut with a sharp object) or *contact of mucous membrane* or *nonintact skin* (e.g., exposed skin that is chapped, abraded, or afflicted with dermatitis) with blood, tissue, or other body fluids that are potentially infectious body fluids.

. . . Feces, nasal secretions, saliva, sputum, sweat, tears, urine, and vomitus are not considered potentially infectious unless they contain blood. The risk for transmission of HBV, HCV, and HIV infection from these fluids and materials is extremely low. (p. 3; emphasis added) *Source: Centers for Disease Control and Prevention [cdc.gov]*

All health care workers should understand what constitutes an exposure and a nonexposure because it is usually the exposed person's own decision to notify the agency's designated infection control officer (DICO) or seek medical attention. Knowing the difference also empowers providers with peace of mind as they encounter blood and body fluids on a daily basis. Such knowledge can save emergency services personnel and their employers significant time and money by avoiding unnecessary medical evaluations. Exposure to blood on intact skin is a nonreportable.

In addition to blood and body fluids questions, if responders have had a reportable exposure, they must immediately report the incident to their DICO and, if appropriate, seek assistance from a qualified practitioner who can objectively assess the potential risks. The immediacy of reporting and potentially being medically evaluated for a blood- or fluid-borne exposure is based on current recommendations, which suggest that PEP with antiviral drugs be started within hours of the exposure to optimize effectiveness in preventing disease transmission to the provider.

Like all other facets of health care, paramedics are also faced with the growing number of superbugs and antibiotic-resistant bacteria that are being seen throughout the United States. In addition to protecting themselves from possible infection, EMS providers must ensure that their vehicles and equipment are adequately cleaned and disinfected so as not to expose future patients. In a study published in *Prehospital Emergency Care*, one department conducted environmental culturing of its ambulances and of 21 ambulances; it found

that 10 were colonized with methicillin-resistant *Staphylococcus aureus* (MRSA; Roline, Crumpecker, and Dunn, 2007). In another study also published in *Prehospital Emergency Care*, the author swabbed 50 stethoscopes of EMS personnel who transported patients to a local emergency department during a 24-hour period and found 16 of the scopes to have been colonized by MRSA (Merlin et al., 2009). Another study tested equipment surfaces most likely to come in contact with patients' skin and found that 57 percent of the equipment tested was identified as still being contaminated with traces of blood despite being identified as ready for reuse (Lee, Levy, and Walker, 2006). Because EMS providers are responsible for cleaning and disinfecting their own ambulance and equipment, an emphasis must be placed on strict policies and procedures in order to protect themselves and future patients who may be suffering from highly transferable and exotic diseases, including avian flu, H1N1 (swine flu), and the newly emerging NDM-1 and Klebsiella pathogens.

RESPIRATORY PROTECTION

Another OSHA standard that is the companion to the blood-borne pathogens requirements and requires significant attention from the EMS safety officer is compliance with 29 CFR 1910.134: the respiratory protection standard. This standard requires all EMS agencies to have a written respiratory protection plan. This plan should require all agency members who have a reasonable chance of being exposed to an airborne pathogen to have an initial and annual fit test for the N95 mask.

The OSHA Respiratory Protection standard 29 CFR 1910.134(f)(2) states in part:

The employer shall ensure that an employee using a tight-fitting facepiece respirator is fit tested prior to initial use of the respirator, whenever a different respirator face piece (size, style, model or make) is used, and at least annually thereafter. *Source: U.S. Department of Labor Occupational Safety & Health Administration, OSHA*

The fit test must be completed using the make and model of N95 mask that will be used by the organization and issued to its members. The standard currently allows for either a qualitative or quantitative fit test. It is not appropriate to accept documentation of a fit-test record from another EMS agency without verifying that make and model of the N95 respirator are the same.

Side Bar

Fit Test: Qualitative versus Quantitative

A qualitative fit test determines whether or not someone can detect various scents or flavors or can experience a negative reaction to a substance that can cause burning, watering eyes.

A quantitative fit test is an assessment of the adequacy of respirator fit that uses numerical measurement of the amount of leakage into the respirator. Quantitative fit tests use a probe inside the facemask often connected to a portacount machine.

Prior to conducting fit testing on an individual, that person must complete a medical questionnaire and evaluation (CFR 1910.134, Appendix C) and be cleared by a licensed health care professional. Every year along with the annual fit test, the employee should complete the Annual Fit Test Evaluation Form (OSHA 1910.134(f)(3). This form should be retained as part of the training record for a year. The medical evaluation only needs to be done once, upon hiring, provided the individual has not experienced a significant weight change, or had a change in significant facial scarring or facial hair, or had major dental changes or reconstructive facial surgery.

During the H1N1 pandemic in 2009, the CDC disseminated guidelines for the transport of potentially infectious patients that are applicable to any patient with a potentially communicable airborne disease.

Side Bar

Guidelines for EMS Transport of Potentially Infectious Patients

If there HAS NOT been swine influenza reported in the geographic area. . ., EMS providers should assess all patients as follows:

1. EMS personnel should stay more than 6 feet away from patients and bystanders with symptoms and exercise appropriate routine respiratory droplet precautions while assessing all patients for suspected cases of swine influenza.
2. Assess all patients for symptoms of acute febrile respiratory illness (fever plus one or more of the following: nasal congestion/runny nose, sore throat, or cough).
   - If no acute febrile respiratory illness, proceed with normal EMS care.
   - If symptoms of acute febrile respiratory illness, then assess all patients for travel to a geographic area with confirmed cases of swine influenza within the last 7 days or close contact with someone with travel to these areas.
     - If travel exposure, don appropriate PPE for suspected case of swine influenza.
     - If no travel exposure, place a standard surgical mask on the patient (if tolerated) and use appropriate PPE for cases of acute febrile respiratory illness without suspicion of swine influenza (as described in PPE section).

Personal Protective Equipment (PPE)

- When treating a patient with a suspected case of swine influenza, the following PPE should be worn:
  - Fit-tested disposable N95 respirator and eye protection (e.g., goggles, eye shield), disposable nonsterile gloves, and gown, when coming into close contact with the patient.

- When treating a patient who is not a suspected case of swine influenza but who has symptoms of acute febrile respiratory illness, the following precautions should be taken:
  - Place a standard surgical mask on the patient, if tolerated. If not tolerated, EMS personnel may wear a standard surgical mask.
  - Use good respiratory hygiene—use nonsterile gloves for contact with patient, patient secretions, or surfaces that may have been contaminated. Follow hand hygiene including hand washing or cleansing with alcohol-based hand disinfectant after contact.
- Encourage good patient compartment vehicle airflow/ventilation to reduce the concentration of aerosol accumulation when possible.

Interim Recommendations

- Pending clarification of transmission patterns for this virus, EMS personnel who are in close contact with patients with suspected, probable, or confirmed swine flu cases should wear a fit-tested disposable N95 respirator, disposable nonsterile gloves, eye protection (e.g., goggles, eye shield), and gown, when coming into close contact with the patient.
- All EMS personnel engaged in aerosol generating activities (e.g., intubation, nebulizer treatment, and resuscitation involving emergency intubation or cardiac pulmonary resuscitation) should wear a fit-tested disposable N95 respirator, disposable nonsterile gloves, eye protection (e.g., goggles, eye shield), and gown, unless EMS personnel are able to rule out acute febrile respiratory illness or travel to an endemic area in the patient being treated.
- All patients with acute febrile respiratory illness should wear a surgical mask, if tolerated by the patient.

Interfacility Transport

EMS personnel involved in the interfacility transfer of patients with suspected, probable, or confirmed swine influenza should use standard, droplet, and contact precautions for all patient care activities. This should include wearing a fit-tested disposable N95 respirator, wearing disposable nonsterile gloves, eye protection (e.g., goggles, eye shield), and gown, to prevent conjunctival exposure. If the transported patient can tolerate a facemask (e.g., a surgical mask), its use can help to minimize the spread of infectious droplets in the patient care compartment. Encourage good patient compartment vehicle airflow/ventilation to reduce the concentration of aerosol accumulation when possible.

EMS Transfer of Patient Care to a Health Care Facility

When transporting a patient with symptoms of acute febrile respiratory illness, EMS personnel should notify the receiving health care facility so that appropriate infection control precautions may be taken upon patient arrival. Patients with acute febrile respiratory illness should wear a surgical mask, if tolerated. Small facemasks are available that can be worn by children, but it may be problematic for children to wear them correctly and consistently. Moreover, no facemasks (or respirators) have been cleared by the FDA specifically for use by children.

Source: Centers for Disease Control and Prevention (2009).

If an agency provides specialized services, including hazardous materials support or tactical EMS, a higher level of respiratory protection will be needed and the individual must be trained on and provided with that device, which may include an air purifying respirator (APR) or self-contained breathing apparatus (SCBA). As with the exposure control plan, documentation of training must be maintained. The plan must also describe the required preventative maintenance schedule for these respirators.

■ ERGONOMICS

A review of the agency's workers' compensation incident reports will give insight to the types of injuries the members receive over the course of a year. The majority will tend to be related to lifting and moving and will most likely involve low-back and shoulder-down injuries. This will be related directly to the environment in which the employee is working. Urban systems tend to have more injuries due to the significant number of patients who need to be carried down multiple flights of stairs.

The EMS safety officer should conduct a review to ensure that the best technology to get the job done is available for use. It is simple to purchase a tracked stair chair, but if more injuries occur trying to remove the device from the ambulance, due to the increased size and weight, then it is not an appropriate tool. Training also must be provided on how and when to use the appropriate lifting and moving device. All training must be documented as it will be called into question in the event of a lawsuit.

In general, things to consider include the following: What is the injury claim rate and cost? Will the reduction in claims cover the cost of investment in new equipment? Power-lift stretchers have been shown to reduce the rate of back injuries and in turn to reduce workers' compensation claims and costs; however, such equipment may cost two to three times as much as a regular stretcher. If the implementation only calls for five units, then the cost is easily justified. However, when an agency is looking at purchasing fifty to a hundred stretchers, what is the return on investment? One of the considerations to be factored in is the cost of training and maintenance.

For one large agency, each hour of in-service time was factored to be nearly $80,000 based on the hourly rate of each individual needing to be trained.

Many states have begun enacting no-lift laws and safe patient handling laws in licensed medical facilities. Although it has not been directly mentioned in the legislation, EMS may be considered a covered entity if owned or operated by a licensed medical facility. Since the tools exist, they should be evaluated to see if they can be adopted for use in EMS. Case in point: If EMS responds to a medical facility for a patient, the EMS personnel should press the staff to provide a Hoyer lift if one is present instead of risking injury to the provider or patient. The ambulances can also be provided with low-friction slide sheets or slide boards that will decrease the friction and make it easier to move the patient (Figure 17.17).

An analysis of call history, patient population and hospital services should be conducted to identify whether or not there is a significant bariatric population in the region, as this may mean the ambulance service needs a specifically

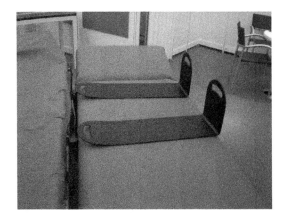

FIGURE 17.17 ■ Agencies that typically move obese patients often implement specialized devices, such as these slide boards, to reduce provider injuries. *Source: Photo courtesy of MONOC Mobile Health Services.*

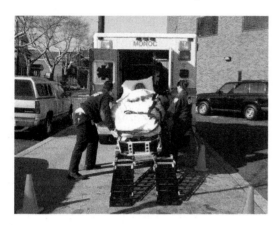

FIGURE 17.18 ■ Some EMS agencies have developed dedicated bariatric transport units and utilize ramps and winches, along with high-capacity stretchers. *Source: Used by permission of MONOC Mobile Health Services.*

designed ambulance that is designed to incorporate equipment intended for the morbidly obese patient. This will include a stretcher that is wider and has a higher weight capacity, larger back boards, and other specialized patient movement equipment (Figure 17.18). The ambulance may have to be redesigned and should contain a ramp and winch system or lifting mechanism so the staff does not have to lift the patient.

Additional training must be provided to staff who will be operating the equipment and moving these patients. This should include an overview of body mechanics, safety precautions, and lifting techniques. Training should also include hands-on skills.

■ RISK MANAGEMENT

Where does safety fit into a service's operational and administrative structure? The answer is often convoluted, but the EMS safety officer should have the authority to cross departmental lines. For example, consider an agency member

who is involved in a motor vehicle collision. The EMS safety officer should ensure that an investigation is conducted in accordance with the standards established by the agency. The EMS safety officer should notify the legal department of the incident and advise legal staff to collect pertinent documents in anticipation of an injury lawsuit. HR staff should review the employee's driver abstract to ensure that it is current and within the guidelines of the agency and the insurance company. Fleet services should be requested to examine the vehicle for damage and the vehicle's service history including tune-ups, brake service, and other issues. The operations manager may be asked to provide documentation of the employee's driving history and training. Depending on the structure or responsibilities, the clinical department may be asked to provide remedial training.

Obviously, all of these actions are not necessarily undertaken for every motor vehicle collision, but in some cases they are automatic. For example, fleet services always will examine the vehicle for drivability and operations will generate an incident report. The EMS safety officer's responsibility is to establish the parameters for the depth of the investigation based on the severity of and exposures resulting from the collision.

The EMS safety officer should work hand in hand with HR staff as the HR department is typically responsible for keeping the required log of workers' compensation incident reports (Figure 17.19). HR will also typically assist in managing insurance issues and will assist in managing insurance issues related to occupational exposures.

In many, cases the EMS safety officers will also assume the role or function of risk managers in that they will examine sentinel events for trends or patterns, conduct investigations into adverse events, and make recommendations to change processes to protect the employee and other assets of the agency. A sentinel event is defined by The Joint Commission on

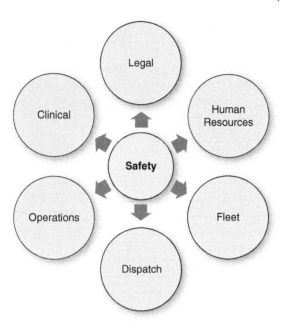

FIGURE 17.19 ■ The safety officer must have inter-action with every department. *Source: Reprinted by permission from MONOC Mobile Health Services.*

Accreditation of Healthcare Organizations (JCAHO) as any unanticipated event in a health care setting resulting in death or serious physical or psychological injury to a patient or patients, not related to the natural course of the patient's illness. Sentinel events specifically include loss of a limb or gross motor function, and any event for which a recurrence would carry a risk of a serious adverse outcome (The Joint Commission on Accreditation of Health-care Organizations, 2013).

Risk management is the process of apply-ing management techniques to the identifica-tion, assessment, and resolution of problems to prevent and/or minimize occurrences that have the potential for injury or loss to patients, employees, visitors, and the organization.

Three risk control options can be applied: exposure avoidance, transfer, and control—each having its own strengths and weakness.

In exposure avoidance, we choose not to engage in a particular activity. The system may choose not to have specially trained EMS per-sonnel for tactical response. This may reduce the likelihood of an occurrence to zero, but it may cause issues within the emergency serv-ices community if you are a sole provider. You may not be able to avoid the exposure in many cases; therefore, you must attempt to control the risk in utilizing other strategies. Segregation of loss exposures involves setting activities and resources in such a way that if an incident occurs, it does not affect the entire organization. This may include using multiple vendors for medication supplies or fleet serv-ices. It may also include storing supplies at individual stations in addition to a centralized warehouse, so in the event of a fire, redundant supplies are on hand. Risk transfer essentially entails getting someone else to do it for you. This strategy may involve outsourcing the public safety answering point (PSAP) func-tions of your dispatch center, thus another agency will assume the liability for call screen-ing. You may also transfer the financial liabil-ity for an activity you wish to retain through the purchase of insurance from a third party. Another option is risk retention, which is deciding how much risk you want to assume. Will you go self-insured and be responsible for first dollar on all losses, but still purchase insurance for excess coverage? Many agencies are becoming self-insured for auto accidents and workers' compensation. The most com-mon non-lawsuit complaints against EMS per-sonnel were for rude behavior, poor technical competency, issues with transportation, and loss of the patient's belongings. The top legal actions against EMS personnel and ambu-lance services include motor vehicle collisions and patient-handling accidents (particularly stretcher tipping and drops).

Every ambulance service should assign an individual who will be responsible for manag-ing a safe medical devices program that involves maintaining patient care equipment, including a preventive maintenance program and a pre-use inspection. In conjunction with the EMS safety officer, the program manager investigates and inspects all equipment involved in patient-related incidents or injuries. In accordance with the Safe Medical Device Act of 1990, an agency shall report to the FDA or manufacturer of the device any information which reasonably suggests that a medical device has caused or contributed to serious illness, serious injury, or death of a patient.

As previously discussed, the Institute of Medicine in its "To Err is Human" report (Kohn, Corrigan, and Donaldson, 1999), estimated that between 44,000 and 98,000 deaths occur annually due to errors in the hospital setting. A similar report does not exist for ambulance services. We do not often know how many near-miss events occur because we typically do not have the resources to identify when an error has occurred. We often rely on a complaint from an outside entity to point us in the right direction. The EMS safety officer should be examining the system for patterns and precursors that will lead to situations that will allow errors to occur. In many cases, under a retrospective review, one can identify the fail points that lead up to a serious or catastrophic event. Most of these fail points are in themselves not critical or even obvious; therefore, all managers need to assist in identifying issues on a daily basis to prevent minor errors from occurring.

For example, a critical care ambulance is performing an interfacility transport with a patient destined for the cardiac catheterization lab. Upon removing the patient from the ambulance, the stretcher collapses to the ground. The patient states he is not injured when questioned. The patient is then brought to the catheterization lab for his scheduled procedure. The agency was notified later that afternoon by the patient's family of the incident. Several weeks later, a notice of claim was received as the patient intended to sue. In addition, the family lodged a complaint with the local department of health, which in turn conducted its own investigation.

An internal investigation revealed a last-minute crew change as the unit went into service. The fleet of critical care ambulances used a different model of stretcher than did the BLS division, and the EMT was not familiar with the loading and unloading process with this stretcher. The crew followed policy and generated an incident report, but they did not notify the supervisor of this sentinel event. Further, they did not obtain a refusal of medical aid (RMA) form from the patient, despite documenting the event in their patient care report. Their documentation did include who at the receiving facility they advised of the incident.

As a result of this event, a management decision was made to standardize all of the stretchers in the fleet. The EMTs were retrained on operating the critical care stretchers, and the staff was in-serviced regarding the reporting requirements of sentinel events.

Most negative outcome events are not the result of a single major failure. Rather, they result from a series of minor events that often go unnoticed until they reach a critical level and result in an injury or negative outcome (Figure 17.20).

In 1931, H. W. Heinrich reported on a study of accidents that he classified according to severity. Heinrich's report showed that for each serious-injury incident, we could expect about 29 minor injuries and 300 near-miss or property-damage incidents. His conclusions are often depicted with a pyramid or triangle indicating a single serious incident at the peak and a broad base of noninjury incidents (Heinrich, 1931; see Figure 17.21). Heinrich promulgated the concept of focusing on controlling hazards in the workplace in addition to changing worker behavior, and this has developed into workplace engineering. For example, staff will often start IVs outside of a controlled setting and away from sharps containers. As managers we

Why do errors occur?

Workload fluctuations

Interruptions

Fatigue

Multitasking

Failure to follow up

Poor hand-offs

Ineffective communication

Protocol violations

Excessive professional courtesy

Complacency

Task fixation/Tunnel vision

FIGURE 17.20 ▪ Publishing a list of the causal factors associated with errors will heighten everyone's awareness. *Source: Reprinted by permission from MONOC Mobile Health Services.*

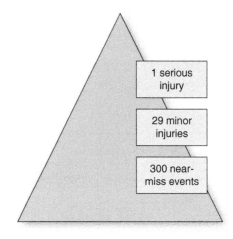

1 serious injury

29 minor injuries

300 near-miss events

FIGURE 17.21 ▪ Heinrich's triangle demonstrates why every near-miss event must be addressed. *Source: Reprinted by permission from MONOC Mobile Health Services.*

must recognize this and adapt. A simple change that can be implemented is the changeover to a needleless IV system and safety catheters.

When applying the ratios suggested by Heinrich, it has been recommended that the focus of safety programs be on preventing less-serious events as an indirect means to prevent a single serious event. Is it always true that serious injuries are caused by the same factors that cause less-serious incidents? This is the basis for near-miss reporting.

When dealing with a limited budget, one must also consider the allocation of resources. How much effort will it take to reduce the base of the pyramid enough to affect the peak? Instead of attempting to change the behavior of all staff members, which can be expensive and time consuming, it may be better to change the environment in which they operate. For example, if we are concerned about fatigue at work, we can modify policies to allow sleeping while on duty and go so far as to provide specific sleeping quarters, or we can limit the

number of consecutive hours we permit staff to work.

Although Heinrich's pyramid theory is interesting and important to understand, perhaps we should consider a more direct approach to accident prevention. Through a risk assessment, operators can identify specific work processes and perform a simple evaluation of the associated risk (a function of the likelihood of a potential incident and level of severity of that incident). The conditions and practices associated with the most risk (most likely to result in severe injury) are addressed first. These represent the peak of the pyramid. Those with a remote possibility of a minor injury or property damage (the base) are assigned lower priority and may be addressed individually when the higher-priority risks are controlled.

A constant review of incident reports, lawsuits, customer complaints, workers' compensation reports, biomedical reports, fleet reports, and clinical counseling files may reveal patterns or trends that can be used to identify potential fail points. Once identified, they can

Special Situations Requiring Standard Operating Procedure	
Helicopter responses	Weapons of mass destruction (WMD)
Large-scale incidents	Large venues
Special populations	Natural disasters
IED responses	Hazardous materials
SWAT requests	Fires

FIGURE 17.22 ■ Every agency should develop a set of standardized operating procedures for special situations to ensure that staff have the proper training and tools needed to mitigate an incident. *Source: Reprinted by permission from MONOC Mobile Health Services.*

be corrected, by either changing a process, piece of equipment, or procedure. So as not to inundate oneself, the corrective focus should be on those specifics that can be labeled as high risk. Simply ask this: How likely is it to happen, and how bad will it be if it does happen (Colwell, Pons, and Pi, 2003)?

SAFETY

As previously discussed, ambulance services provide complex services and operate in complex environments. Most agencies involving 9-1-1 responses have some type of requirement or obligation to provide support services to the municipality or other public safety agencies in the region. The agency safety officer has an obligation to ensure that the staff is properly equipped to deal with these types of responses, which include the appropriate training, access to appropriate PPE, and SOPs (Figure 17.22).

In addition to having administrative functions, the EMS safety officer will often respond to events of such a nature that an incident command system will be established. This may be dictated by the agency's policies or procedures.

When deployed to a scene or site of an ongoing event, the EMS safety officer will assume the role of the ISO and function to develop and recommend site-specific measures for ensuring personnel safety and to assess and/or anticipate hazardous and unsafe situations. The ISO reports directly to the incident commander and has the authority and obligation to alter, delay, suspend, and terminate any and all operations immediately dangerous to life and health of any personnel.[5]

Only one primary ISO will be assigned for each incident. The ISO is often assigned assistants, depending on the complexity of the incident. The assistant safety officer (ASO) may be representing other agencies or task-specific functions, such as air operations, hazardous materials (HAZMAT), or maritime operations, etc. The ISO should be certified or qualified to the level of operations being performed so he/ she is familiar with the potential hazards that may be encountered and may stop operations if the tasks being performed are not in compliance with the approved training (Figure 17.23). NFPA 1521, section 2.5.1 states, "At an emergency incident where activities are judged by the Incident Safety Officer (ISO) to be unsafe or involve an imminent hazard, the ISO shall

---

[5]Supervising ambulance officers (first-line supervisors) should have appropriate general ICS training (ICS 100, 200, and 300), knowledge of the National Response Framework (ICS 700 and 800), and specialty courses for EMS branch director, operations section chief, and logistics section chief, in accordance with agency plans. Managing and executive ambulance officers should add ICS 400 training, major incident management training (e.g., The Texas Engineering Extension Service—TEEX—Enhanced Incident Management/Unified Command Course), as well as emergency operations center general and position-specific training.

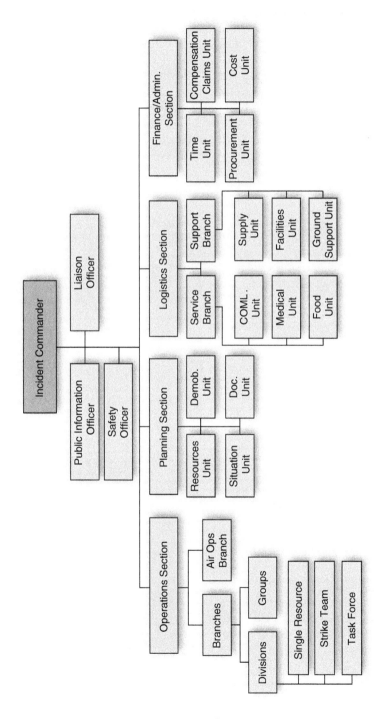

FIGURE 17.23 ■ The safety officer is part of the command staff and reports directly to the incident commander. *Source: Reprinted by permission from MONOC Mobile Health Services.*

have the authority to alter, suspend, or terminate those activities. The ISO shall immediately inform the Incident Commander of any actions taken to correct imminent hazards at an emergency scene (National Fire Protection Association, 2009a).

In general, the ISO should be in a position to monitor and assess safety hazards or unsafe situations at an incident scene and develop protective measures for ensuring EMS personnel safety. They should address the safety of responders at every emergency and function. The ISO needs to have knowledge of safety standards and hazards and the safety procedures enacted by the agency. The ISO is responsible for ensuring compliance with policies and standards, including wearing the appropriate PPE when deployed.

At the scene of an incident or preplanned event, the ISO should do the following:

* Wear an identify vest.
* Ensure personnel know that an EMS safety officer is on scene.
* Conduct safety briefings.
* Understand the incident action plan.
* Develop the incident safety plan—ICS215a.
* Perform a 360-degree walkaround.
* Ensure that all personnel are wearing appropriate safety equipment.
* Risk a lot only to save a lot.
* Risk only a little to save a little.
* Risk nothing to save what is already lost.
* Ensure that safety zones are established.
* Ensure that rapid intervention teams are available.
* Ensure that rehab/prehab are established.
* Commit a transport unit under logistics.
* Consider assigning additional safety officers.

The ISO should not be confused with the EMS safety officer. Although the ISO and EMS safety officers are often the same person, they operate with different priorities. The ISO is responsible for the safety of personnel and operations during a specific incident.

The ISO is responsible for activities during a specific incident or event. The EMS safety officer holds primarily an administrative position and is responsible for coordination of safety and wellness activities and managing the general safety program. They will develop SOPs for high-risk activities, as previously listed, and will deliver safety training programs and manage injury and exposure documentation programs.

The EMS safety officer should also seek to ensure that the agency is in compliance with all regulatory requirements and standards that may not be readily apparent, as previously mentioned. An example of this is ensuring that all oxygen and compressed air cylinders are stored in compliance with the Compressed Gas Association's requirement that all tanks must be secured by a chain or contained in storage racks (Figure 17.24).

Other standards that the EMS safety officer may have to follow depend on how the agency operates. If hospital based, The Joint Commission will play a large part. Fire-based agencies are often governed by the National Fire Protection Association. Municipal or private agencies may be responsible to OSHA or PEOSHA. Those agencies seeking accreditation will have to comply with standards set

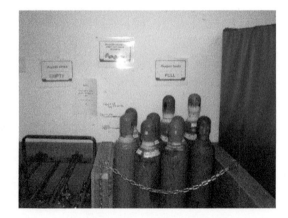

FIGURE 17.24 ■ Oxygen tanks must be properly secured at all time, as even "empty" tanks are under pressure. *Source: Used by permission of MONOC Mobile Health Services.*

forth by the Commission on Accreditation of Ambulance Services (CAAS) or the Commission on Accreditation of Medical Transport Systems (CAMTS).

CAAS has established a standard for employee safety—202.02.01 Employee Safety—which requires the agency to have a policy or procedure addressing the safety of its employees. At a minimum, this policy/procedure shall include facility safety, exposure control, safety at scenes, safe lifting, hazardous materials, employee wellness programs, employee duty and rest cycles, and any applicable local, state, or federal requirements for employee safety (Commission on Accreditation of Ambulance Services, 2010).

Both CAAS and CAMTS also require the formation of a safety committee. This committee should be endorsed by management and have the authority to implement a safety program. Membership on the safety committee should include the following:

* The EMS safety officer
* The medical director
* The quality improvement or quality assurance coordinator
* Field EMS personnel
* A representative from the communications center
* Appropriate members of the management team

As part of its mission, the safety committee should address issues related to safety including these:

* Equipment
* Specific incidents and sentinel events
* Training and education
* Data collection and review
* Laws, regulations, standards, and procedures

The safety committee can use as a resource the NFPA 1500 Standard on Fire Department Occupational Safety and Health Program, CAAS/CAMTS standards, and OSHA regulations, among others. Work product should be kept confidential, as should findings of investigation. Recommendations should be presented to management for implementation.

CHAPTER REVIEW

Summary

In general, the answer to the question "What is the EMS safety officer responsible for?" will include risk management, motor vehicle collisions, blood-borne pathogens, respiratory protection plan, OSHA and regulatory compliance, training issues, ergonomics, employee wellness, legal and management issues, and everything else.

WHAT WOULD YOU DO? Reflection

What are your agency's policies for reassigning staff from unit to unit?

Your policy should ensure that all EMS personnel are trained to use the equipment that is assigned to them.

What is your protocol for dealing with equipment failures?

Your agency should have a checklist that dictates the process to be followed, including removing the piece of equipment from service and having it tested by an authorized vendor, having staff generate incident reports, and being retrained on the piece of equipment.

What documentation do you maintain for proof of training and for retraining staff on the use of equipment?

Copies of certifications and training records, as well as any documentation pertaining to being in-serviced on new procedures, policies, and equipment, should be kept in the employee's clinical file.

What policies do you have in place for notification of sentinel events?

Your agency should have a process that is clearly conveyed to all employees as to the definition of a sentinel event, which manager should be notified within what time frame, and what documents should be collected at the time of the event.

Review Questions

1. What are the differences between an EMS safety officer and an incident safety officer?
2. Define risk management, and list the three main components of limiting risk.
3. What technology can be leveraged to reduce the rate of ambulance collisions?
4. Why would an ambulance service want to create a position for an EMS safety officer?
5. Explain the purpose of the OSHA's General Duty Clause.
6. How does the Safe Medical Device Act help improve the quality of patient care?
7. List three challenges to implementing a safety program.
8. List five reasons errors occur.
9. Who should promote safety in an organization?

References

American Ambulance Association. (2007). "Ambulance Facts." See the organization website.

Brown, L. H., C. L. Whitney, R. C. Hunt, M. Addario, and T. Hogue. (2000, January–March). "Do Warning Lights and Sirens Reduce Ambulance Response Times?" *Prehospital Emergency Care 4*(1), 70–74.

Calkin, S. (2011, August 9). "Ambulance Crews Attacked During London Riots." See the Health Service Journal website.

Center for Leadership, Innovation and Research in EMS. (2013). "E.V.E.N.T.—EMS Voluntary Event Notification Tool." See the organization website.

Centers for Disease Control and Prevention. (2001, June 29). "Updated U.S. Public Health Service Guidelines for the Management of Occupational Exposures to HBV, HCV, and HIV and Recommendations for Postexposure Prophylaxis." *Morbidity and Mortality Weekly Report 50*(RR-11).

Centers for Disease Control and Prevention. (2003). "Ambulance Crash-Related Injuries Among Emergency Medical Services Workers—United States, 1991–2002." *Mortality Morbidity Weekly Report (MMWR) 52*(8), 154–156.

Centers for Disease Control and Prevention. (2009, August 5). "Interim Guidance for Emergency Medical Services (EMS) Systems and 9-1-1 Public Safety Answering Points (PSAPs) for Management of Patients with Confirmed or Suspected Swine-Origin Influenza A (H1N1) Infection." See the organization website.

Centers for Medicare & Medicaid Services. (2007, January). "Ref S&C-07-10." See the organization website.

Colwell, C. B., P. Pons, J. H. Blanchet, and C. Mangino. (1999, November–December). "Claims Against a Paramedic Ambulance Service: A Ten-Year Experience." *Journal of Emergency Medicine 17*(6), 999–1,002.

Colwell, C. B., P. T. Pons, and R. Pi. (2003). Complaints against an EMS System." *Journal of Emergency Medicine 25*(4), 403–108.

Commission on Accreditation of Ambulance Services. (2010, January). "CAAS Standard 202.02.01 Safe Operations and Managing Risk." CAAS Standards for the Accreditation of Ambulance Services, version 3.0. Glenview, IL.

EMS Magazine. (2006, December). "4th Annual National EMS Systems Survey." See the organization website.

Emergency Nurses Association. (2010). "ENA Workplace Violence Toolkit." See the organization website.

EMS World. (2009). "Small-Town Shootings Claim Providers in Montana, New York State." See the organization website.

Harrison, P. (2004). "High Conspicuity Livery for Police Vehicles." Publication No. 14/04. Home Office, Police Scientific Development Branch. See the organization website.

Heinrich, H. W. (1931). *Industrial Accident Prevention: A Scientific Approach*. New York: McGraw-Hill.

Kahn, C. A., R. G. Pirrallo, and E. M. Kuhn. (2001, July–September). "Characteristics of Fatal Ambulance Crashes in the U.S: An 11-Year Retrospective Analysis." *Prehospital Emergency Care 5*(3), 261–269.

Kohn, L., J. Corrigan, and M. Donaldson. (1999, November). "To Err Is Human: Building a Safer Health System." Institute of Medicine. See the organization website.

Kollek, D., M. Welsford, and K. Wanger. (2010). "Canadian Operational and Emotional Prehospital Preparedness for a Tactical Violence Event." *Prehospital Disaster Medicine 25*(2), 164–169.

Larson, J. (2009, November 14). "Paramedic Who Beat Patient Sentenced to Prison." 9news.com: A Gannett Company. See the organization website.

Lee, J. B., M. Levy, and A. Walker. (2006). "Use of a Forensic Technique to Identify Blood Contamination of Emergency Department and Ambulance Trauma Equipment." *Emergency Medicine Journal 23*(1), 73–75.

Levick, N. R., and J. Swanson. (2005). "An Optimal Solution for Enhancing Ambulance Safety: Implementing a Driver Performance Feedback and Monitoring Device in Ground Emergency Medical Service Vehicles." *Annual Proceedings of the Association of Automotive Medicine 49,* 35–50.

Maguire, B. J., K. L. Hunting, G. S. Smith, and N. R. Levick. (2002). "Occupational Fatalities in Emergency Medical Services: A Hidden Crisis." *Annals of Emergency Medicine 40* 625–632.

Mayhew, C., and Chappell, D. (2009). "Ambulance Officers: The Impact of Exposure to Occupational Violence on Mental and Physical Health." University of Wollongong Research Online. See the organization website.

Merlin, M. A., M. L. Wong, P. W. Pryor, K. Rynn, A. Marques-Baptista, et al. (2009). "Prevalence of Methicillin-Resistant *Staphylococcus aureus* on the Stethoscopes of Emergency Medical Services Providers." *Prehospital Emergency Care 13*(1)71–74.

National Association of Emergency Medical Technicians. (2013). "EMS Statistics." See the organization website.

National Association of State EMS Officials. (2009). "EMS Occupational Risks." See the organization website.

National Fire Protection Association. (2009a). "NFPA 1521: Standard for Fire Department Safety Officer," 2008 ed. Quincy, MA.

National Fire Protection Association. (2009b). "NFPA 1901: Standard for Automotive Fire Apparatus," 2009 ed. Quincy, MA.

National Fire Protection Association. (2011). "NFPA 1917: Standard for Automotive Ambulances," proposed 2013 ed. Quincy, MA.

National Institute for Occupational Safety and Health. (2010, April). "Preventing Exposures to Bloodborne Pathogens among Paramedics." DHHS (NIOSH) Publication No. 2010-139. See the organization website.

O'Brien, D. J., T. G. Price, and P. Adams J. (1999, April). "The Effectiveness of Lights and Siren Use During Ambulance Transport by Paramedics." *Prehospital Emergency Care* 3(2), 127–130.

Rajasekran, K., R. J. Fairbanks, and M. N. Shah. (2008). "No More Blame and Shame: Developing Event-Reporting Systems May Go a Long Way to Reducing Patient Care Errors in EMS." *EMS Magazine* 37(9), 61–67.

Roline, C. E., C. Crumpecker, and T. M. Dunn. (2007, April–June). "Can Methicillin-Resistant Staphylococcus Aureus Be Found in an Ambulance Fleet?" *Prehospital Emergency Care 11*(2) 241–244.

The Joint Commission on Accreditation of Healthcare Organizations. (2013). "Sentinel Event." See the organization website.

U.S. Department of Labor, Occupational Safety & Health Administration. (n.d.). "Healthcare-Wide Hazards: Needlestick/Sharps Injuries." See the organization website.

U.S. Department of Transportation. (2009). *Manual on Uniform Traffic Control Devices.* See the organization website.

U.S. Federal Motor Carrier Safety Administration. (2009). "A Motor Carrier's Guide to Improving Highway Safety." See the organization website.

U.S. Fire Administration. (2009, August). "Emergency Vehicle Visibility and Conspicuity Study." See the organization website.

U.S. Fire Administration. (2010, July). "Firefighter Fatalities in the United States in 2009." See the organization website.

Wang, H. E, R. J. Fairbanks, M. N. Shah, B. N. Abo, and D. M. Yealy. (2008, September). "Tort Claims and Adverse Events in Emergency Medical Services." *Annals of Emergency Medicine* 52(3), 256–262.

Key Terms

DART rate OSHA uses the incidence rate for days away from work, days of restricted work activity or job transfer (DART) to target high-risk work sites for inspection. A high DART rate could mean that a company needs to improve safety procedures. A low DART rate could mean noncompliance with OSHA reporting regulations.

EMS safety officer Individual who handles day-to-day administrative functions related to improving the safety aspects of the agency.

EMS voluntary event notification tool A data collection tool designed to improve the safety and quality of the provision of EMS by providing an anonymous method of collecting information pertaining to near-miss and actual sentinel events.

exposure control plan An OSHA-required document that details how employees will be trained in identifying the proper personal protection equipment, when they will use it, how it will be disposed of, and who will be responsible for following up on exposures.

incident safety officer (ISO) Individual responsible for monitoring and assessing safety hazards or unsafe situations and for developing measures for ensuring personnel safety.

National Fire Protection Association (NFPA) An agency that develops and promotes scientifically based consensus standards.

near miss An event that produces no measurable loss but has the exact parameters of an event that does involve a loss.

Occupational Safety and Health Administration (OSHA) Division of the U.S. Department of Labor tasked with promulgating and enforcing standards that affect safety in the workplace.

personal protective equipment (PPE) Equipment provided to the employee that is used to prevent exposures to biological hazards as defined by OSHA in its blood-borne pathogen and respiratory protection standards.

risk management Process of applying management techniques to the identification, assessment, and resolution of problems to prevent and/or minimize occurrences that have the potential for injury or loss to patients, employees, visitors, and the company using several techniques, including exposure avoidance, risk transfer, and retention.

Ryan White Comprehensive AIDS Resources Emergency (CARE) Act Act intended to improve the quality and availability of care for low-income, uninsured, and underinsured individuals and families affected by HIV and AIDS. A section of the act requires hospitals to provide notification to EMS providers in the event of an exposure to a blood-borne pathogen.

sentinel event Any unanticipated event in a health care setting resulting in death or serious physical or psychological injury to a patient.

Ambulance Service Activities in Support of the Community

Skip Kirkwood, M.S., J.D., NREMT-P, EFO, CEMSO

Objectives

After reading this chapter, the student should be able to:

18.1 Describe the range of roles that an ambulance service may play in its community.

18.2 Discuss the benefits to an ambulance service of taking a broad view of its role in the community.

18.3 List six areas where common processes may be beneficial to the ambulance service and the patients it serves.

18.4 Discuss considerations surrounding ambulance service involvement in providing medical support to community mass gatherings.

18.5 Discuss considerations involved with the provision of medical support to fire service and law enforcement special operations teams and activities.

18.6 Describe the benefits to the ambulance service and the community from involvement in efforts to control illnesses, reduce injuries, and provide nontraditional care to special populations in the community.

Overview

Ambulance services in the United States range in size from one ambulance operated by volunteers and managed by a community board of directors to large governmental agencies and even larger, private, for-profit corporations. This text presents information that the manager of an ambulance service, large or small, needs in order to keep the business solvent and provide clinically excellent service to the community.

Key Terms

community
  paramedicine
first responders

mass gatherings
special operations

WHAT WOULD YOU DO?

You are the operations manager for a large, community-owned, not-for-profit ambulance service. Your agency serves seven municipalities with a combined population of nearly 1,000,000 people. Your agency provides both emergency response and scheduled interfacility transportation throughout your community—some 100,000 calls per year. From time to time, rumors circulate that several local fire departments plan to "go into the EMS business," and a large national ambulance company has been discovered courting some of your more lucrative nonemergency transportation clients. Three months ago, you assigned a committee of employees to discuss ways to enhance the company's visibility and standing in the community. They are expected to deliver a report to you in 30 days, and you want to prepare yourself for what they might present. Are you aware of unmet needs in your community and among your allied public safety and public health agencies? Is there a larger or different role that your ambulance service might play in the community?

■ INTRODUCTION ————————

An ambulance service may play a variety of different roles in the community and EMS systems it serves. The scope of those roles may range from serving as the lead agency for the system, with statutory responsibility for all aspects of EMS activity in the system, all the way to serving as a contract provider only of ambulance transportation, with all other responsibilities performed by other system players.

Nonetheless, the prospective ambulance service manager should constantly be scanning the environment, looking for opportunities to expand and enhance the services provided by his agency. To identify those opportunities, an ambulance service manager must be aware of opportunities that have come to others in the ambulance industry and be able to think outside of the conventional silo, usually circumscribed by whether an effort will produce an increased volume of billable transports. Programs or projects that enhance the market position of the ambulance service, whether or not they will result in a direct increase in transport volume, may improve the image of the ambulance service in the community; provide for better relationships with first response agencies, other public safety agencies, and community and public health and medical care organizations; and may aid in recruitment and retention of personnel. A broad view of what constitutes the best interests of the ambulance service is recommended.

WORKING WITH FIRST RESPONDERS

It's becoming more evident that good relationships between first response EMS personnel and ambulance transport personnel facilitate quality patient care and thus better outcomes for those patients requiring emergency medical care. At the other extreme of this continuum, poor relationships between **first responders** and ambulance personnel, with constant threats of takeover and difficult on-scene interactions, result in decreased quality of patient care.

It may not be within the purview of the ambulance service to set the tone of the relationship. Other players, including organized labor, first response agency management, and the media exert strong influence. However, to the extent that it is possible, ambulance service management should strive to take the high road, and to ensure that whatever competition may exist between the ambulance service and its first responders takes place at the boardroom level and does not translate into unpleasantness once units are dispatched.

Where possible, the following actions or attributes can contribute to good on-scene interactions between first responders and ambulance medics:

* *Common medical direction* can ensure that all on-scene efforts focus on treating the patient in the best evidence-based manner, rather than sorting out differences in approaches to patient care. Where that is not possible,

* *Common patient care protocols*, agreed upon by physicians independently providing medical direction to first response and transport agencies, can smooth at-scene delivery of patient care.
* *Common operational protocols* can facilitate smooth scene operations. For example, if protocols clearly delineate who is supposed to play what roles in the incident command system at multiple patient scenes, time lost in organizing the scene and completing incident management tasks can be minimized.
* *Common medical equipment* can speed transitions of patient care. For example, if both first response and transport agencies utilize the same brand of monitor-defibrillator, then cables and defibrillator pads can be quickly exchanged during patient transfer, rather than requiring complete removal and reattachment of pads, electrodes, and wires. Common configuration (and even shared ownership) of medical equipment, such as splints and backboards can facilitate operations and reduce logistical overhead for all involved in the system.
* *Common medical supplies* can likewise prevent patient care errors. Packaging of dissimilar drugs in similar packaging is a common contributor to drug administration errors, whereas standard packaging, standard placement, and even standardized medication bags or kits can help the patient by ensuring that when one medic reaches for a particular drug, it is the drug that is actually desired.
* *Common continuing education* can keep all personnel on the same page, and interactions in the classroom may improve at-scene interactions.

MEDICAL SUPPORT OF SPECIAL EVENTS

Historically, the approach of ambulance services to special events was one that allowed event organizers to rent the services of ambulance and personnel, typically on an hourly basis. Although

Best Practice

Mass Gatherings Special Operations in Boston

In order to quickly respond to and treat patients during special events and major emergencies, Boston EMS utilizes resources beyond traditional ambulance units.

For example, the Special Operations Division operates Defibrillator Bicycle Units at various events throughout the year. EMS bike teams are able to maneuver through congested areas and crowds, reaching patients quickly and delivering initial care more rapidly than would be possible with traditional ambulances (Figure 18.1). EMS bike units often operate in conjunction with EMS all-terrain vehicles which can transport patients through crowds and areas inaccessible by ambulance. In addition, during major events and emergencies, the Special Operations Division will often deploy fixed medical stations to care for injured and ill victims on-site. Boston EMS EMTs and/or Paramedics are also assigned to the Boston Police Harbor Unit during the City's active boating season from April through October as well as during special events such as the Tall Ships or the 4th of July Celebration. *Source: Reprinted by permission from UMDNJ University Hospital-EMS*

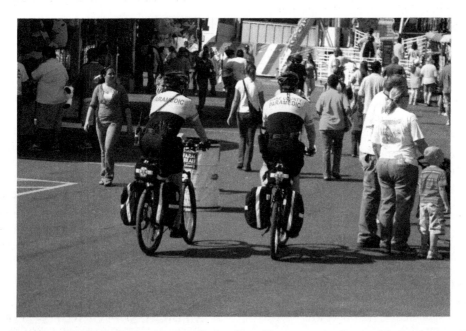

FIGURE 18.1 ■ An EMS bike team may ease the burden of large community special events on an EMS system, while showcasing the ambulance service in a positive manner. *Source: Official Wake County EMS photo by Mike Legeros. Used by permission.*

often sufficient, a more proactive approach to medical support of special events may benefit the ambulance service, the EMS system as a whole, and the citizens of the community.

Some special events, particularly those involving sales of alcohol, produce more need for EMS and ambulance transportation than might be expected. If not properly prepared and accounted for, these events may place an extra, unanticipated burden on the community's 9-1-1 system, drawing resources that are intended for the community at large, increasing response times, and worsening system performance.

A progressive ambulance service manager may find it advantageous to devote more resources to an event than a promoter believes are necessary—after all, the event promoter may have profits foremost in mind, not the safety of the public. Rather than waiting for a promoter to determine a level of EMS involvement, the ambulance service manager may find it advantageous to inject himself or his organization into the event planning process, working to ensure that adequate medical resources are assigned to the event. The ambulance service might decide it wise to assign additional resources to the event, or to the 9-1-1 system, in anticipation of increased and unanticipated demand for service. Such participation can cast

In many communities, local permitting processes may be nonexistent, or may not include the ambulance provider. For example, in New York State (New York State Sanitary Code, Part 18), **mass gathering** permits are issued by state officials, and consultation with county and municipal officials is not required. While specifying requirements for an emergency venue, Part 18 does not require that a local ambulance provider be involved. An ambulance service may consider the creation of a medical intelligence officer whose job it is to monitor sources of information, and to ensure that the ambulance service is not taken by surprise when a substantial event occurs in its service area." For more on this concept, see www.emsworld.com/article/10320241/the-medical-intelligence-officer.

the ambulance service in a favorable light, making it appear to be a positive contributor to the health and safety of the community.

■ MEDICAL SUPPORT OF LAW ENFORCEMENT AND FIRE SERVICE SPECIAL OPERATIONS———

Law enforcement and fire service **special operations**[1] entail special risks to the personnel who undertake to deliver them. The response activities of these special teams also

Side Bar

Know What's Happening in Your Community: The Medical Intelligence Officer

It is important that a community's ambulance providers are aware of what's going on throughout that community for two significant reasons:

- Community events may create additional patient load, particularly where adult beverages are available.
- Community events may disrupt normal patterns of travel, including ingress and egress routes around hospitals.

---

[1] *Special operations* include atypical response activities undertaken in response to unusual situations. In the law enforcement community, special operations include special weapons and tactics (SWAT) responses, negotiations in hostage situations, and the management of clandestine drug laboratories. In the fire service, special operations includes the activities of hazardous materials teams, urban search-and-rescue teams, high-angle rescue, swift-water rescue, and a host of others. This list is representative but by no means exhaustive.

Best Practice

Tactical Emergency Medical Support in Newark, New Jersey

University Hospital (Newark, New Jersey) EMS provides medical support for the Newark Police Department Emergency Response Team (ERT) and Emergency Services Unit (ESU) operations. UH-EMS Tactical Medical Specialist members of the ERT are carefully selected to participate in tactical training with the sworn members of the

Newark Police Department. All members of ERT are required to pass the same rigorous physical standards as their police counterparts and provide on-site tactical medical support for a multitude of law enforcement and tactical entry operations. The UH-EMS medical component of the ERT was initiated in 1994 and includes representatives from the BLS, ALS, Rescue, Supervisor, and Management divisions. Check them out at www.uh-ems.org/ert.html.

---

entail additional risk to the members of the EMS team who support them. Moreover, the history of these teams reveals that it is far more likely for members to be injured during the extensive, physically demanding training that is required to prepare a special team for service.

Medical support for special operations activities, like the activities of the teams themselves, is of a different nature than daily EMS and ambulance activities. Rather than the community at large being the consumer of medical services, special operations medical support involves a primary focus on caring for the members of the special team, as they train, deploy, and operate. It involves activities that are different from those of an ordinary EMS response medic, including preventative care, supportive injury care (so that the team member can continue to work), and an ongoing personal relationship between medic and team member.

Historically, medical support for law enforcement and fire service operations has been relatively easy in the public sector, but fraught with challenges when the private (including the nonprofit) sectors have been involved. Public agencies, often part of the

same or concurrent jurisdictions, are able to share resources with relatively little difficulty. The challenge comes when strong, private EMS agencies, funded on a fee-for-service basis, approach the subject of special operations support—which involves a tremendous commitment of time but produces a very limited number of revenue-producing events. These agencies (with some justification) often ask "Who is going to pay us for this service?"

One of the solutions that frequently surfaces when a law enforcement or fire suppression agency has limited organic (internal) EMS capabilities, but requires medical support for special operations and is supported by a private agency, is the suggestion that the team send a police officer or firefighter team member for EMT or paramedic training. This is a less-than-optimal solution. Special operations team members require the support of clinically competent, excellent medics. It is unlikely that an individual who obtains an EMS credential as an additional duty, who does not work in the field on a regular basis, will have the knowledge, experience, and proficiency to provide excellent care in a complex and difficult solution. This option provides an illusion of EMS care rather than a solid foundation of EMS care for special operations team members.

Ambulance service executives interested in building a firm place for their agency in the community would be well advised to find a way to fund special operations medical support to the communities that they serve as part of the ongoing operational budget of the agency. Supporting the notion that public safety special operations units receive care from the most experienced EMS personnel in the community is the right thing to do. In addition, it is one more way to ensure that the ambulance service is not viewed as a one-trick pony that can easily be replaced by the next low bidder.

■ INJURY PREVENTION AND ILLNESS CONTROL——————

Another group of useful services—often discussed and less often undertaken as a core component of the service mix of a typical ambulance service—is the prevention of injury and the control of illnesses. Public education, injury prevention, and illness control have been part of the activities of an EMS system for the past 40 years. However, given the fragmented nature of EMS systems in the United States and the fee-for-service funding method endured by many ambulance services, there has been a strong economic incentive to avoid (or at least to perform at the lowest possible level) direct, strong organizational participation in prevention and control activities.

Ambulance services obtain a wealth of data about the health needs of the community. Electronic patient care reporting (ePCR) systems record information about cause of illness, nature of injury, location, and much more.

That information can be used to identify a wide variety of unmet community health needs. It is a natural progression for an ambulance service that wishes to be proactive to take the accumulated data, identify particular community health needs that are amenable to intervention, and build programs that can improve the health status and the health economics of the community.

These programs appear to represent a conundrum to a transport revenue-funded ambulance service. At first blush, it would appear that these programs, if successful, would reduce billable transports and thus be harmful to the ambulance service. That is true if one only looks at the gross revenue of the service: the amount billed to the patients and insurance companies, regardless of whether it is ever collected or not. However, a more in-depth look can reveal that in communities with poor health status, in which prevention and control programs find target-rich environments, bills for transportation to the hospital emergency department are rarely paid, and even more rarely are they paid at face value. Patients transported for chronic diseases, "frequent flyers," and repeated falls often are uninsured or underinsured, resulting in a net loss to the ambulance company. Simple, lesser-cost in-field interventions could reduce the economic burden to the ambulance company of serving the community, while providing a more positive community image, more tight integration into the public health and medical care communities, and a more positive work environment for ambulance personnel (Ferno, n.d.). Although not widespread, these **community paramedicine** programs represent a bright spot of innovation throughout not only the United States but also the international EMS community. San Francisco's HOME program (Mund, 2010), MEDSTAR's (Fort Worth, TX) Community Paramedic program (MedStar Emergency Medical Services, 2010), Wake County (NC) EMS's Advanced Practice Paramedics program (Wake.gov, 2012), and the rural Community Health and Emergency Cooperative (CHEC) in Minnesota (Community Paramedic, 2008–2012) are all representatives of progressive EMS systems seeking solutions for community health problems outside the box of conventional ambulance calls resulting in transportation to a hospital emergency department (Figure 18.2). These programs all seek a common result: a more appropriate end point that is better for the patient and more economically efficient for the health care system and the community as a whole.

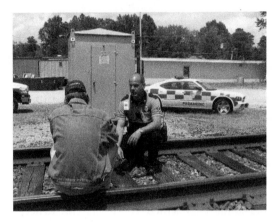

FIGURE 18.2 ■ A Wake County Advanced Practice Paramedic works with a homeless individual to determine the most appropriate destination for his immediate and ongoing difficulties. *Courtesy of the Author.*

CHAPTER REVIEW

Summary

A variety of important, positive, and highly visible activities can be undertaken by an ambulance company to enhance the role that it plays in the community it serves. The opportunities in each community may vary, and it is important for the forward-thinking ambulance service leader to be alert to the opportunities in his or her community, as well as the work that has been done in other communities to develop successful models for alternative, particularly nontransport, service delivery. Some examples include enhanced cooperation with first responders, proactive involvement in providing medical support to special events (mass gatherings), providing medical support to law enforcement and fire service special operations programs, and community paramedicine. These programs may be helpful in developing a positive community image and limiting the ability of other ambulance providers to displace an existing provider.

WHAT WOULD YOU DO? Reflection

Your employee committee reported to you with a detailed report suggesting several initiatives. At first, you were taken aback at the quantity and potential cost of these proposals. After reflection, and discussion with your senior management, you begin to see that there are opportunities to implement some of these proposals without a huge investment of corporate funds—you see grants, partnerships, and expense avoidance as possibilities.

You go back to your employee committee with your prioritized list of its initiatives, and ask the members to spend the next 30 days discussing several proposals with local agencies, with a special group assigned to explore grant funding opportunities for a program that would provide alternatives (instead of just transporting to the local ED) for the care of diabetics, chronic inebriates, and asthmatics who frequently call 9-1-1.

Review Questions

1. Why should an ambulance service executive constantly be scanning the environment for opportunities outside the agency's core ambulance transportation service?
2. What are some possible consequences of poor relationships between first responders and ambulance medics?
3. Why might an ambulance service want to provide more protection to a mass gathering than a promoter is willing to pay for?
4. If your local police agency approached you about sending a new SWAT team member to paramedic school, how would you respond?
5. How might a community paramedicine program developed with ambulance service funding provide financial benefit to that ambulance service?

References

Community Paramedic. (2008–2012). "The Community Paramedic Program: a New Way of Thinking." See the organization website.

Ferno. (n.d.). "Innovations in Prevention, Public Health and Community Outreach." See the organization website.

MedStar Emergency Medical Services. 2010, July 23). "MedStar Receives Glowing Review." See the organization website.

Mund, E. (2010, October 31). "Grounding Frequent Flyer." *EMS World.* See the organization website.

Wake.gov. (2012, October 1). "Advanced Practice Paramedics." See the organization website.

Key Terms

community paramedicine A model of care whereby paramedics apply their training and skill, in community-based environments (outside the usual emergency response/transport model). The community paramedic may practice within an expanded scope (applying specialized skills/protocols beyond that which he was originally trained for), or an expanded role (working in nontraditional roles using existing skills).

first responders Medically trained individuals who respond to EMS calls in advance of transporting ambulances. In communities where ambulances are dynamically deployed, first responders are sometimes called co-responders because ambulances sometimes arrive first. Typically, first responders are firefighters, police officers, lifeguards, park rangers.

mass gatherings Events where relatively large numbers of people gather on a short-term basis, such as concerts, demonstrations, rallies, festivals, marathons, state fairs, and similar events. Sometimes called special events.

special operations Include transport and activities such as providing medical support for mass gatherings, tactical emergency medical support for law enforcement special operations units, incident rehabilitation for fires and other large incidents, deployment of ambulance strike teams and EMS task forces to support other jurisdictions, and providing medical support to hazardous materials and urban search-and-rescue teams.

Ambulance Operations in Support of Disaster Operations

Lawrence Nelson, M.Sc., EMT-P (Ret.), NMCEM

Objectives

After reading this chapter, the student should be able to:

19.1 Utilize the National Incident Management System and the incident command system when operationally engaged.

19.2 Develop the capacity to coordinate, communicate, and collaborate prior to, during, and following critical incidents involving ambulance services and other agencies.

19.3 Describe the emergency management continuum of mitigation, preparedness, response, and recovery as it relates to planning of ambulance operations in a natural, technological, or criminal disaster situation.

19.4 Delineate the elements necessary to develop and execute a successful memorandum of understanding and mutual aid agreement.

19.5 Conduct a needs analysis, hazard/threat survey, and a gap analysis to improve the organization's potential response to a disaster.

19.6 Conduct a post-incident debriefing (after-action conference) and develop an after-action report and improvement plan.

19.7 Explain the roles and responsibilities (within the incident command system) of the incident commander in the initial phases of an incident or for the totality of a smaller incident; of the EMS branch director at larger incidents involving multiple casualties; of a division/group supervisor at an incident of any size; and of a task force/strike team leader for an out-of-jurisdiction response to a major event.

Overview

Ambulance services in the United States range in size from one ambulance operated by volunteers and managed by a community board of directors to large governmental agencies and even larger, private, for-profit corporations. This text presents information that the manager of an ambulance service, large or small, needs in order to keep the business solvent and provide clinically excellent service to the community.

Key Terms

mass casualty incident (MCI)	mitigate	preparedness	strike team
memorandum of understanding (MOU)	mutual aid agreement (MAA)	recovery	task force
	National Response Framework (NRF)	response	

WHAT WOULD YOU DO?

The beginning of spring marks the onset of severe weather and fire season in your operational area. In a few weeks, hurricane season will start. Since last fall, a new nursing home housing eight-four residents of mixed mobility has opened, you have added two 24-hour ambulances to your current deployment of nine, and your community's emergency manager has received a new State Homeland Security Grant. Part of the emphasis for this year's grant is developing an evacuation plan for special populations in your community. Your service's chief executive has assigned you as liaison to the emergency management office. At the first meeting of the plan development team, you are asked to provide several items for reference at the next meeting: a list of the types of resources you have, a copy of any memorandums of understanding (MOUs) with the local health care facilities, and mutual aid agreements (MAAs) with nearby ambulance services. You are also asked if you have a continuity of operations (COOP) plan and an emergency operations plan. You return to the EMS administration building wondering about what you had been asked to provide.

1. For what number of patients could you adequately care?
2. What internal resources do you have, and where would you obtain more in the event of a disaster?
3. Are you prepared to continue operating immediately after a disaster, or how long would it take for you to return to service?
4. Are the field personnel trained, equipped, and prepared for a major incident?

■ INTRODUCTION

Thankfully, disasters, catastrophes, pandemics, and other high-visibility, high-impact, and high-publicity incidents are rare. However, with increased populations, incident complexity, and community/consumer awareness, the need to approach incidents and events in a more systematic manner has become more important. As resources change and more organizations and jurisdictions are supporting each other, having a common operating system becomes more important. The phrase "The right hand has to know what the left hand is doing" becomes even more significant. To accomplish this, the components of planning, organizing, operational concept, communications, control, and mission support must be considered and made as uniform as possible. This will reduce waste, duplication, and risk to all involved.

Ambulance operations in support of disaster management are key to the overall goals of emergency management: saving lives, protecting property, and preserving the environment (Figure 19.1). Ambulance operations are an essential activity, and understanding the various roles of ambulance services in disasters makes ambulance services a significant partner in the emergency management continuum.

> ### Side Bar
>
> Ambulances are key to supporting the goals of emergency management.

■ COMMAND, CONTROL, AND COMMUNICATIONS——————

Any incident with a growing number of affected persons, jurisdictions, and complexity requires increased levels of organization. Unity of command, adequate control of resources, and the ability to communicate accurately and quickly can be lifesaving. Through trial and error, EMS has a variety of tools to use to reduce chaos and risk during incidents.

NATIONAL INCIDENT MANAGEMENT SYSTEM

The National Incident Management System (NIMS) is a systematic approach that guides

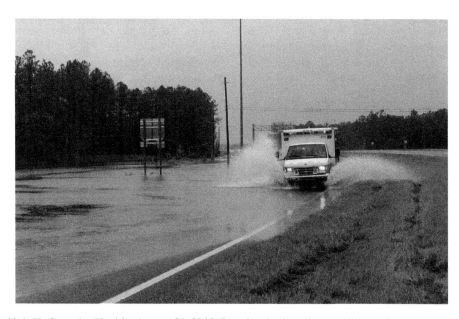

FIGURE 19.1 ■ Osceola, Florida, August 21, 2008. Despite the flooding conditions, this Seminole County Emergency Response ambulance makes a run during Tropical Storm Fay. Local and state emergency/first responders have braved all conditions for their communities' safety. *Source: FEMA*

agencies at all levels of government, the private sector, and nongovernmental organizations in working seamlessly to prevent, protect against, respond to, recover from, and **mitigate** the effects of incidents, regardless of cause, size, location, or complexity, in order to reduce the loss of life, destruction of property, and harm to the environment.

NIMS has been evolving over many years, but the catalyst for its introduction was the terror attacks of September 11, 2001. Following the attacks and upon creation of the Department of Homeland Security (DHS), President George W. Bush signed Homeland Security Presidential Directive 5 (HSPD-5) (Maniscalco and Christen, 2011), which mandated that all federal agencies would use NIMS to manage activities during emergencies. NIMS consists of command and control—including the incident command system (ICS)—resource typing, **preparedness**, communications/information technology, and ongoing development. In order to encourage participation at all government levels, grants and other funding sources are tied to levels of compliance in training, planning, and resource management. All responders should participate in some level of NIMS/ICS training, based on their level of leadership. This training is available both live (classroom) and online through the DHS/FEMA Emergency Management Institute.

NIMS works hand in hand with the **National Response Framework (NRF)**. NIMS provides the template for the management of incidents, whereas NRF provides the structure and mechanisms for national-level policy for incident management (FEMA, 2013).

Resource Management

Resource management includes resource typing, which is the categorization of assets (human and material) by capabilities. Certification, credentials, and capacity are used in this typing process. It reduces ambiguity. If you (as an incident commander) ask for an "ambulance," you don't know exactly what you are going to get. What is the highest level of medical training of the personnel assigned? What type of equipment is available on the ambulance? Are you getting a vehicle that can transport patients, or do you get the crew to operate it as well? Are they ALS or BLS capable? Are they capable of operating in a hazmat environment? Are they a unit capable of transporting patients? Resource typing clarifies communication by defining the asset.

Preparedness consists of the training, planning, and exercises involved in making an organization (either a governmental entity or a nongovernmental organization) ready to respond to any incident Figure 19.2). Outside of the basic medical training involved in EMS, additional training may involve awareness/operations level in weapons of mass destruction (WMDs), hazardous materials release, pandemic disease **response**, mass evacuation and sheltering from natural/human-made disasters, mass gathering events, or mass casualty/fatality incidents. Planning should involve developing **memorandums of understanding** between agencies, incident action plans, operational policies and procedures, demobilization plans, after-action reviews, and improvement plans. Use of the Homeland Security Exercise and Evaluation Program (HSEEP) integrates all these activities and also makes the capture of lessons learned and best practices easier to use and share.

Incident Command System

Most responders are familiar with the ICS component of NIMS. ICS was originally developed as part of Firefighting Resources of California Organized for Potential Emergencies (FIRESCOPE). FIRESCOPE was the result of "lessons learned" recommendations

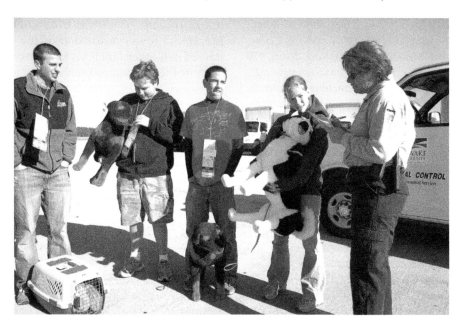

FIGURE 19.2 ■ A well-designed drill will test all of the capabilities that might be required during an actual event. Here, an animal control officer demonstrates the ability to deal with companion animals arriving on a National Disaster Medical System flight. *Source: Official Wake County EMS photo by Lee Wilson. Used by permission.*

following wildfires in California in the 1970s (Maniscalco and Christen, 2011). The desired goal was a seamless, event-agile, command structure capable of expanding and contracting with the complexity and size of the incident.

Side Bar

The incident command system improves operations.

Key Management Objectives
The following are the key management objectives for command, control, and communications, as well as their implementation and evaluation:

+ *A system of command, within which a single individual (or unified command team) is responsible for the ultimate outcome of the incident.* This objective is generally resolved. Communities have codified in forms of ordinance, standard operating procedures (SOP)/ standard operating guidelines (SOG), and memorandums of understanding. The incident commander is designated by the responsible agency for the type of incident.

+ *A system of common terminology.* All agencies should understand each other. FEMA and the National Fire Academy (NFA) have developed a dictionary of terms, and common terms are included in all levels of ICS/IMS training produced by FEMA, NFA, and individual study programs.

* *A system of coordination among diversified agencies.* Fire service and EMS are generally coordinated. Law enforcement is less coordinated, but it should reach parity with fire/EMS because of implementation of NIMS.

* *A communications system with shared frequencies and common radio language.* This remains a problem, as illustrated in the "9/11 Commission Report." If larger cities, such as New York, are having a problem reaching common ground (usually because of fiscal and bureaucratic stumbling blocks), then what are smaller cities doing? Some positive signs are the 800 phone trunking system and ease in programming of large numbers of radios in the field. Unfortunately, the 800 system is heavily computer reliant and potentially susceptible to crashing due to power failure or cyber attack. Losses of relay towers also are potential weak links in the chain. Clear text and voice are mostly implemented in the fire/EMS services. Law enforcement agencies generally continue to use the APCO 10 codes, whereas some West Coast jurisdictions still use their codes and signals method internally. Generally, in an interagency event, clear text is used.

* *A system for resource allocation, including prioritizing and staging.* Most fire/EMS agencies are well adapted in the use of resource allocation. Where the friction occurs is when law enforcement agencies want to reposition units. This can generally be resolved quickly, but the use of time and effort to do so detracts from dealing with the overall situation. This problem occurs less frequently when a unified command team is implemented, or when a law enforcement agency liaison is present at the command post to deal with such issues.

OPERATIONS

Operations is the function that produces the end results, be it making widgets, building

house trailers, or, in the EMS context, the preservation and protection of the sick and injured. All other functions in an organization support the operations branch.

Major Operational Responsibilities

The major operational responsibilities of ambulance services in a disaster are divided between pre-incident and post-incident phases. In the immediate pre-incident phase, such as when some warning is available, the focus is on preservation of the service and evacuation of special populations that require ambulance transport. The post-incident phase focuses on dealing with multiple casualties and dealing with transport of patients to facilities that are out of the disaster area.

Mass Casualty Incident

In *Advanced Disaster Medical Response*, Briggs and Brinsfield (2008) defined the term **mass casualty incident (MCI)**. This is sometimes referred to as a multiple casualty incident. Regardless, an MCI is an event resulting from human-made or natural causes that results in illness and/or injuries that exceed the EMS capabilities of a hospital, locality, jurisdiction, and/or region (Figure 19.3).

MCI management goals include the following:

1. Do the greatest good for the greatest number.
2. Make the best use of personnel, equipment, and facility resources.
3. Do not relocate the disaster.

MCIs fall into one of the following four categories:

* An *expanded medical incident* requires the use of local resources and/or mutual aid to manage it. The scale of this incident can be managed by an incident commander and the designated functions of staging, extrication/rescue, triage, treatment, and transportation.

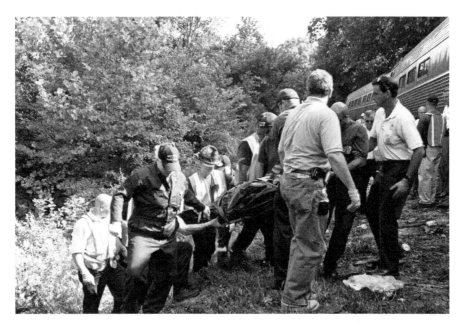

FIGURE 19.3 ▪ Multiple-patient or mass-casualty incidents require strong interagency cooperation at all levels. Here, a multidisciplinary team extracts an injured person in the wake of a train versus dump truck collision. *Source: Official Wake County EMS photo by Lee Wilson. Used by permission.*

An EMS/medical would be appointed by and report to the incident commander. In a small incident, one person may assume more than one function. In a larger incident, the functions are assigned. In accordance with many local jurisdiction protocols, this would be considered a Level I MCI.

* A *major medical incident* requires the use of regional and/or multiregional resources to manage the incident. This depicts a larger incident with multiple agency response and may deploy a fully developed EMS/medical group. An expanded incident on this scale also requires an increase in the number of functions (e.g., the addition of a liaison or information officer). In some jurisdictions, this would be considered a Level II or higher MCI.

* A *disaster* requires the use of state and/or federal resources to manage the incident. This is an even larger incident that requires the addition of functions such as planning, logistics, and finance. This may be dictated by incidents covering large areas or of extended duration. This may be referred to as a Level III MCI.

* In a *catastrophe*, there is destruction and loss of local infrastructure, so outside resources are required.

Disaster Incident

Operational organization in a disaster may sound like an oxymoron, but integration, coordination, collaboration, and communications occur through preplanning and using ICS models during tabletop, functional, and full-scale exercises.

Resource Configurations

In addition to ambulances as single resources, ambulances and their crews might be used in other resource configurations. The most common of these are the **strike team** and the **task force**.

Strike teams are groups of personnel or similar types of assets, usually intended to strongly supplement currently engaged resources. They may be from a single organization or mixed in a staging area. An example might include a team of five Type II ambulances and a strike team leader in a nontransport vehicle (e.g., a large sport-utility vehicle or a sedan) assigned to evacuate an assisted care center.

Task forces are mixed resources assigned to perform a specific task. They may be from a single organization or multiple agencies. An example might include a medical rescue task force, consisting of a Type II ambulance from an EMS agency, a Type 1 engine from a fire/rescue service, a piece of Type II snow-removal equipment from a public works department, and a mass-transit passenger bus assigned to check stranded vehicles on a snow-clogged freeway.

EMS Functional Positions

During an EMS-focused incident, the position of EMS branch director (BD) is in charge of initiating care and transporting patients. The BD is mobile and in the thick of the situation. Despite this, the BD is nonclinical. The BD has to function as a servant-leader, working with the logistics team to ensure that necessary resupply, additional personnel, and transport are available to meet the needs of the treating medics and the patients. At the same time, the BD is keeping the incident commander informed on numbers of patients, fatalities, assets needed, and status of the tempo of operations.

As patients are removed from the scene, their distribution is noted and advised. As the initial issues of patient evacuation are resolved, EMS then starts to serve as logistical support for fire services (firefighter treatment or rehab) or law enforcement (special team support or rehab).

To accomplish the mission, tasks within the operational branch are delegated. Officers are assigned to implement a part of the total EMS operations process (Figure 19.4).

The triage officer is responsible for the initial actions taken after assurance of scene safety and donning appropriate personal protective equipment (PPE). *Triage*, from the French meaning "to sort," was first implemented by Napoleon's surgeon to preserve the most viable wounded soldiers from the battlefield. The task is implemented to do the most good for the most viable patients.

> **Side Bar**
>
> Triage is intended to do the most good for the most viable patients.

Triage can be accomplished in less than 1 minute per patient, using the Simple Triage and Rapid Treatment (START) method. No definitive care is given, aside from repositioning the head to open an airway, or having the patient/bystander apply direct pressure to continuous bleeding. The triage officer (and assistants) continue on their way through the scene, designating patients immediate/most critical (red), delayed/generally lacking self-mobility but relatively stable (yellow), minor/walking wounded (green), or fatalities (black). Follow-up personnel then move patients to the treatment areas, according to triage level. Fatalities are left in place.

As the triage process progresses and additional personnel arrive, the BD designates three treatment areas (sectors) to correspond with the color codes in use (red, yellow, green). In these areas, patients are treated and stabilized and "packaged" for transportation. Treatment officers coordinate with the BD for resupply and transport to move patients to receiving facilities and with the triage officers to determine future needs. The next resource issue becomes skill level of the providers, and where they should be assigned. The more critical patients are assigned to the more skilled and experienced personnel. However, delayed and minor patients may need further reassessment

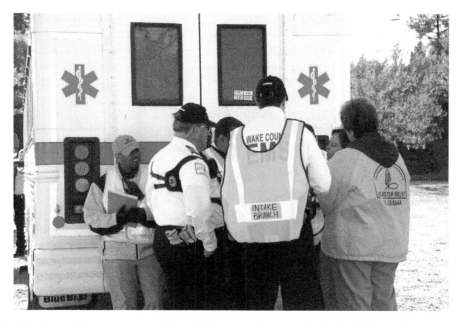

FIGURE 19.4 ▓ Branch directors play a key role in managing complex EMS incidents. *Source: Official Wake County EMS photo by Lee Wilson. Used by permission.*

and movement to a higher-level treatment area or immediate transport. EMT-Basics can handle the majority of the patients in the minor category (bandaging, splinting, oxygen, epinephrine, DuoDote Auto Injector, and bronchodilator administration) but should be overseen by an individual with a higher skill level. A paramedic or R.N. should be assigned as the treatment green or treatment yellow officer.

Transportation determines bed availability and sends patients to designated hospitals, attempting to prevent overwhelming a few ERs with the most critical patients. After initial triage, there may now be a location problem. Incidents can happen anywhere, so there may be limited options at the scene. Transporting the patients from the scene becomes an issue. How large is the area necessary for treatment of the patients in each category? How close to the scene is it, and is there a clear ingress–egress route? Consideration should be given for need and location of a helistop.

When a MCI occurs, by definition it outstrips the available resources. Mutual aid for both scene response and coverage of temporarily underserved areas of the involved community must be negotiated in advance and included in the agency SOP/SOG. Personnel on ambulances may have varied skill levels, so this must be considered when selecting the patients to be transported by each unit. City buses might be considered for delayed-level patients. These considerations must be addressed with the BD, who in turn relays these needs to the incident commander, who then contacts the emergency operations center (EOC) to request those assets.

As ambulances arrive, staging is implemented, and patients are again triaged (which is really an ongoing process). Hopefully, a mix of treatment-leveled patients can be transported from the scene and receive prompt care at the receiving facility. Arriving units may also bring additional supplies and personnel, which the transport team then directs to treatment. A staging officer will manage ambulances that are assembled away from the incident site to reduce the congestion that frequently occurs during an operation of significant size. This requires close coordination and communications between the treatment and transportation officers.

LOGISTICS

Logistics is the primary support for MCI and high-impact operations. It consists of four critical functions: medical supply, communications, facilities, and security.

Medical Supply

Initial supplies are pushed through existing stock on responding ambulances. As this stock is used, additional pushed supplies arrive at the scene on second, third, and subsequent units. These arrive as prepackaged, stored kits.

Occasionally, special items are pulled (drawn from stock and special called to the scene). These might include pediatric-size supplies, as in a school bus accident, or Duo-Dote Auto Injector kits in the event of a hazmat situation involving organophosphate poisoning or nerve agents in a terrorism event.

Caches are preplanned sets of equipment that can either be pushed to a scene or used in place in the event of a disaster. Larger or specialized caches, such as the Metropolitan Medical Response System caches or the Centers for Disease Control and Prevention (CDC) mobile medical caches in secure storage, can be pushed to or near the scene of a medical disaster.

Communications

Communications is the link necessary to provide continuity and connectivity between and through levels in the ICS. Radios are the most common; runners may also exist.

Change of position, especially IC, requires face-to-face relief. The outgoing IC gives the incoming IC a brief report of the incident, tasks in progress, condition and disposition of patients, and assets available and en route.

Facilities

Facilities provides infrastructure for large events or those of long duration. Areas covered include food, water, sanitation, auxiliary power, and rehab areas.

Security

The primary duty of security is to protect medics. That duty is usually performed by law enforcement officers. This may be a strike team to provide perimeter and interior security, but it may include canine (K-9) and explosive ordnance disposal (EOD) task forces, especially at vehicle-borne improvised explosive device/improvised explosive device (VBIED/IED) incidents where a secondary device may be present. An example is the Atlanta bar bombing that resulted in public safety casualties when a remotely detonated secondary device exploded.

HAZARDOUS MATERIALS INCIDENTS

During an active hazardous materials event, an EMS unit should be dedicated to providing support to the hazmat team and leader. The EMS unit is not assigned to the operations EMS branch but, rather, is part of the fire/rescue branch. Among the tasks performed by EMS unit personnel are these:

- Practice self-protection by remaining in the uncontaminated "cold zone"
- Coordinate with the safety and decontamination officers
- Assess, plan, implement treatment, and evaluate care for hazmat team members and victims
- Monitor hazmat team members in the rehab area, looking for heat stress–related injuries, fatigue, chemical contamination, and trauma

◆ Consult with the resource/reference officer for specific treatment requirements and information on the chemicals involved

MANMADE DISASTERS/TERRORIST ACTS

Terrorism is defined by the Code of Federal Regulations as "the unlawful use of force and violence against persons or property to intimidate or coerce a government, the civilian population, or any segment thereof, in furtherance of political or social objectives" (28 C.F.R. Section 0.85). To achieve these ends, terrorists— either in cells (groups) or individually ("lone wolf operations")—will use whatever weapon they can obtain to inflict maximum casualties. "Kill one, terrorize a thousand" is an old anarchist saying that is the keystone of the terrorist's choice of tactics.

Statistically, 70 percent of all terrorist attacks involve the use of explosives, followed by small arms. As of this writing, there has been no successful employment of chemical, biological, or radiation-related weapons in the United States. Although hybrid (combined use of explosives and chemicals) attacks have been attempted in the United States (cyanide gas and explosives at the first World Trade Center bombing) and overseas (mixing of anticoagulants with shrapnel in suicide vest/belt bombs in Israel), thus far they have proven ineffective (Briggs and Brinsfield, 2008).

Side Bar

Of all terrorist attacks, 70 percent involve the use of explosives, followed by small arms.

Situational awareness will give medics early warning of terrorist acts. Explosions are obvious, but once on the scene, be observant for secondary explosive devices. These are designed to kill and maim responders. Recall the effects on the public when first responders were killed on September 11. Those deaths overshadowed the other losses of life because of the psychological effect on the public.

Be aware of situations that may be called in as "difficulty breathing" or "seizures"; if the number of these events escalates over a short period of time, it may be warning of a chemical agent release. When arriving on the scene, ambulance personnel should look at the surroundings. Dead insects, birds, and animals may be an early warning that the ambulance has entered a hot zone. Chemical agents were originally designed to be insecticides. It has been said that a chemical attack is a hazmat situation with a bad attitude.

Also, consider an uptick of flu-like symptoms in patients and co-workers, especially 2 to 3 days after a large event in an enclosed venue. This may be a harbinger of a developing biological weapons attack. Most of the probable agents are viral and present in similar fashion (Ryan and Glarum, 2008).

These events may provide extreme challenges to ambulance operations. It is necessary to plan ahead and to be ready to acquire additional assets when the incident is characterized by sudden surges of patients, overload of the medical infrastructure, and the necessity to employ alternate care standards. Become familiar with programs that support the medical and health functions. These might include, depending on the location, the Metropolitan Medical Response System, Cities Readiness Initiative, and Urban Area Security Initiative. Further information on these programs is listed in "Your Web Connection" at the end of this chapter.

■ PLANNING

The old axiom "You don't plan to fail, you fail to plan" holds true for ambulance services and becomes most glaring during a disaster.

Although many ambulances are completely divorced from the emergency management function in their community, no responsible ambulance service manager should allow that gap to continue. Engagement is essential to success—an ambulance service will be expected to perform in a disaster, regardless of its level of engagement prior to the disaster.

To prevent failure, ambulance services can take some specific steps. A service will never know when a disaster will occur, so the process of planning is continuous. Leaders must plan, develop a training schedule, improve durable medical equipment and rolling stock inventories, and determine an alternative location (or locations) from which to operate. If these actions have not been initiated, the following provides a suggested framework to use:

- *Establish an internal disaster committee.* Determine the stakeholders and participants who would be involved in logistical, planning, and operational functions. Involve them in the planning, organizing, directing, and coordinating. Moderate differences and facilitate improved cooperation among agencies.
- *Become familiar with Emergency Support Function #8 (ESF #8).* Using the Federal Response Framework, EMS will function under the ESF #8, Public Health and Medical Services, which provides the mechanism for coordinated federal assistance to supplement state, tribal, and local resources in response to a public health and medical disaster, potential or actual incidents requiring a coordinated federal response, and/or a developing potential health and medical emergency.
- *Develop memorandums of understanding between emergency management and other emergency support function (ESF) agencies.* MOUs codify the actions, contact points, procedures, and planning among agencies. In addition to MOUs, develop mutual aid agreements to share services with other providers in a disaster.

- *Have the disaster committee conduct a community threat assessment.* Work with the local emergency management agency to determine the direction and priorities for planning, training, and logistical needs, based on the probability of various natural or human-made disasters.
- *Schedule quarterly meetings of the disaster committee.* Maintain interaction among agencies, plan exercises, and familiarize new representatives from the agencies. "Put a name to a face"—an incident is not a place to be exchanging business cards.
- *Respond to the next disaster like you own it.* Do realistic training ("Train like you fight"). Plan for contingencies. Create subsets ("Plans B, C, and D"). Debrief energetically, using lessons learned from both your exercises and actual events, as well as other jurisdictions.
- Reevaluate your plans, and modify them as necessary.

■ MEDICAL SUPPORT UNIT

A disaster of any type overwhelms the local capacity to resolve the situation. In a medical disaster, this usually extends to a region's incapacity to deal with the incident. In this scenario, a state health department or the U.S. Public Health Service will come in and set up a medical support unit (MSU) to assist the local jurisdiction.

The MSU is parallel in structure to the IMS. It may be co-located with the EOC, or may be in a separate venue (Figure 19.5). The MSU deals with the public health issues until the disabled local infrastructure can be repaired or replaced. Among these services are personnel, equipment, surveillance, nuclear/biological/chemical (NBC) hazards, occupational safety, mental health, inpatient care, and other public health functions (vector control, potable water, information, etc.).

The MSU serves as a master EOC for subordinate incidents. During Tropical Storm

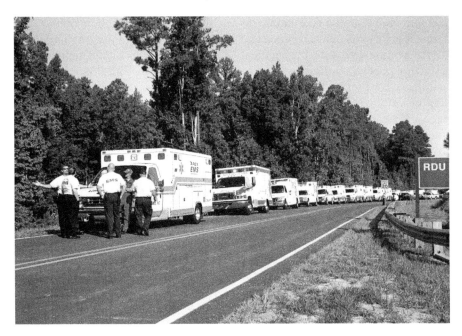

FIGURE 19.5 ▨ Ambulances staged for the National Disaster Medical System receiving point at the Raleigh–Durham Airport in the weeks following Hurricane Rita, September 2005. *Source: Official Wake County EMS photo by Lee Wilson. Used by permission.*

Allison in Houston, the Texas Medical Center received heavy rainfall and a bayou flooded, with the overflow incapacitating the two level I trauma centers for a population of 3.5 million. These two hospitals (Memorial Hermann and Ben Taub) were evacuated, displacing 700 hospital beds to community hospitals. Several other hospitals suffered lesser damage and were able to continue to operate on a restricted basis.

An MSU was activated and controlled a disaster medical assistance team (DMAT) at the Houston Astrodome, another in east Harris County, at two other evacuation shelters, and at the airlift support by a company of U.S. Army Reserve and a company of Texas National Guard UH-60 helicopters. Each of the DMATs functioned as a clearing station and urgent care. Patients requiring hospitalization were transported, either by air or ground, to outlying hospitals that were supplemented by staff from the affected hospitals in the medical center.

For several weeks following the flooding, during which the hospitals were undergoing repairs (Memorial Hermann Hospital had enough water in it to fill the Houston Astrodome), the MSU coordinated the activities of the DMATs. The MSU and the last DMAT secured 5 weeks after the event. The MSU concept proved itself in the Allison event and has led to some changes in the infrastructure and operational planning for future medical disaster events in Houston.

▨ NATIONAL DISASTER MEDICAL SYSTEM

Sometimes the results of a disaster come to you. The National Disaster Medical System (NDMS) is a federally coordinated system that augments the nation's medical response capability. The overall purpose of the NDMS is to supplement an integrated national medical response capability for assisting state and local authorities in dealing with the medical impacts of major peacetime disasters and to provide support to the military and the Department of Veterans Affairs medical systems in caring for casualties evacuated back to the United States from conventional armed conflicts overseas.

The National Response Framework utilizes the National Disaster Medical System (NDMS), as part of the Department of Health and Human Services, Office of Preparedness and Response, under Emergency Support Function #8 (ESF #8), Health and Medical Services, to support federal agencies in the management and coordination of the federal medical response to major emergencies and federally declared disasters.

Side Bar

NDMS is part of both the military and civilian casualty evacuation plans.

NDMS was utilized during Hurricanes Katrina and Rita (2005) and again during Hurricanes Dean (2007) and Ike (2008) to evacuate already hospitalized patients to areas away from the disaster, or potential disaster zones. Following the earthquake in Haiti in 2010, patients were transported by the U.S. Department of Defense (DoD) aeromedical evacuation system to Florida, where patients were then dispersed to hospitals throughout the southeastern United States.

The lead federal agency for the NDMS is the Veterans Administration (VA), as NDMS was originally designed to move wartime casualties from foreign combat zones to hospitals (military, VA, and civilian) in the United States, the premise being that the surge of casualties would quickly outstrip in-theater military medical resources. The VA is supported by the DoD, which provides aeromedical transport through existing DoD resources.

At the disaster site, patients are stabilized for transport. Patients will be transported from the disaster area to cities with Federal Coordinating Centers, usually the VA hospital, or to non-VA hospitals that are members of the NDMS system, closest to the reception point. At the airport of the NDMS reception area, patients will be met by a local medical team that will reassess, triage, and match patients to participating hospitals, according to procedures developed by local authorities and the local area's NDMS Federal Coordinating Center. Patients will be transported to participating hospitals using locally available ground and air transport (U.S. Department of Health and Human Services [HHS], 2011).

Under most circumstances, the reception point will serve as the triage area (usually staffed by physicians and nurses from the VA or a teaching hospital), where patients are reassessed (some may have deteriorated, due to the stress of flight), immediately necessary treatment is rendered, and the transportation sector assigns a unit (in the staging area) to transport the patient to a care facility. This may be a predetermined facility, but if the patient's acuity has changed, the destination facility may be revised. Occasionally, there is a death in flight, so an area for morgue operations must be designated, away from the treatment and transport areas.

■ FINANCE AND ADMINISTRATION——————

In the preparedness phase, plans must be developed to obtain additional ambulances and crews, based on the need for evacuation of nonambulatory patients and to stage ambulances within a 4-hour normal drive. These resources can be planned for through the use of MOUs and **mutual aid agreements (MAAs)**.

MOUs, as described, outline support to be provided between organizations, usually as an intergovernmental document. At the very least, the contents of an MOU specify the agencies involved, the mutual services to be provided, issues of liability, insurance, pay, workers' compensation, and medical protocols (especially in the case of an ALS service).

When local resources are completely engaged in an incident, additional resources may be available through an MAA. These are similar to MOUs, but they generally involve county, regional, or tribal groups of like resources. For example, a county might develop an MAA among independent fire departments within the county. The same content is gener-

ally found in an MAA as in an MOU, but it can be more complex as more governmental entities and jurisdictions are involved. Usually, implementation of an MAA is done through the county emergency manager.

If an incident has utilized to capacity all local, regional, and state resources, then the resources of nearby states may be utilized. These would be requested by the state level EOC to adjoining states through the Emergency Management Assistance Compact (EMAC). EMAC was established in 1996, following Hurricane Andrew. EMAC is the first national disaster-relief compact since the Civil Defense and Disaster Compact of 1950. Since its ratification by Congress, all fifty states, the District

Best Practice

American Medical Response

After Hurricanes Katrina and Rita, the inconsistency and unavailability of ambulances and self-deployment were noted as areas for improvement. To correct this deficiency, FEMA developed and implemented a plan to establish a comprehensive EMS response to federally declared disasters and placed a request for proposals for contractors interested in providing ambulance services. American Medical Response (AMR) was awarded the contract in 2007. During Hurricane Dean later that year, AMR dispatched 300 ground ambulances, 25 air (rotor and fixed wing) ambulances and paratransit assets to transport 3,500 persons. These were not all AMR units; agreements between AMR and subcontractors were also in place. At the time, FEMA described this deployment as one of the largest mobilizations of EMS resources in the history of the United States. AMR's Hurricane Dean deployment was evaluated by FEMA, and the results have been posted publicly (American Medical Response, 2013). AMR attained either "outstanding" or "excellent"

evaluation scores from FEMA and the U.S. Dept. of Health and Human Services in all categories. One lesson learned from various ambulance deployments is that ambulance companies should familiarize employees with deployment issues before a disaster happens (as a part of ongoing training), because when an event occurs, it is too late to train for it. Ambulance service should also keep in mind that employees selected for employment should be motivated, physically fit paramedics who will not, because of their personal needs, become a burden to the deployment operation.

During 2008, Hurricanes Gustav, Hanna, and Ike struck southern Louisiana, South Carolina, and the area of Galveston, Texas, respectively, within 3 weeks of each other. This was the most massive deployment of ambulances (600) on record. A Public Health Service officer compared the deployment as "grossly equivalent to a U.S. Army Armored Division deployed across an area more than twice the size of Iraq" (American Medical Response, 2013; Pound and Gould, 2010) of Columbia, Puerto Rico, Guam, and the U.S. Virgin Islands have enacted legislation to become EMAC members. EMAC is administered through the National Emergency Management Association. The EMAC Articles of Agreement clearly spell out responsibilities and procedures for the signatories (National Emergency Management Association, 2013).

FEMA also has a nationwide contract to provide ambulances and crews. As of March 2011, this contract was with American Medical Response.

This example of private and public collaboration, cooperation, and communication continues to evolve as lessons are learned and areas for improvement are noted and acted upon. Among these are the following:

- *Ambulance equipment.* Essential equipment for ambulances varies from state to state. AMR assisted HHS in establishing minimum equipment standards for ALS and BLS ambulances deploying to federally declared disasters.
- *Bariatric ambulances.* Hurricanes Gustav and Ike underscored the need for these specialized services. FEMA and AMR modified the national response to include bariatric ambulances in the arsenal of EMS disaster services.
- *Scope of practice for federal disasters.* Due to variations in EMS scope of practice between states, AMR established a nationwide "EMS Scope of Practice, Protocols and Medical Control and Direction for AMR/FEMA Federal Disaster Deployments" (American Medical Response, 2010). The National EMS Scope of Practice Model (National Highway Traffic Safety Administration, 2007) and National EMS Core Content were used to develop this standard.

■ RECOVERY

Following the immediate response to the disaster comes the **recovery** period. This is defined as the period following stabilization

of the emergency until normal operations resume. Activities during this period may include relocation of patients from damaged facilities, performing rehabilitation services for persons engaged in debris removal, or reconstituting the business operations of the ambulance services.

Continuity of operations plans (COOPs) include determining alternate operations and administrative locations, lines of succession, and workforce relocation. This plan is developed in the pre-incident phase to ensure that the private or public operation can continue.

■ REIMBURSEMENT OPPORTUNITIES

A presidentially declared disaster opens reimbursement opportunities. Eligible applicants may include state, local, and tribal governments and private nonprofit organizations or institutions that provide ambulance services. State, local, and tribal governments may provide ambulance services directly, or may contract with other ambulance service providers for such services, including mutual aid agreements and emergency memoranda of understanding. Private for-profit ambulance providers are not eligible for direct reimbursement from FEMA. However, state, local, or tribal governments that contracted with the private ambulance providers may submit a claim for reimbursement to FEMA. Reimbursement will be subject to cost sharing requirements.

If required as a result of an emergency or major disaster declaration, eligible ambulance service provider costs include, but are not limited to, the following:

- The costs of activating ambulance contracts and staging of ambulances (contract or publicly owned) prior to the impact of an incident, such as landfall of a hurricane, typhoon, or tropical storm. Contracts for staging ambulance services must be part of the state or regional evacuation plan. The costs of staging ambulances are eligible even if the incident does not directly impact the staging area, provided the president declares an emergency or major disaster. Reasonable costs incurred in advance of or as the result of an emergency or major disaster declaration for transporting disaster victims to a hospital or other medical facility are also covered.

Side Bar

Reimbursement for response during a presidentially declared disaster is available when specific criteria are met.

* Ambulance services supporting shelter operations or on site at shelter locations are also reimbursable. These may include the reasonable costs for ambulance services used to transport a congregate shelter evacuee/shelteree, ambulances used for distributing immunizations, staffing shelters and emergency departments, setting up mobile medical units, and responding to hazards.
* The costs to staff congregate shelters with medical practitioners to provide assistance to evacuees, as are symptom surveillance and reporting, and transporting and redistributing patients to make necessary hospital bed space available.
* Equipment costs incurred by the ambulance provider, including fuel and medical supplies capable of providing basic and advanced life support are reimbursable. The costs for using applicant-owned equipment while conducting eligible work are reimbursed.
* The ambulance transportation service provided should be customary and appropriate for the work required. Emergency air and ground ambulance services may be required to transport disaster victims and/or evacuees

requiring emergency medical care to medical facilities. Paratransit transportation services (such as vans, minibuses, and buses) may be required as an alternative transportation mode for individuals including senior citizens, individuals with disabilities, individuals in nursing homes and assisted living facilities, and homebound individuals impacted by a disaster. Eligible costs will be limited to a period of up to 30 days from the date of the emergency or major disaster declaration, or as determined by the federal coordinating officer.

An eligible applicant may not seek reimbursement from FEMA for any ambulance service costs that are covered by private insurance, Medicare, Medicaid, or a preexisting private payment agreement. States must use due diligence in determining whether a prohibited duplication of benefits has occurred and must return such funds to FEMA at a project's final inspection and closeout.

FEMA reimbursement for activating, staging, and using ambulance services will end when FEMA and the state determine that the incident did not impact the ambulance staging areas; or evacuation and repatriation of medical and special needs patients is complete; or the immediate threat caused by the incident has been eliminated and the demand for services has returned to normal operation levels.

Eligible labor costs include overtime pay for regular full-time employees performing eligible work and regular time and overtime pay for extra hires specifically hired to provide additional support as a result of the emergency or declared disaster.

If volunteer emergency medical technicians perform eligible work essential to meeting immediate threats to life and property resulting from a major disaster or emergency, FEMA will credit the donated labor toward the non-federal share of the grant costs under the public assistance program.

CHAPTER REVIEW

Summary

Disasters can overwhelm even the best ambulance services. The extent to which service is interrupted is directly dependent on how well prepared a service is before the incident. By developing internal plans, such as emergency operations plans, business continuity/continuation of operations plans, and preplanning for alternate facilities, the confusion and chaos normally associated with disasters can be reduced.

Additional resources are available through the use of memorandums of understanding and mutual aid agreements. If the disaster is large enough, the implementation of EMAC and the FEMA/AMR contract will provide additional resources.

Working with local emergency managers as part of the emergency preparedness committee will pay dividends during a disaster by clarifying a clear position from which to perform duties safely and effectively, both operationally and logistically.

WHAT WOULD YOU DO? Reflection

You return to the EMS administration building and find the documents required. Most of the documents have not been reviewed in a couple of years and do not match your current resources. There is no COOP, plan and the mutual aid agreements include a private ambulance service that went bankrupt and closed last year. You sit down with the EMS administrator, describe the deficits, and work out a plan to work with the emergency manager to develop, update, and improve the plans.

You develop a disaster planning team with members from throughout your organization. You assess your system and find the need for training, additional equipment, and exercises. You work with the emergency manager to identify vulnerable facilities and persons. This results in a plan for vulnerable individuals to register for transport in the event of a disaster. You also develop a mutual aid agreement with two new ambulance services in the county.

You work with the office administrator and your department chief to locate an alternative business office in the event of damage to the primary headquarters. You find the solution in an unoccupied city warehouse near your department's shop and supply facility. A memorandum of understanding is signed with the city, with permission to preposition some office equipment that is surplus to the primary office.

About 3 months later, a levee collapses upstream of your community, and the resultant flooding turns the new nursing home's property into an island. You are part of the unified command, and when requested, your organization activates a task force. Using high-profile fire department and National Guard vehicles, the residents are extracted from the facility to an assembly point. There, the residents are triaged, evaluated by public health and community hospital staff, and treated for hypothermia and rehydrated, with most of the residents taken to a temporary shelter by city bus. Another dozen are taken to other nursing homes for temporary housing and continued skilled care until the water recedes and power is restored. None require hospitalization.

Review Questions

1. What are some of the attributes of using the incident command system?
2. Define the EMS specific functional positions used in a mass casualty incident.
3. What are the management goals of a mass casualty incident?
4. Describe the functions of an ambulance crew assigned to the rehab sector.
5. Describe the documents that provide a means of obtaining additional assets in the event local resources are exhausted.
6. Describe the most common weapon used by terrorists and for what additional risks responders must be alert.
7. Describe how ambulance services are reimbursed in a presidentially declared disaster.
8. Describe the purpose of a continuity of operations plan.

References

American Medical Response. (2010). "EMS Scope of Practice, Protocols, and Medical Control and Direction for AMR/FEMA Federal Disaster Deployments." See the organization website.

American Medical Response. (2013). "AMR Disaster Response Team Recent Disaster Responses." See the organization website.

Brennan, J., and J. Krohmer, Eds. (2006). *Principles of EMS Systems*, 3rd ed. Boston: American College of Emergency Physicians/Jones and Bartlett.

Briggs, S. M., and K. H. Brinsfield, Eds. (2003). *Advanced Disaster Medical Response*. Boston: Harvard Medical International.

Canton, C. (2007). *Emergency Management: Concepts and Strategies for Effective Programs*. Hoboken, NJ: Wiley.

National Emergency Management Association. (2013). "EAC Emergency Assistance Compact. AMAC Articles of Agreement." See the organization website.

Evans, B., and J. Dyar. (2010) *Management of EMS*. Upper Saddle River, NJ: Prentice Hall.

FEMA. (2008). "Emergency Support Function #8." See the organization website.

FEMA. (2009). "Public Assistance for Ambulance Services." See the organization website.

FEMA. (2013). "National Incident Management System." See the organization website.

Maniscalco, P., and H. Christen. (2011). *Homeland Security: Principles and Practice of Terrorism Response*. Boston: Jones and Bartlett.

National Association of State EMS Officials. (2010). "Overview of AMR/FEMA Federal National Disaster Emergency Medical Services." See the organization website.

National Highway Traffic Safety Administration. (2005, July). "National EMS Core Content." See the organization website.

National Highway Traffic Safety Administration. (2007, February). "National EMS Scope of Practice Model." See the organization website.

Perry, R., and M. Lindell. (2007) *Emergency Planning.* Hoboken, NJ: Wiley.

Pound, P., and M. Gould. (2010). "Effective Emergency Management: Making Improvements for Communities and People with Disabilities." Conference Presentation, National Council on Disability, February 4, 2010.

Ryan, J., and J. Glarum. (2008). *Biosecurity and Bioterrorism: Containing and Preventing Biological Threats.* Oxford, UK: Elsevier.

U. S. Department of Health and Human Services. (2011). "National Disaster Medical System." See the organization website.

Key Terms

mass casualty incident (MCI) An event resulting from human-made or natural causes that results in illness and/or injuries that exceed the EMS capabilities of a hospital, locality, jurisdiction, and/or region.

memorandum of understanding (MOU) An agreement between agencies of a single governmental entity or between governmental entities that delineates the actions and establishes control, financial considerations, and legal protections of the signatory parties.

mitigate The actions taken to reduce or eliminate a natural, technological, or human-induced threat.

mutual aid agreement (MAA) Similar to MOUs, but generally involve county, regional, or tribal groups of like resources.

National Response Framework (NRF) Developed as a lesson learned after Hurricane Katrina, the NRF is designed to give guidance to federal, state, tribal, county, and municipal governments; nongovernmental organizations; and private businesses regarding the scope of services.

preparedness Planning, training, equipping, and conducting exercises to ensure mission readiness for all hazard incidents.

recovery Activities undertaken after stabilization of the incident to return life activities, the community, and the economy to pre-incident status.

response Conducting operations during an incident from the time of first warning until the situation is declared stable. These operations are focused on the safe preservation of life, protection of property, and conservation of the environment.

strike team A group of like resources performing a single function. An example would be five ambulances and a supervisor assigned to evacuate a nursing home.

task force A group of mixed resources assigned a task. An example might include a public works snowplow, a fire department engine company, an ALS ambulance, and a municipal transit bus assigned to conduct search-and-rescue operations in a blizzard on a freeway.

Glossary

accounting The systematic recording, reporting, and analysis of financial transactions of a business according to a set of rules.

accounts payable Any amount owed to another business as the result of a purchase of goods or services on a credit basis.

accounts receivable Any amount owed from another business as the result of a purchase of goods or services on a credit basis.

advanced life support (ALS) Enhanced assessment, invasive life support techniques provided by EMT-Paramedics who have completed a 1,000- to 1,500-hour vocational/technical certification course.

advocacy Working to influence a legislative body, public officials, or public policy individually or on behalf of a group.

Air and Surface Transport Nurses Association (ASTNA) Formerly the National Flight Nurses Association (NFNA). The professional association that represents a large number of nurses involved in AMS and critical care ground transport.

air medical services (AMS) Refers to the provision of medical transport services with the use of aircraft.

ambulance A vehicle (automotive, airborne, or waterborne) used for transporting medical personnel and equipment to the location of a sick or injured person, and for transporting sick or injured individuals to a location where further care can be provided.

American Red Cross Beginning as the Sanitary Commission during the Civil War, this private organization provided necessary items, such as blankets, food, medicines, and so on and aided in the establishment of field hospitals. It also trained and provided nurses for the army. Its most important contribution may have been its codifying of criteria to be used by medical personnel for the maintenance of sanitary conditions in the treatment of soldiers and the environment of the hospitals.

American Society for Testing and Materials (ASTM) An international standards organization that develops and publishes voluntary consensus technical standards for a wide range of materials, products, systems, and services.

Americans with Disabilities Act (ADA) Federal legislation that expanded the scope of discrimination protection initially provided by the Civil Rights Act to include individuals with disabilities. Disability is defined as any physical or mental impairment that substantially limits a major life activity.

angle of departure Angle between the ground and a line running from the rear of the rear tire (where the tire meets the ground) to the lowest hanging vehicular component to the rear of that point. The angle of departure addresses the ability of a vehicle to drive off of a ramp, curve, and so on without the further-to-the-rear component impacting the ground.

applicable requirements and regulations Govern ambulance design, construction, and equipment in a particular jurisdiction or specified in a particular contract for service.

Association of Air Medical Services (AAMS) An international trade association that represents a large segment of AMS providers.

Association of Public-Safety Communications Officials (APCO) International The world's largest association of communications professionals, providing professional development, technical assistance, outreach, and advocacy.

audit An examination of an organization's records conducted by the organization, a regulatory agency, or a third party to assess compliance with one or more sets of laws, regulations, or other standards.

automatic call distribution (ACD) A device with which inbound calls are routed to specific persons based on a routine programmed into the telephone system.

automatic vehicle location (AVL) System that makes use of the GPS to enable an ambulance service (or other agency) to remotely track the location of its vehicle fleet. AVL systems combine GPS technology, cellular or radio frequency communications, street mapping, and computer software to connect the pieces to a computer where vehicle location is displayed.

average cost curve A graph of the average cost per call as volume increases. This accounts for the effect of variable or marginal costs decreasing the average cost per call as volume increases up to a limit.

average cost per call The total fully loaded expense for the service for a period of time divided by the number of calls run during the same time period. This accounts for both fixed and variable costs per unit of service.

aviation maintenance technician An individual with special expertise and training to maintain aircraft. The technician is required, in most cases, to maintain certification by the proper authorities to provide this service.

balance sheet A statement of the financial position of a business on a specified date.

Baron F. P. Percy Introduced the idea of a regular corps, specially trained in and equipped for the transport of injured, using stretchers and educated in a formal, regimented course of instruction. The corps accompanied a large medical wagon to the scene of the battle wounded, striking out in a radial fashion to rapidly retrieve the injured. Once returned to the mobile hospital wagon, the surgeons would immediately provide medical care to the wounded, treating them sufficiently until they were either ambulatory or could be transported in the wagon.

basic life support (BLS) Basic assessment and noninvasive clinical techniques provided by basic-level EMTs who have completed a 110- to 200-hour vocational/technical certification course.

Board for Critical Care Transport Paramedic Certification (BCCTPC) The professional body that awards special certification to paramedics who operate in the AMS and/or critical care ground environment.

budget Inclusive list of proposed expenditures and expected receipts of any person, enterprise, or government for a specified period, usually 1 year. Budget estimates are based on the expenditures and receipts of a similar previous period, modified by any expected changes.

business intelligence The computerized collecting and analyzing of data in such a way that business decisions can be made. Business intelligence is most valuable when it can identify and trend otherwise seemingly useless data.

business logic Coding with a particular ePCR program that recognizes the relationship between certain data elements within an ePCR document and adjusts the document based on input in certain key data elements. For example, if the "no patient found" call disposition is selected, the name and other demographic fields may become disabled in that form.

call disposition The outcome of a call for service or an individual response.

certification Attesting to a truth; in the EMS context, it represents that a minimum standard has been met by a person or organization.

Certified Flight Paramedic (FP-C) A special certification issued to paramedics who are or seek to be involved in the AMS industry.

Certified Flight Registered Nurse (CFRN) A special certification issued to nurses who are or seek to be involved in the AMS industry.

Certified Medical Transport Executive (CMTE) A certification acknowledging satisfactory mastery of leadership materials and concepts. It is offered at the successful completion of the Medical Transport Leadership Institute.

charity care Care provided to individuals who do not have sufficient insurance or financial means to pay for their care, which accounted for as a loss (written off) by the organization providing care.

chart of accounts A list of numbered accounts containing account names and numbers showing classifications and subclassifications that are affected by the financial transactions of a business.

chief complaint A very brief summary of the most serious aspect of the patient's assessment, usually in five words or less. It should reflect the patient's condition more than the patient's verbally stated complaint.

Civil Rights Act Federal legislation that outlawed discrimination in schools, the workplace, and public facilities on the basis of race, color, religion, sex, or national origin.

code of conduct A written set of rules governing the behavior of an organization and its employees or members.

community paramedicine A model of care whereby paramedics apply their training and skill, in community-based environments (outside the usual emergency response/transport model). The community paramedic may practice within an expanded scope (applying specialized skills/protocols beyond that which he was originally trained for), or an expanded role (working in nontraditional roles using existing skills).

compliance committee An interdepartmental committee bringing together managers and resources from various areas of the organization to address risk areas and concerns specific to regulatory issues and to provide a route for disseminating information to and from the compliance officer on a regular basis.

compliance officer A senior manager responsible for operation of the compliance program.

compliance program An organized set of procedures and personnel tasked with ensuring that regulatory requirements are met.

computer-aided dispatch (CAD) system; computer-aided dispatching (CAD) A suite of software used to initiate public safety calls for service, dispatch, and maintain the status of responding resources in the field. CAD systems consist of multiple modules including call input, dispatching, vehicle status maintenance, field unit status and tracking, and call disposition. CAD systems often include interfaces that permit the software to provide services to dispatchers, call takers, and field personnel.

cooperative hospital service organization (CHSO) A nonprofit organization owned by two or more nonprofit hospitals, designed to provide shared services to participating hospitals.

corporate integrity agreement (CIA) An agreement between the Office of Inspector General and a health care provider as part of a settlement for alleged civil wrongdoing relating to federal health care laws.

cost per call The annual cost of providing service divided by the number of ambulance calls.

cost shifting The practice of raising prices in reaction to underpayment of fees charged to government payers and bad debts from patients without insurance or the means to pay their bills.

critical care transport (CCT) Specialized clinical care transport provided by specially trained paramedics or registered nurses during transport from one facility to another facility.

DART rate OSHA uses the incidence rate for days away from work, days of restricted work activity or job transfer (DART) to target high-risk work sites for inspection. A high DART rate could mean that a company needs to improve safety procedures. A low DART rate could mean noncompliance with OSHA reporting regulations.

data dashboard Collection of data compiled into one or more visual representations that can be interpreted rapidly.

data element An individual piece of data collected on a form or in a report, typically in the form of a question or a field that must be filled in by a provider.

days sales outstanding (DSO) An analysis that provides general information about the number of days on average that customers take to pay invoices.

delivery models The ways in which EMS systems are designed in order to provide service to the public. Some types include fire department agencies and hospital-based and commercial services.

deployment simulation software Integrates computer technology with operations research methods and techniques quickly and accurately.

Dominique-Jean Larrey Chief surgeon for Emperor Napoleon Bonaparte, who conceptualized and implemented a cogent, comprehensive prehospital care system that, for the first time, triaged the injured, provided immediate, temporary medical care and transported the injured from the site of injury to medical aid stations in a formal, regulated way using special apparatus.

dual-role, cross-trained member A firefighter/paramedic who is trained, licensed, and authorized to provide both firefighting services and emergency medical care.

duplex A radio system that uses a repeater to boost signals.

economic market Describes any one of a variety of systems, institutions, procedures, social relationships, or infrastructures that describe or facilitate parties in commerce.

emergency medical dispatch (EMD) The use of specific, script-based call-taking protocols to determine appropriate levels and modes of response and providing pre-EMS arrival medical instructions to callers.

emergency medical services (EMS) The provision of medical care by specially trained and authorized personnel to the suddenly ill or injured prior to, and in the absence of, a hospital setting.

EMS safety officer Individual who handles day-to-day administrative functions related to improving the safety aspects of the agency.

EMS Systems Act of 1973 Federal law that determined an EMS system provides for the arrangement of personnel, facilities, and equipment for the effective and coordinated delivery of health care services in an appropriate geographical area under emergency conditions.

EMS voluntary event notification tool A data collection tool designed to improve the safety and quality of the provision of EMS by providing an anonymous method of collecting information pertaining to near-miss and actual sentinel events.

Enhanced 9-1-1 (E 9-1-1) A class of 9-1-1 service that delivers both the location and number of the calling party.

Eugene Nagel, M.D. The visionary who blended the training of surrogate quasi-physicians with radio technology to invent the paramedic using telemetry communication to receive real-time medical command from a doctor at a hospital.

exposure control plan An OSHA-required document that details how employees will be trained in identifying the proper personal protection equipment, when they will use it, how it will be disposed of, and who will be responsible for following up on exposures.

Fair Labor Standards Act (FLSA) Federal legislation that established employer responsibilities and national standards with regard to employee compensation and child labor.

False Claims Act A federal law designed to combat fraud against the government and governmental programs.

Family Medical Leave Act (FMLA) Federal legislation that provided for unpaid leave for employees experiencing certain qualifying medical or family related issues.

Federal Aviation Administration (FAA) The primary arm of the U.S. government with jurisdiction over aviation-related matters. Many other countries have equivalent entities.

Federal Communications Commission (FCC) A government agency responsible for assigning radio licenses and promulgating rules for communications.

Federal Register The daily publication in which federal agencies publish regulations.

federal sentencing guidelines A detailed set of instructions for judges to determine appropriate sentences for federal crimes.

field EMS Those components of the EMS system that concern the direct provision of care to patients, beginning with the dispatch of first responders and ambulance services through the transport of the patient to the hospital, or other appropriate disposition of the patient.

final inspection Performed by representatives of the ambulance service prior to the ambulance leaving the production facility to ensure that the vehicle is built completely to specification. This inspection should utilize checklists to ensure that that every vehicle system and feature is functional before the vehicle is accepted by the buyer.

finance The management of revenues; the conduct or transaction of money matters generally, especially those affecting the public, as in the fields of banking and investment.

financial accounting Used primarily by those outside of a company or organization. Financial reports are usually created for a set period of time, such as a fiscal year or period. Financial reports are historically factual and have predictive value to those who wish to make financial decisions or investments in a company.

first responders Medically trained individuals who respond to EMS calls in advance of transporting ambulances. In communities where ambulances are dynamically deployed, first responders are some-times called co-responders because ambulances sometimes arrive first. Typically, first respond-ers are firefighters, police officers, lifeguards, park rangers.

fixed wing Airplanes.

fraud 1. A knowing misrepresentation of the truth or concealment of a material fact to induce another to act to his detriment. 2. A misrepresentation made recklessly without belief in its truth to induce another to act. 3. An unintentional deception or misrepresentation that causes injury to another. 4. Fraud that has been made illegal by statute and that subjects the offender to criminal penalties.

Generally Accepted Accounting Principles (GAAP) Rules that accountants are required to follow when tracking and reporting financial transactions.

geospatial demand Occurs in a particular location in a service district such as a city or county.

global positioning system (GPS) Satellite-based navigation system that allows users to determine their exact location, velocity, and time 24 hours per day, in all weather conditions, anywhere in the world. GPS is used to support a broad range of mili-tary, commercial, and consumer applications.

gross vehicle weight rating (GVWR) Maximum operating weight of a vehicle, as specified by the manufacturer. The weight of an ambulance, includ-ing equipment, fuel, crew, patients, and so on may not safely exceed the GVWR.

health information exchange (HIE) An effort to standardize elements of patient electronic health records.

Health Insurance Portability and Accountability Act (HIPAA) A federal law dealing with patient privacy and the handling of medical records that has particular implications for EMS services and their documentation practices.

horizontal consolidation The expansion of service geographically under a single provider or network.

hospital A permanent structure that houses the appropriate facilities, equipment, and personnel necessary to provide immediate diagnostic serv-ices and emergent, definitive, and sustaining medi-cal care for those patients who arrive, by whatever means.

incident safety officer (ISO) Individual responsi-ble for monitoring and assessing safety hazards or unsafe situations and for developing measures for ensuring personnel safety.

income statement An accounting of income and expenses that indicates a firm's net profit or loss over a certain period of time, usually 1 year.

interfacility The transportation of a patient between two independently licensed health care facilities.

intermediate life support (ILS) Assessment and limited invasive treatment provided by EMT-Intermediates who have completed a 250- to 300-hour certification course.

International Association of Flight & Critical Care Paramedics (IAFCCP) Formerly the National Flight Paramedics Association (NFPA). The profes-sional association that represents a large number of paramedics involved in AMS and critical care ground transport.

Internet A computer network consisting of a World Wide Web of connected computers sharing information.

interoperability The ability of disparate users or systems to seamlessly communicate.

intrafacility The transportation of a patient between two facilities licensed under the same license.

intranet A computer network that is typically lim-ited to sharing among employees in an individual organization.

in-vehicle navigation (IVN) Composed of a GPS receiver and specialized software that provides directions to a particular destination.

J. Frank Pantridge, M.D. Researched and scien-tifically established both the need and the efficacy of prehospital emergency medical services for myo-cardial infarction cases, through a landmark study entitled "Mobile Intensive Care Unit Management of Myocardial Infarction."

job descriptions Written documents that establish roles and responsibilities, minimum and preferred qualifications, and reporting structure with regard to other positions.

Jonathan Letterman, M.D. Established an effec-tive ambulance corps and included techniques in the loading and unloading of patients on stretchers into and out of ambulance wagons. He ordered that all ambulances be staffed with dedicated attendants at all times and be prepared to move immediately and quickly when called upon.

kickback Offering anything of value in return for services that can be billed to Medicare or Medicaid.

KSAs Knowledge, skills, and abilities, usually used with regard to a job description or job posting.

licensure Formal permission from a governmental or other official body to conduct business or perform a profession.

lost unit hours The number hours in a period of time that an ambulance is unavailable to respond to calls for service for some reason, such as mechanical problems, crew issues, administrative issues, or patient off-load delays at a hospital that are longer than expected.

managerial accounting Used primarily by those within a company or organization. Reports can be generated for any period of time, such as daily, weekly, or monthly. Reports are considered to be future looking and have forecasting value to those within the company.

marginal cost per call Represents the direct additional average cost per call of running additional volume. This represents variable costs, but does not include fixed costs.

mass casualty incident (MCI) An event resulting from human-made or natural causes that results in illness and/or injuries that exceed the EMS capabilities of a hospital, locality, jurisdiction, and/or region.

mass gatherings Events where relatively large numbers of people gather on a short-term basis, such as concerts, demonstrations, rallies, festivals, marathons, state fairs, and similar events. Sometimes called special events.

maximal coverage model Holds the number of vehicles fixed, then locates the vehicles to cover as many calls as possible within a given response-time requirement.

medical director The physician designated to authorize medical care administered by out-of-hospital EMTs and paramedics.

medical necessity The determination of a patient's need for medical transportation services.

medical transportation The provision of medical care or medical monitoring during transport of a patient.

medical transportation systems The movement of patients to, from, or between medical facilities of any kind, including physicians' offices, ambulatory care centers, and such specialized medical facilities as dialysis centers and hospitals.

Medicare A federal system of health insurance for people over age sixty-five and for certain other people. Federal legislation established ambulance transportation as a covered beneficiary service. In so doing the federal government had established a long-term funding mechanism for EMS and medical transportation.

memorandum of understanding (MOU) An agreement between agencies of a single governmental entity or between governmental entities that delineates the actions and establishes control, financial considerations, and legal protections of the signatory parties.

mentoring The process of an experienced or senior member of an organization working with a less experienced or new employee to develop knowledge, skills, and abilities.

Mickey Eisenberg, M.D. Published the results of a study he conducted on the effects of rapidly instituted cardiopulmonary resuscitation (CPR) and definitive medical care provided to patients suffering sudden cardiac arrest in the field, prior to arrival at a hospital.

minimum qualifications The lowest knowledge, skills, or abilities necessary to perform a job.

mitigate The actions taken to reduce or eliminate a natural, technological, or human-induced threat.

mobile data computers (MDC) Mounted in or used in vehicles, typically as the remote end of the CAD system data stream, as well as for storage, manipulation, and input of incident and response data.

mutual aid agreement (MAA) Similar to MOUs, but generally involve county, regional, or tribal groups of like resources.

National Emergency Number Association (NENA) A professional organization solely focused on 9-1-1 policy, technology, operations, and education issues.

National EMS Information Systems (NEMSIS) A program developed by the federal government to advance information collection within EMS, thereby creating a single national database of EMS information for the purpose of EMS research and system development.

National Fire Protection Association (NFPA) An international nonprofit organization dedicated to reducing the worldwide burden of fire and other hazards on the quality of life by developing and advocating for scientifically based consensus codes and standards, research, training, and education.

National Highway Safety Act Federal law passed in 1966 that highlighted emergency medical care as a necessary element to reducing death and disability associated with traffic accidents. Extensive regulations promulgated pursuant to the act created the first comprehensive description of an EMS system, components, and standards.

National Highway Traffic Safety Act (NHTSA) On November 9, 1966, the National Traffic Safety Agency (authorized by the National Traffic and Motor Vehicle Safety Act of 1966; PL 89-563) and the National Highway Safety Advisory Committee (authorized by the National Highway Safety Act of 1966; PL 89-564), both in the Department of Commerce, were merged. Because both acts included many overlapping items, many of their components were eventually merged or consolidated. Both acts are now collectively referred to as the "National Highway Safety Act."

National Response Framework (NRF) Developed as a lesson learned after Hurricane Katrina, the NRF is designed to give guidance to federal, state, tribal, county, and municipal governments; nongovernmental organizations; and private businesses regarding the scope of services.

National Street and Highway Safety Conferences A series of conferences focused on the planning and design of roadways and the creation and implementation of uniform codes of vehicle rules. They were associated with the prevention of vehicle-caused injury and deaths and did not address emergency medical services.

near miss An event that produces no measurable loss but has the exact parameters of an event that does involve a loss.

negligence Conduct that falls below the standard of behavior established by law or industry for the protection of others against unreasonable risk of harm.

Next Generation 9-1-1 (Next Gen & NG 9-1-1) The next level of 9-1-1 service that will include enhancements such as texting, video, and telematic data.

nonmedical transportation Transportation provided without medical care or medical monitoring.

Occupational Safety and Health Administration (OSHA) Division of the U.S. Department of Labor tasked with promulgating and enforcing standards that affect safety in the workplace.

patient A person in need of medical care or medical monitoring during transportation.

patient care report (PCR) Document that is currently evolving from its traditional, written format, which has existed for more than a generation, to the electronic format of the future.

PCR narrative A free-form, paragraph-style aspect of the PCR that often serves as the primary summary and explanation of the events of the patient encounter.

performance improvement A method of bettering productivity (human or business) by establishing metrics and then providing feedback based on those metrics.

personal protective equipment (PPE) Equipment provided to the employee that is used to prevent exposures to biological hazards as defined by OSHA in its blood-borne pathogen and respiratory protection standards.

Physician Certification Statement A written statement from a physician attesting to the need for medical care or medical monitoring during transportation.

policies Courses of action established by an organization in order to carry out its objectives.

prebuild conference Meeting between the ambulance service representative(s), ambulance vendor, and ambulance manufacturer, during which a complete review of the buyer's specifications is conducted, and during which any questions about any vehicle details are resolved, prior to beginning construction of the ambulance.

preferred qualifications Knowledge, skills, or abilities a supervisor/manager would like a candidate to have for a position.

preparedness Planning, training, equipping, and conducting exercises to ensure mission readiness for all hazard incidents.

President's Commission on Highway Safety This commission's final report listed emergency care and transportation of the accident victim as an important community action program.

progressive discipline A method of modifying employee performance though escalating steps of penalty for unacceptable performance or behavior.

public switched telephone network (PSTN) Conventional wire line telephony; the system of trunks and switches that deliver calls.

public utility economics Describes the interaction of market forces in a public service in which the majority of the cost of producing the product or service is incurred in the development of the distribution system required to deliver it to the consumer and the marginal cost of delivering each individual product or service is relatively low.

public utility model (PUM) A model of EMS system design popularized in the 1980s, utilizing a governmental authority, which contracts with an operations contractor to actually operate ambulances on behalf of the authority. A typical PUM has exclusive operating rights for all emergency and nonemergency ambulance activity in the area it serves.

"Accidental Death & Disability: The Neglected Disease of Modern Society" Published by the National Research Council of the National Academy of Sciences in 1966, this report provided an overview of the woefully inadequate medical care given to victims of vehicle accidents. It scientifically established the need for specialized emergency medical services for patients suffering trauma from motor vehicle accidents.

recovery Activities undertaken after stabilization of the incident to return life activities, the community, and the economy to pre-incident status.

regulation Establishing conformity with rules, principles, or common practice.

response Conducting operations during an incident from the time of first warning until the situation is declared stable. These operations are focused on the safe preservation of life, protection of property, and conservation of the environment.

retained earnings/equity The portion of net income that is retained by the corporation rather than distributed to its owners as dividends.

risk management Process of applying management techniques to the identification, assessment, and resolution of problems to prevent and/or minimize occurrences that have the potential for injury or loss to patients, employees, visitors, and the company using several techniques, including exposure avoidance, risk transfer, and retention.

rotary wing Helicopters.

Ryan White Comprehensive AIDS Resources Emergency (CARE) Act Act intended to improve the quality and availability of care for low-income, uninsured, and underinsured individuals and families affected by HIV and AIDS. A section of the act requires hospitals to provide notification to EMS providers in the event of an exposure to a blood-borne pathogen.

scope of practice The defined medical procedures authorized by state regulatory authorities to be administered by EMTs and Paramedics.

scripting validation Commonly known as closed call rules, these parameters define what data elements in a PCR must be completed before that report can be considered complete.

self-pay A person who pays out of pocket for a health-related service in absence of insurance to cover the costs of that service.

sentinel event Any unanticipated event in a health care setting resulting in death or serious physical or psychological injury to a patient.

set covering model Seeks to minimize the number of vehicles needed to cover all specified ambulance response zones.

simplex A radio system with which users talk radio to radio without a repeater.

social media Media designed to be shared through social interaction, typically via the Internet.

special (EMS) operations Include transport and activities such as providing medical support for mass gatherings, tactical emergency medical support for law enforcement special operations units, incident rehabilitation for fires and other large incidents, deployment of ambulance strike teams and EMS task forces to support other jurisdictions, and providing medical support to hazardous materials and urban search-and-rescue teams.

stakeholder A person or group of people who have an interest or concern in an ambulance service due to direct or indirect involvement.

statement of cash flows A financial statement that shows how changes in balance sheet accounts and income affect cash and cash equivalents, and breaks the analysis down to operating, investing, and financing activities.

statute An enactment of a legislative body expressed through a formal document or law.

strike team A group of like resources performing a single function. An example would be five ambulances and a supervisor assigned to evacuate a nursing home.

Structured Query Language (SQL) A database computer language designed for managing data in relational database management systems (RDBMS), and originally based on relational algebra and calculus. Its scope includes data insert, query, update and delete, schema creation and modification, and data access control.

submarket A geographic, economic, or specialized subdivision of a market.

succession planning The process of developing programs designed to identify and prepare employees to step into key positions within an organization.

syndromic surveillance (SS) systems Monitor ambulance (or other health) data sources in real time, and they alert users to sudden increases in specified levels of activity, with the intention of making authorities aware that there has been a sudden up-tick in a particular syndrome. For example, a sudden uptick in calls for service due to respiratory emergencies might be an indicator of the deployment of a chemical weapon.

system A group of objects or subsystems interacting in an organized manner to produce an intended outcome.

system deployment (or deployment) The process by which EMS units are placed in the field for response to EMS calls.

task force A group of mixed resources assigned a task. An example might include a public works snowplow, a fire department engine company, an ALS ambulance, and a municipal transit bus assigned to conduct search-and-rescue operations in a blizzard on a freeway.

temporal demand Volumetric demand or demand that occurs in a specific hour of the day or day of the week irrespective of the geographic location of the demand.

third party An organization other than the patient (first party) or health care provider (second party) involved in the financing of personal health services.

total task time The amount of time the ambulance resource is committed to a call for service until the ambulance resource is completed with the current call and available for another call for service.

traditional media Communication venues such as television, cable television, radio, newspaper, and magazines.

traffic preemption system Allows the normal operation of traffic lights to be preempted or reordered to assist emergency vehicles, stopping conflicting traffic and allowing the emergency vehicle the right-of-way.

trunked A radio system using smart radios that are assigned by computer to an open channel among a pool of frequencies.

unit hour Measurement based on an hour when an ambulance is staffed and on duty.

unit hour utilization The ratio of the number of transports per period divided by the total number of hours staffed per period.

U.S. Public Health Service Established on July 16, 1798, through the Act for the Relief of Sick and Disabled Seamen, creating the Marine Hospital Service, which became the U.S. Public Health Service. The act established a network of medical care, with a system of hospitals, for the aid of American merchant seamen, beginning along the northeast coast and eventually proliferating to the Great Lakes and the Gulf and Pacific Coasts.

vehicle local area networking (V-LAN) Usually wireless, based in a vehicle, and allows computers and other devices on the vehicle to communicate with each other and remote sites (via the Internet or other media).

vehicle on-board monitoring and driver feedback systems (black boxes) Record vehicle operating parameters, communicate those parameters beyond the vehicle for later analysis, and provide feedback (usually audible) when a driver approaches or exceeds specified parameters.

vertical consolidation The consolidation of services under a single production strategy. For example, the same ALS ambulances respond to all ALS and BLS emergency and nonemergency calls.

virtual meetings Any form of video face-to-face communication that allows individuals or groups communication greater than audio alone.

Voice over Internet Protocol (VoIP) The transfer of telephony over the Internet.

Web presence The impact or visibility that a particular organization may have on the Internet.

wholesale competition Periodic competition *for* the market rather than constant retail competition *within* the market.

Index

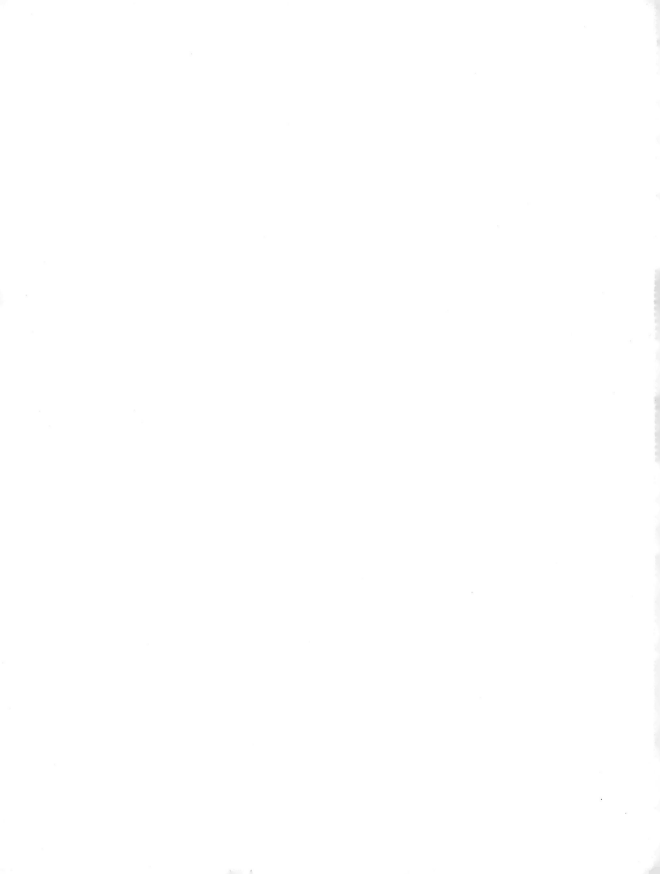